The Body Embarrassed

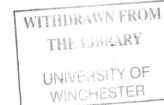

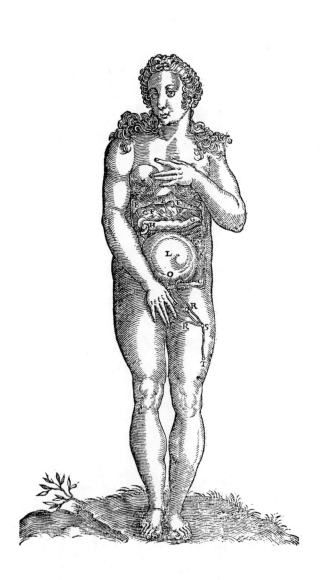

THE BODY
EMBARRASSED

DRAMA AND THE
DISCIPLINES OF SHAME
IN EARLY MODERN ENGLAND

GAIL KERN PASTER

Cornell University Press

ITHACA, NEW YORK

Frontispiece: Figure of a woman, viscera partially exposed. From Helkiah Crooke, *Microcosmographia: A Description of the Body of Man* (London, 1615), title page detail. By permission of the Folger Shakespeare Library.

First published 1993 by Cornell University Press.

International Standard Book Number 0-8014-2776-2 (cloth)
International Standard Book Number 0-8014-8060-4 (paper)
Library of Congress Catalog Card Number 92-36855

Printed in the United States of America

Librarians: Library of Congress cataloging information appears on the last page of the book.

⊗The paper in this book meets the minimum requirements of the American National Standard for Information Sciences—Permanence of Paper for Printed Library Materials, ANSI Z39.48-1984.

For Howard

CONTENTS

ILLUSTRATIONS

ACKNOWLEDGMENTS

In writing this book, I have experienced an embarrassment of assistance in many forms—from the fortuitous leavings of others' scholarly endeavors ("grist for your horrid mill," as one friendly contributor memorably scrawled on a photocopy) to no less essential but more substantial institutional support. The Folger Shakespeare Library, scene and center of my scholarly life for more than two decades, awarded me an O. B. Hardison, Jr., Fellowship in 1988–1989. By naming me a Fellow in 1990–1991, the John Simon Guggenheim Memorial Foundation made this book's completion possible. For their timely generosity, I am extremely grateful to both these institutions, as I am to George Washington University for twice granting me leave. Special thanks are due to those knowledgeable retrievers, the Folger Reading Room staff under Betsy Walsh. An earlier version of Chapter 1 appeared under the same title in *Renaissance Drama* n.s. 18 (1987), published by Northwestern University Press. An earlier version of Chapter 3, titled "'In the Spirit of Men There Is No Blood': Blood as Trope of Gender in *Julius Caesar*," was published in *Shakespeare Quarterly* 40 (1989). I am grateful to the publishers for permission to make use of this material. For permission to reprint photographs from its collection, I am grateful to the Folger and for permission to photograph and reproduce her sieve portrait of Queen Elizabeth, I thank Mrs. Francis T. P. Plimpton.

The time line of my personal indebtedness to others in this project begins with invitations from Carol Leventen and R. L. Widmann to speak at Modern Language Association special sessions in 1986 and 1987. The plenitude of other listeners in subsequent years I owe to the good offices of Karen Newman, David Bevington, Suzanne Gossett, Lynne Magnusson, and C. Edward McGee. Graduate student and faculty groups at Columbia University, the University of Virginia, the University of Maryland, Dartmouth College, and the Bread Loaf School of English have also heard more than they ever wished to know about purging, bleeding, and other forms of excretory discipline. Thanks go to Jean Howard, Katharine Maus, Marion Trousdale, Lynda Boose, James Maddox, and Paul Cubeta for making available such apparently willing victims. Listening to, hearing out, even coming to share my growing obsession with the early modern body has been the equivocal fate of many. Nostalgic thanks to those unsurpassable redcoats, my fellow Folger Fellows of 1988–1989—A. R. Braunmuller, Linda Levy Peck, and Michael Neill. Mary Beth Rose, Jean Howard, and Frank Whigham were early, unflagging supporters, joined by Lynda Boose, Michael Bristol, Darryl Gless, Susan Snyder, Barbara Traister, and Jeanne Roberts, who said decisively and by no means tautologically, "This is a book." I am grateful to Eugene Waith for tempering his skepticism with loyal affection, to Virginia Callahan for sending along classical source material, to Paul Werstine for patience, more patience, and understanding. Werner Gundersheimer, another unabashed shame maven, has cloaked this project in his own inimitable respectability, while Peter Blayney has never failed to shed light on archaeologically dark corners. Thomas L. Berger, Boyd Berry, Theodore Leinwand, Miranda Johnson Haddad, Donald Nathanson, and David Cressy each came to my rescue at least once. And Louis Conte, from another sphere of my existence, provided the altogether helpful affirmation of a practicing psychoanalyst. Catherine Belsey and Coppélia Kahn, though they did not plan to, arrived at the Folger just in time to read not insubstantial portions of the manuscript. Barbara Mowat has read all of it more than once, with an acuity and generosity impossible to overstate or fully repay. And finally, to Bernhard Kendler, my thanks for marshaling my efforts to what I trust is a timely end.

Over the years of this book's composition, my family has, of necessity, become inured to dinner-table gatherings increasingly infiltrated with its source materials and bodily preoccupations. While it cannot be said that Emily and Timothy Paster have failed to notice accompanying breakdowns of the shame threshold in their midst or the steady deterioration of their mother's conversation (if not also of her character), their grace under this most peculiar pressure has proved both a reality check on the nature of embarrassment and a constant source of inspiration. Howard Paster, of course, tries to save me from all the embarrassments he can, for which any thanks at this point would be shamefully meager indeed.

G.K.P.

NOTE ON TEXTS

When quoting from primary texts in original or facsimile editions I have retained original orthography except for silently modernizing i, j, u, v, and expanding contractions. Wherever possible for ease of reference, I have tried to cite period documents in facsimile editions even when the original was available to me. In all cases, I have included standard reference numbers (abbreviated STC and Wing) from *The Short-Title Catalogue of Books . . . 1475–1640*, ed. A. W. Pollard and G. R. Redgrave, 2d ed. (London: Bibliographic Society, 1986), and *The Short-Title Catalogue of Books . . . 1641–1700*, ed. Donald Wing, 2d ed. (New York: Modern Language Association, 1972). Quotations from Shakespeare throughout are from *The Riverside Shakespeare,* ed. G. Blakemore Evans (Boston: Houghton Mifflin, 1974), and will be cited parenthetically. Quotations from non-Shakespearean texts are given full bibliographic citation in individual chapters.

The Body Embarrassed

INTRODUCTION

Civilizing the Humoral Body

The bodies whose embarrassments I retrace in this book are those of early modern English men, women, and children and their representations in the drama. That these embarrassments take historically specific forms and thus have heuristic importance is the assumption underlying all that follows and the heart of the matter it intends to specify. This assumption owes much of its conviction and embellishment to recent theoretical developments in intellectual and material history, the most important of which is the legible history the body has been accorded. It has been placed at the center of a decidedly new discursive domain, influenced by Michel Foucault, to which practitioners in academic departments of anthropology, philosophy, history, and literature, both ancient and modern, have contributed.[1]

1. For examples of the growing bibliography in the history of the early modern body following upon Michel Foucault's *History of Sexuality*, vol. 1: *An Introduction*, trans. Robert Hurley (New York: Vintage, 1980), see Francis Barker, *The Tremulous Private Body: Essays on Subjection* (London: Methuen, 1984); Peter Stallybrass, "Patriarchal Territories: The Body Enclosed," in *Rewriting the Renaissance: The Discourses of Sexual Difference in Early Modern Europe*, ed. Margaret W. Ferguson, Maureen Quilligan, and Nancy J. Vickers (Chicago: University of Chicago Press, 1986), pp. 123–42; Frank Whigham, "Encoding the Alimentary Tract: More on the Body in Renaissance Drama," *ELH* 55 (1988), 333–50. On the currency of the body's history generally, see Scott Heller, "The Human Body and Changing Cultural Conceptions of It Draw Attention of Humanities and Social Science Scholars," in *Chronicle of Higher Education*, 12 June 1991, pp. A4–9.

At the same time, though usually independent of the new histories of the body, there has been an awakening of psychoanalytic interest in shame, the most body-centered of affects. Its origins in intrapsychic time and space, its psychological meaning and importance, its social determinations and significance, its triggering mechanism, its bodily *naturalness*—all these aspects of shame have emerged from an occlusion caused by the greater attention paid to guilt and anxiety by Freud and the ego psychologists and object-relations theorists who came after him.[2]

This study of the early modern body's embarrassments is informed throughout by two preoccupations of my own which have developed both within and apart from these larger enterprises. One such preoccupation is a revisionary deployment of two accounts of the body which have been influential in establishing its new history: Norbert Elias's *History of Manners*, the first of three remarkable volumes of *The Civilizing Process*, and Mikhail Bakhtin's *Rabelais and His World*.[3] The other preoccupation involves an investigation, in part by means of those histories, of the experience *as from within* of bodies that understood themselves and were understood by others in terms of humoral physiology. What connects these two preoccupations is that they have *not* been connected in any previous account of the early modern subject. From their work on bodily paradigms and behaviors there is no evidence that Elias or Bakhtin had any analytic interest in the role of physiological theory in determining either the social contours of the signifying body or the psychic contours of the signifying subject. Foucault, although interested in the reciprocal effect of medical regimes and social organization, is also silent on the humors. But in early modern Europe, despite the challenges to Galenism posed in the sixteenth century by Paracelsus and his followers, the dominant physiological paradigm was the classical theory of the four humors upon which ancient biology and hence the practice of medicine were based for centuries. This introduction and the chapters that follow are much concerned with Elias's description of the advance of the threshold of shame as a control mechanism of the civilizing process and Bakhtin's brilliant diachronic contrast between the two bodily canons

2. On this history see Andrew P. Morrison, *Shame: The Underside of Narcissism* (Hillsdale, N.J.: Analytic Press, 1989), pp. 21–47.

3. Norbert Elias, *The History of Manners* (1939), vol. 1 of *The Civilizing Process*, trans. Edmund Jephcott (New York: Pantheon, 1978); Mikhail Bakhtin, *Rabelais and His World*, trans. Helene Iswolsky (Bloomington: Indiana University Press, 1984).

he labels grotesque and classical. But I want to argue here for the place of physiological theory in the social history of the body. Specifically I want to outline the difference humoralism, or *any other* influential account of human physiology, makes to the subjective experience of being-in-the-body and thus to such matters as the inescapable, though by no means historically uniform experience of bodily shame or its somewhat diminished variant—embarrassment.

In one sense, my project applies and seeks to historicize ethnographic distinctions between the "two bodies," social and physical, about which Mary Douglas has written.[4] But I wish further to complicate her distinctions between physical and social by theorizing a connection between the history of the outer body—physical *and* social, the body visible in different ways to self and other—and that of the inner body, the physical and social body perceived, experienced, and imaged from within. The distinction between them is, in part, an analytic construct. As Douglas has suggested, "There is no reason to assume any primacy for the individual's attitude to his own bodily and emotional experience, any more than for his cultural and social experience."[5] But in order historically to theorize the connection between outer and inner, I propose an internal division within the conception of the bodily habitus—that ensemble of gestures, bearing, behaviors, and techniques described by Marcel Mauss.

"These 'habits' do not just vary with individuals and their imitations," Mauss notes, "they vary especially between societies, educations, proprieties and fashions, prestiges. In them we should see the techniques and work of collective and individual practical reason rather than . . . merely the soul and its repetitive faculties."[6] As Mauss demonstrates with unforgettable examples of the Masai asleep standing up, the rise and fall of the breast stroke, and teaching a young girl from a family of nonspitters how to spit, evident contrasts between the uniformity of bodily experience within a culture and the variety of experience between cultures argue powerfully for the cultural determination of the body's apparently natural possibilities of expression and technique. Here, however, I wish to specify the ensemble of techniques Mauss writes about as the body's *external* habitus,

4. Mary Douglas, *Natural Symbols: Explorations in Cosmology* (New York: Pantheon, 1970), pp. 65–81.

5. Mary Douglas, *Purity and Danger: An Analysis of the Concepts of Pollution and Taboo* (1966; rpt. London: Ark, 1984), p. 121.

6. Marcel Mauss, "Techniques of the Body," *Economy and Society* 2 (1973), 73.

its socially and self-perceptible details of dress, bearing, gesture, bodily behavior. In order to imagine the formative effects of physiological theory on the subject, we need to conceptualize an equally formable, if not equally visible, *internal* habitus. This is the enshrouded domain of the body's internal workings and the locally determined explanatory framework within which those workings are always understood.

It would be naïve to argue that bodies at any given moment in a complex culture are understood socially or felt experientially in only *one* way. But just as Mauss has argued for a decisive uniformity of bodily techniques, so for bodily function we may theorize a decisive uniformity that is to be understood not merely as part of the order of nature (whatever that might be) but as part of the order of culture. At one level this uniformity can be understood to occur because of the physical fact that bodies are composed and function in predictable, naturally limited ways. But conceptually this uniformity occurs because no matter what the physical facts of any given bodily function may be, that function can be understood and experienced only in terms of culturally available discourses. These discourses may be more or less technical, more or less empirically accurate, more or less close to us in historical time and cultural space. No one can really dispute that science is bringing us to an understanding of human physiology that is progressively more accurate and complete. But from the point of view of ideological efficacy and historical determination, historians of the body have no business distinguishing between physiological theories on empirical grounds.

The interaction between bodily self-experience and its discursive realization, then, takes place in and through culture or its more politically conceptualized cognate, ideology. In fact, dominant physiological paradigms should be expected to produce an ideological effect if we understand ideology in Jean Howard's lucid quasi-Althusserian formulation to be a conditioning experienced as "the obviousness of culture, what goes without saying, what is lived as true."[7] The work of ideology includes the social formation of the body because of the "obvious" physical and psychological inseparability of the subject from his/her bodily envelope—no matter how internally divided and self-alienated the subject may be. The body is materially at the center of "what is lived as true." But the operations of ideology upon the body may be even harder to detect than the operations of ideology

7. Jean E. Howard, "Scripts and/versus Playhouses: Ideological Production and the Renaissance Public Stage," *Renaissance Drama* n.s. 20 (1989), 37.

upon emerging subjectivity because we experience our bodies as natural and because we experience them as belonging to us—we
"proprio-percept" them—*all the time*. Often what goes on within the
body "goes without saying" because it goes on daily, habitually, involuntarily, and universally; in this respect, bodiliness is the most rudi-
mentary form of self-presence. Hence it seems to fall beneath the
threshold of significance into the domain of the *merely* natural.

Precisely because what is lived as true will approach conscious understanding only incompletely and intermittently, if at all, the silent
and invisible effects of what might be termed the bodily insignificant
may be among the most powerful of social operations. As Pierre
Bourdieu has argued,

> If all societies . . . that seek to produce a new man through a process of
> "deculturation" and "reculturation" set such store on the seemingly most
> insignificant details of *dress, bearing,* physical and verbal *manners,* the
> reason is that, treating the body as a memory, they entrust to it in abbre-
> viated and practical, i.e. mnemonic, form the fundamental principles of
> the arbitrary content of the culture. The principles em-bodied in this
> way are placed beyond the grasp of consciousness, and hence cannot be
> touched by voluntary, deliberate transformation, cannot even be made
> explicit; nothing seems more ineffable, more incommunicable, more
> inimitable, and therefore, more precious than the values given body,
> *made* body by the transsubstantiation achieved by the hidden persuasion
> of an implicit pedagogy, capable of instilling a whole cosmology, an ethic,
> a metaphysic, a political philosophy through injunctions as insignificant
> as "stand up straight" or "don't hold your knife in your left hand."[8]

Bourdieu is arguing here for the silent and invisible formation of the
external habitus (though, as we shall see, the conduct books that appeared in the sixteenth century, designed to codify behaviors, offer an
important qualification to his thesis). But we can reasonably infer an
equal or even greater hiddenness and efficacy in the social formation
of the internal habitus, in, as Mary Douglas says, the "continual exchange of meanings between the two kinds of bodily experience."[9]
Society's cumulative, continuous interpellation of the subject includes
an internal orientation of the physical self within the socially available

8. Pierre Bourdieu, *Outline of a Theory of Practice,* trans. Richard Nice (Cambridge:
Cambridge University Press, 1977), p. 94.
9. Douglas, *Natural Symbols,* p. 65.

discourses of the body—an orientation in terms of current standards of attractiveness and acceptable behaviors and also in terms of current standards of bodily self-mastery and internal regulation. As part of this orientation, of his or her acculturation, the child comes to attach differential meanings to the contents, products, and workings of his or her own body, never in isolation but always in a complexly articulated, hierarchized relation to the bodies of others. In the continuous series of negotiations by which the body is inscribed as a social text, it also becomes a social *sub-* or *infra-*text, the outward manifestation of and container for dense inner workings, less visible than the external habitus but no less subject to social formation and judgment.

This is precisely the ideological freight borne by humoral theory, a system of explanation of the body's composition and functioning which held sway for centuries from the classical period until the start of a slow and incomplete disintegration in the seventeenth century. As an explanation of human physiology, humoral theory no longer compels belief, its social and scientific instrumentality having been gradually replaced by the empirically based orthodoxies of the modern biological sciences.[10] And to the literary or social historian for whom medical or scientific history is a specialized field of inquiry with a narrative divisible from the sociopolitical mainstream, it is tempting to relegate humoralism to the marginal place of intellectual "background." It belongs with the astrological chart or the concentric spheres of the Ptolemaic heavens in the nostalgic space of quaint, mistaken beliefs, an ancestral lore replaced by more efficacious, if less colorful, truths. The four humors are traditionally enumerated in a footnote to the texts of canonical authors from Chaucer to Milton in order to gloss references to choleric characters, to describe the affective vogue of melancholy in early seventeenth-century courtly and literary coteries, or to explain the workings of outmoded theories of disease and contagion. But in English the symptomatological effects of the humors remain like archaic sediments in the ordinary language of the body: we catch "cold," are "filled with" our emotions, are "sanguine" or not about the weather (the stock market, the state of Western culture), are said to be in a good or bad humor.

10. For an accessible brief account of the collapse of Galenism in the seventeenth century, see Lester S. King, "The Transformation of Galenism," in *Medicine in Seventeenth Century England*, ed. Allen G. Debus (Berkeley: University of California Press, 1974), pp. 7–31. On the humors, see Nancy G. Siraisi, *Medieval and Early Renaissance Medicine: An Introduction to Knowledge and Practice* (Chicago: University of Chicago Press, 1990), pp. 104–6.

Because such phrases no longer fit the facts of our bodies as we come to know and experience them, the signifiers of humoralism could easily be dismissed as dead metaphors or inconsequential idioms that distort their signifieds whether they appear in earlier texts or contemporary utterances. They are the residuum of error. But for the reason that to employ the language of an otherwise outmoded bodily self-experience is to be formed in part *by* it, the subjective effect of humoral theory is still very much worth scrutiny, particularly in relation to the men and women of early modern Europe, who grew up within its domain. As Nancy Siraisi points out, "Humoral theory is probably the single most striking example of the habitual preference in ancient, medieval, and Renaissance medicine for materialist explanations of mental and emotional states."[11] Humoral materialism lingers in our propensity to describe ourselves as—and, I suggest, *feel* ourselves to be—"filled" with emotion, but the subjective effects of humoralism in an earlier time that lived it as true were far more pervasive.

Even as they suffered and died from the effects of purges, bleedings, and the other common practices of humoral medicine, the men and women of early modern Europe understood their mortality, described their sensations and bodily events, and often experienced physical and psychological benefit in humoral terms. More subtly, they experienced such basic social interpellations as their engenderment in humoral terms, since, as I shall argue in detail, humoral theory was instrumental in the production and maintenance of gender and class difference as part of what Foucault has called "the hysterization of women's bodies."[12] When they were required to master their bodies for the sake of "the civilizing process," the various disciplinary regimes Foucault has seen as characteristic of emergent modernity, the bodies to be mastered were humoral bodies. And the embarrassed bodies of wives, whores, rustics, and children, who predictably failed in such tasks, suffered humoral forms of embarrassment.

Humoral theory, however empirically inaccurate—not *true*, in the ordinary sense of the word—is a matter entirely separate from its ideological efficacy and meaning. During humoralism's long cultural reign, the body was thought to be composed of four humors—blood,

---

11. Siraisi, *Medieval and Early Renaissance Medicine*, p. 106.
12. Foucault, *History of Sexuality*, p. 104.

phlegm, choler or yellow bile, and black bile. They were, says Siraisi, "real bodily fluids to which largely hypothetical origins, sites, and functions were ascribed."[13] Since, as Lucinda Beier notes, "all healers and sufferers subscribed to a humoral view of disease and therapy," no significant differences existed between the medical beliefs of learned and unlearned practitioners or the medical self-understanding of learned and unlearned patients.[14] Every subject grew up with a common understanding of his or her body as a semipermeable, irrigated container in which humors moved sluggishly. People imagined that health consisted of a state of internal solubility to be perilously maintained, often through a variety of evacuations, either self-administered or in consultation with a healer.[15] As the work of Thomas Laqueur, Ian Maclean, Caroline Bynum, and others has demonstrated, this body had a distinct set of internal procedures dependent on a differential caloric economy (most men being hotter than most women) and characterized by corporeal fluidity, openness, and porous boundaries.[16]

"For the matter of mans body," says Helkiah Crooke, the king's physician, in 1615, "it is soft, pliable and temperate, readie to follow the Workeman in every thing, and to every purpose; for man is the moystest and most sanguine of all Creatures."[17] John Donne's image in a 1623 Lenten sermon that "every man is a spunge, and but a spunge filled with teares," which sounds startling, vivid, even grotesque to modern readers, works by embroidering upon a fundamen-

13. Siraisi, *Medieval and Early Renaissance Medicine*, p. 105.
14. Lucinda McCray Beier, *Sufferers and Healers: The Experience of Illness in Seventeenth-Century England* (London: Routledge and Kegan Paul, 1987), p. 31.
15. I am indebted to L. J. Rather's description of the humoral body as a system of irrigated canals in "Pathology at Mid-century: A Reassessment of Thomas Willis and Thomas Sydenham," in *Medicine in Seventeenth Century England*, p. 73. On the question of solubility, see Beier, *Sufferers and Healers*, p. 61.
16. See Thomas Laqueur, *Making Sex: Body and Gender from the Greeks to Freud* (Cambridge: Harvard University Press, 1990), pp. 19–20. My disagreements with Laqueur on various matters become clear in Chapters 2 and 4. Indebted to Laqueur's work in its early stages, Caroline Bynum writes powerfully of the interpretative problems posed by a failure to understand ancient physiological theory and hence to historicize gender. See "The Body of Christ in the Later Middle Ages: A Reply to Leo Steinberg," *Renaissance Quarterly* 39 (1986), 421. Also useful here are Ian Maclean, *The Renaissance Notion of Woman: A Study in the Fortunes of Scholasticism and Medical Science in European Intellectual Life* (Cambridge: Cambridge University Press, 1980), pp. 28–46; and Siraisi, *Medieval and Early Renaissance Medicine*, pp. 78–114.
17. In Helkiah Crooke, *Microcosmographia: A Description of the Body of Man* (London, 1615; STC 6062.2), p. 5.

tal humoral truth for the sake of pathos.[18] I suspect that its striking-ness for Donne's audience would have resided less in the idea of human soddenness—the moist sponginess of "man" which Crooke regarded as factual truth—than in man's humoral reduction to tears alone, to a passive and feminized state inclusive here of both genders. (Donne did not go on to add, with Crooke, that "our life is nothing else but a drying of the spermaticall parts."[19] Perhaps the mental picture of a dried-up sponge/man would ruin the sermon's admonitory agenda and its cultivation of Lenten pathos.)

Galenic physiology proposed a body whose constituent fluids, all reducible to blood, were entirely fungible. Not only did blood, semen, milk, sweat, tears, and other bodily fluids turn into one another, but the processes of alimentation, excretion, menstruation, and lactation were understood as homologous and hence were less conceptually differentiated than they may be in popular medical understanding now.[20] Besides being open and fungible in its internal workings, the humoral body was also porous and thus able to be influenced by the immediate environment. Crooke cites the Hippocratic aphorism, "All bodies are *Transpirable* and *Trans-fluxible*, that is, so open to the ayre as that it may passe and repasse through them," though not, he hastens to add, "so aboundantly as it doth by the windepipe."[21] Solubility, the sine qua non of bodily health, was a function of internal and external economies potentially fraught with peril. Bodies were always filled with humors, but the quantity of humors not only depended on such variables as age and gender but also differed from day to day as the body took in food and air, processed them, and released them. The humors moved with greater or less fluidity within the bodily container and exited the body with varying degrees of efficiency. The key differentials were heat, which in the mean promoted solubility, and cold, which hampered it. Achieving the ideal internal balance and movement of humoral fluids was also a function of the individual body's capacity for transpiration and evacuation—the exchange of elements with the surrounding air and water.

Because the workings of the humoral body were dependent upon regulation of internal temperature, micro- and macroclimatic changes

18. *The Sermons of John Donne*, ed. George R. Potter and Evelyn M. Simpson, vol. 4 (Berkeley: University of California Press, 1959), p. 337. This line is cited in the *OED*, s.v. *sponge.*
19. Crooke, *Microcosmographia*, p. 55.
20. See Laqueur, *Making Sex*, pp. 35–36.
21. Crooke, *Microcosmographia*, p. 175.

were always significant. "Such is the air," states Robert Burton aphoristically, "such be our spirits; and as our spirits, such are our humours."[22] This sense of climatic vulnerability rationalizes the seasonal timing of bodily events—which months were considered advisable or not for purging, bleeding, even bathing.[23] Here too Burton is helpful: "Joh. Struthius contends, *that if one stay longer than ordinary at the bath, go in too oft, or at unseasonable times, he putrefies the humours in his body.*" Since foods were thought of in thermal terms—variously promoting cooling and heating within the body or aiding in the regulation of body temperature and solubility through retentive or eliminative properties—the diet of the humoral body was in the ideal to be adjusted seasonally. The pursuit of venery, too, was included in the regimen of the seasons since the release of bodily fluid in intercourse was part of the general economy of bodily solubility. Burton cites Galen's authority that melancholy was one of those diseases "which are *exasperated by venery: . . .* because *it infrigidates & dries up the body, consumes the spirits.*"[24]

Other descriptions of the functional humoral body, as we shall see in chapters to come, build narrative potential into its openness and exquisite sensitivity to atmospheric change. The point to be made here is that when the early modern subject became aware of her or his body (however we wish to problematize that process) and when that body came more and more formally under the auspices of specific cultural regimes, the body in question was always a humoral entity. The corporeal flux Laqueur has seen as characteristic of this body implies not only that its internal procedures were versions of one another but also that they were unstable, full of variation, unpredictable. More crucial for my argument here, insofar as bodily self-experience becomes knowable and communicable as a reciprocal function of sensation and language, the language of the humoral body constructs a bodily self-experience that is often tumultuous and dramatic even when function is normal. Humoral physiology ascribes to the workings of the internal organs an aspect of agency, purposiveness, and plenitude to which the subject's own will is often decidedly irrelevant.

22. Robert Burton, *The Anatomy of Melancholy*, ed. Floyd Dell and Paul Jordan-Smith (New York: Tudor, 1938), p. 206.
23. Georges Vigarello, *Concepts of Cleanliness: Changing Attitudes in France since the Middle Ages*, trans. Jean Birrell (Cambridge: Cambridge University Press, 1988), pp. 9–20.
24. Burton, *Anatomy of Melancholy*, p. 205.

Crooke's description of the functional anatomy of the digestive process is especially vivid in this regard: "Appeareth the Maze or labyrinth of the guts wheeled about in manifold foulds & convolutions, that neither the aliment should so suddenly passe away, and so the wombe of man become an insatiate Orque voyding whilst it doth devour, neyther yet the noisom steame of the Faeculent excrements have free and direct ascent to the upper parts, but be intercepted and deteined within those Meanders, & so smothered in those gulphs of the Guts."[25] Here, because of the length and dilatory action of the alimentary tract, the ordinary internal protocols of digestion prolong the transformation of food into aliment and excrement, thus deferring a specter of monstrous appetite, of ingestion and excretion in endless, horrible simultaneity. The guts swell to oceanic proportions, smothering in their "gulphs" the "steam" that arises from their midst. In the process digestion assumes an ethical meaning, a social coding, as the steam of the lower body is providentially diverted from improper access to the noble organs above.

Body parts are even imbued with their own affective capacity. Crooke declares that the stomach is not itself nourished by the aliment it concocts, "but only delighted with his presence." He justifies the need to relieve the body of an excess of choler by imbuing the humor with a madcap personality and rebellious proclivities. Choler, "being a mad and hare-brain'd humour, had neede at the first generation of it be sent away, least it should set all the body in an uprore."[26] The dramatic narratives of even more emotionally charged body parts such as the uterus will provide the arguments of later chapters. Here I want only to note the color, vividness, and animation that the vernacular medical literature ascribed to the internal workings of the humoral body even when it was more or less healthy and functioning normally.

All parts of the humoral body were capable of containing fumes and smoky "fuliginous" vapors that could rise from the guts to the cranium, winds that roared and rumbled, sharp and vehement gripings, belchings, gross and clammy crudities, fluids that putrefied and stank or, burning up, became "adust," seed that sent up poisoned vapors to the brain. The humoral body's ability to regulate and release these vapors was critical to its solubility. Among the four reasons the Tudor surgeon Thomas Vicary enumerates for why the head has hair

25. Crooke, *Microcosmographia*, pp. 94–95.
26. Ibid., pp. 162, 135.

is that "the fumosities of the brayne might assend and passe lyghtlyer out by them" than they might were the head covered with a harder substance.[27] Bodily events that in the absence of disease we ordinarily regard as trivial—nosebleeds, for instance, or splinters—might in the humoral body be fraught with significance as unwilled alterations of the body's internal state, as exceptional evacuations or perilous invasions of this porous and fragile envelope. Release of the internal winds was thought so important that well after the advent of powerful excretory disciplines, farting was governed by rules of health rather than behavior. Erasmus discusses the matter fully:

> There are some who lay down the rule that a boy should refrain from breaking wind by constricting his buttocks. But it is no part of good manners to bring illness upon yourself while striving to appear "polite." If you may withdraw, do so in private. But if not, then in the words of the old adage, let him cover the sound with a cough. Besides, why do they not rule in the same way that boys should not purge their bowels, since it is more dangerous to refrain from breaking wind than it is to constrict the bowels?[28]

The vigorous, even turbulent activity that a physician such as Crooke finds in the normal workings of the humoral body is in large part a rhetorical function of the aggressive active verbs he uses to describe normal digestive processes we tend neither to notice nor to be able to experience. The effect of such language, however, is to locate a form of selfhood, analogous with agency, within. Similarly, the behavioral syndromes Burton describes in the body given over to one of the many forms of melancholy construct a humoral body within of meteorological force and scope. Indeed, the clinical language of most disease states in the humoral body is particularly florid and hence, I would argue, full of affective power and coloration. Here, for example, is Burton's description of "windy hypochondriacal melancholy":

27. Thomas Vicary, *A Profitable Treatise of the Anatomie of Mans Body* (London, 1577; STC 24713; rpt. Amsterdam: Da Capo Press, 1973), sig. C3r.
28. I quote from Erasmus, *On Good Manners for Boys (De civilitate morum puerilium)*, trans. Brian McGregor, *Collected Works of Erasmus*, vol. 25, ed. J. K. Sowards (Toronto: University of Toronto Press, 1985), pp. 277–78. This passage is also quoted by Elias, *History of Manners*, p. 130. We find Erasmus's thoroughness and seriousness odd or endearing, Elias tells us, not simply because the control of flatus is no longer considered a vital function of health but because it has become a matter of elementary conditioning within the first years. While farting remains a shame-laden behavior, it is no longer thought to be a matter of life or death.

Besides fear and sorrow, *sharp belchings, fulsome crudities, heat in the bowels, wind and rumbling in the guts, vehement gripings, paine in the belly and stomach sometimes, after meat that is hard of concoction, much watering of the stomack, and moist spittle, cold sweat, . . . unseasonable sweat*. . . . Some againe are black, pale, ruddy, sometimes their shoulders, and shoulder blades ache, there is a leaping all over their bodies, sudden trembling, a palpitation of the heart, and that grief in the mouth of the stomack, which maketh the patient think his heart itself acheth, and sometimes suffocation, short breath, hard wind, strong pulse, swooning.[29]

To a twentieth-century reader accustomed to the affectlessness of technical bodily discourses, what strikes us pleasantly as the colloquialism and quaint inaccuracy of seventeenth-century medical writing in the vernacular makes the multiplication of such examples tempting. In this discourse symptoms seem to grow in affect, to proceed from mighty internal convulsions or errant humors, to represent bodies so porous, vulnerable, various, or even bizarre that they seem to be created out of alien substance. Peculiar objects—pins, hairballs, monsters, serpents—emerge from the humoral body; its blood, according to the phlebotomists who drew it, came in twenty colors from palest white to raven black. In the strange materiality of medical texts, such bodies have forms of self-experience no longer possible for us. This alterity is true not only for the humoral body suffering diseases we no longer suffer but for the humoral body experiencing its own normal function, its own health. Even though male and female grew up differently within humoralism, all being-in-the-humoral-body involved a turbulent interior plenitude capable of absorbing and being physically altered by the world around it and, like Donne's human sponge, not distinctly separable from it.

But if the insubstantial margins of the humoral body open that body to the world, the cultural meaning of that openness remains indeterminate. As Douglas notes, "The body can stand for any bounded system. Its boundaries can represent any boundaries which are threatened and precarious."[30] For the humoral body, *all* boundaries were threatened because they were—as a matter of physical definition and functional health—porous and permeable. What they may have threatened most of all was the psychic economy of the humoral subject in an age newly preoccupied with corporeal self-

29. Burton, *Anatomy of Melancholy*, pp. 350–51.
30. Douglas, *Purity and Danger*, p. 115.

discipline. Here is where humorality comes into conflict with Elias's assertion that canons of bodily propriety underwent a significant transformation in sixteenth-century Europe as a self-reinforcing mechanism of social (and, I would add, gender) differentiation. Increased expectations of bodily refinement and of physical and emotional self-control worked to lower thresholds of shame at the same time they promoted what Foucault and others have seen as a reform movement directed toward inculcating self-discipline. What I infer from this history of bodily regulation is the structure of a contradiction between a popular medical practice authorizing experiences of somatic uncontrol in the form of humoral evacuation and an emergent ideology of bodily refinement and exquisite self-mastery. As Stephen Greenblatt has suggested, "Eventually all of the body's products, except tears, become simply unmentionable in decent society."[31] Those products were the visibly issuing effects of the body's humorality, crossing the borders of the body and taking on the character of what, according to Julia Kristeva, the subject experiences more or less powerfully as defilement.[32]

At this point, readers of Bakhtin will have noticed that my emphasis upon the humoral body's corporeal flux and openness to the world distinctly resembles Bakhtin's description of the grotesque body, which "is not separated from the rest of the world. It is not a closed, completed unit; it is unfinished, outgrows itself, transgresses its own limits. The stress is laid on those parts of the body that are open to the outside world, that is, the parts through which the world enters the body or emerges from it, or through which the body itself goes out to meet the world."[33] Those parts are the bowels, the belly, the genitalia, the excretory organs, the mouth—the sites of consumption and evacuation, the body's thresholds and its sites of pleasure. Like the humoral body, the grotesque body is a plenitude, full of activities apart from mind through which it expresses its unity with and sense of belonging to the natural world.

If there remain significant contrasts between the humoral and grotesque bodies, they have in part to do with theoretical perspectives. Bakhtin conceptualizes the canon of the bodily grotesque from within popular festive celebrations of the body's pleasures; I have con-

31. Stephen Greenblatt, "Filthy Rites," *Daedalus* 111 (1981), 11.
32. Julia Kristeva, *Powers of Horror: An Essay on Abjection*, trans. Leon S. Roudiez (New York: Columbia University Press, 1982), p. 69.
33. Bakhtin, *Rabelais and His World*, p. 26.

structed the humoral body here by way of its textual instantiations in vernacular medical writing. But similarities between the humoral and grotesque bodies could not be coincidental, because the medieval culture Bakhtin reads in order to construct his grotesque bodily canon understood the body in humoral terms. In part, then, the humoral body offers historical corroboration of the Bakhtinian grotesque from another part of the culture. But the humoral body's self-experience also works as critique and correction of Bakhtin, insofar as Bakhtin promotes the heuristic construction of a collective body in order to make a politically emancipating argument about class struggle. Not only does Bakhtin associate this bodily canon with a specific, if prolonged, cultural moment already passing when Rabelais wrote the novel that serves as Bakhtin's textual point of departure. But he also identifies it with plebeian culture and hence with a leveling, anti-hierarchical impulse in which the body is a centrally important political instrument of the carnivalesque. The grotesque body is a popular-festive body that, outgrowing itself, threatens forms of established order for the sake of its own immediate self-celebration and for the long-term goal of promoting social cohesion and purposiveness from below.

For this reason, Bakhtin identifies the grotesque body as a collective form, not only separate from the individual body but antithetical to any claims to be made on its behalf. The grotesque body is a thematizing image of the popular body which by definition cannot belong to or be identified with selfhood, with the discrete, pathetically finite boundaries of the individual life in time. Although Bakhtin introduces an opposition to the grotesque body in the form of the classical bodily canon, he does not do so in order to make connections to the history of the subject or to structural changes in the psychic economy of early modern Europe. If the classical body—opaque, closed off, finished, a body all surface and no interior—instantiates the body ideal of Renaissance absolutism, it does so more as a denial of common bodiliness *tout court* than as a new form of bodiliness individualized. For Bakhtin the body's concrete materiality—or lack of it—remains primarily symbolic. He is interested neither in actual bodily practices over time nor in the body's changing modes of self-experience but in the body as instrument of political critique.

In its populist aspect Bakhtin's contrast of bodily canons would thus seem to have little or nothing to contribute analytically to the history of the subject. But in the grotesque body's structural resemblance to the humoral body, the history of the subject may in fact be reinserted. Because humoralism was the governing paradigm of function within which any individual perceived his or her own body in the early modern period, humoral theory can be used heuristically to connect Bakhtin's totalizing narrative of the contrasting bodily canons with subjective economies and to locate the subject's being-in-the-body within the long-term historical changes with which Bakhtin is most directly concerned. In addition, humoral theory can serve to connect the Baktinian bodily canons with Norbert Elias's history of the civilizing process, "by which Elias means," writes Roger Chartier, "the pacification of behaviour and the control of emotions."[34] The permeability, volatility, and especially the insistent interiority of the humoral body helps to motivate and rationalize the changing thresholds of embarrassment and shame seen by Elias as punctuating the history of the social body. He insists, for example, that an overt, unembarrassed interest in the body's secretions and evacuations—now "normally" only visible in children—"shows itself as an earlier stage of the historical process," a stage we might denominate as humoralism. The suppression and silencing of the body's functions—first from view, then from mention—is also a gradual suppression and silencing of the evidence of its humorality, agential interiority, and physiological porousness. Thus, as Elias points out, the only substantive opposition to emerging constraints on bodily function came from medicine and even that opposition was repressed and transformed over time: "In the nineteenth century, [medical arguments] nearly always serve as instruments to compel restraint and renunciation of instinctual gratification."[35]

Finally, humoralism provides a fertile theoretical groundplot for psychoanalytically motivated revision of both Bakhtin and Elias. As I shall suggest in detail in the chapters that follow, the materials of early modern humoral theory encode a complexly articulated hierarchy of physiological differences paralleling and reproducing structures of social difference. Prime among these, of course, is the structure of gender difference, the most basic social category of the body and one that both Bakhtin and Elias silently subsume. Thomas Laqueur has

34. I quote here from Roger Chartier's preface to the new French edition of *The Court Society* (1985), reprinted as "Social Figuration and Habitus: Reading Elias," in *Cultural History: Between Practices and Representations*, trans. Lydia G. Cochrane (Ithaca: Cornell University Press, 1988), p. 74.

35. Elias, *History of Manners*, pp. 149, 135.

subordinated the importance of gender difference in Galenic physiology to a one-sex, one-flesh model where "the boundaries between male and female are of degree and not of kind." Because male and female genitalia were understood within classical anatomy and physiology to be inversions of each other in structure and homologous in function, Laqueur argues, the Greeks and those who came after them conceptualized male and female as difference without opposition until well after William Harvey's discovery of the female ovum in 1651 and Regnier de Graaf's discovery of the ovarian follicle in 1672.

But despite the breadth of his learning and the long sweep of his narrative, Laqueur's interest in the body inscribed by Galenic humoralism is narrowly focused on the history and theory of genital difference, as he himself implicitly acknowledges: "I am saddened by the most obvious and persistent omission in this book: a sustained account of experience in the body."[36] To some degree this book begins to fill in that omission, but it does so by departing in crucial ways from Laqueur's paradigm. My contrary assumption is that humoralism had broad and pervasive effects on the discourse, experience, and expression of bodiliness and on the enculturation process in general. In enculturation the hierarchical differences effaced by Laqueur's one-sex, one-flesh paradigm become the key bodily signifiers of social and subjective experience, centrally organized by the continuously formative processes of engenderment.

Tutored by Lacanian psychoanalysis, we look for the beginnings of enculturation in the mirror stage, that moment which "turns the I into that apparatus for which every instinctual thrust constitutes a danger." Where Lacan's presentation of the mirror stage most closely approximates the issues of social formation inflected so differently by Elias and Bakhtin is in identifying as psychically formative the momentous contrast between the baby's perception of his/her bodily exterior—"the total form of the body . . . given to him only as *Gestalt*"—and "the turbulent movements that the subject feels are animating him." Perceiving the "total form of the body" is the baby's cognitive path to a self-possession that is, of course, also self-alienation. The mirror enacts only one early stage in the baby's gradual expulsion from the Imaginary preoedipal unity with the mother into culture, into the self-alienating conditions of subjectivity, gender, and organized sexuality. But the mirror moment's contrast between

36. Laqueur, *Making Sex*, pp. 25, 171–74, 23.

the baby's perception of symmetrical, opaque, and completed exteriority at variance with his experience of a turbulent, uncontrollable set of drives within—what Lacan calls "intestinal persecutions"—inserts the Lacanian subject into the Bakhtinian contrast between the bodily canons and Elias's history of the civilizing process. For Lacan describes the power of the mirror moment as a "spatial captation," a seduction by surface, which leaves the baby aware "of an organic insufficiency in his natural reality."[37] Thus, since neither Bakhtin, Elias, nor Lacan imagines individuals as free and unique, the mirror stage is also the conceptual moment within the life of the subject that begins to instantiate centuries-long civilizing processes.[38] The image returning the baby's gaze seems to inhabit a body in a greater state of self-possession than the baby feels his/her own insufficient body to be. The state of bodily self-control, like other claims to the self in Lacanian thought, occurs as an illusory object of desire constituted by the subject's lack-in-being. This may not be the baby's *first* experience of bodily shame, since some psychoanalysts in contemporary practice have recently identified shame as one of several innate affects working to stabilize the infant's organization of and response to stimuli.[39] And Lacan himself identifies the mirror stage as occurring "even before the social dialectic."[40] But crucially for my argument, the mirror stage does locate shame socially, in the gaze of a desirable other, and thus brings it within the dynamic agencies of theater.

For Lacan the demand (or desire) for self-control arises within the individual life out of the subject's projective identification of the fic-

37. Jacques Lacan, "The Mirror Stage," in *Ecrits: A Selection*, ed. and trans. Alan Sheridan (New York: Norton, 1977), pp. 5, 2, 4.

38. According to Chartier, this is precisely where Elias begins to differ with liberal historians. See "Social Figuration and Habitus," p. 72.

39. See Silvan S. Tomkins, "Shame," *The Many Faces of Shame*, ed. Donald L. Nathanson (New York: Guilford Press, 1987), pp. 133–61. Tomkins has identified shame-humiliation as an innate negative affect to be distinguished from other negative affects, which he labels disgust and dissmell. With other innate affects, positive and negative, it works axiologically to inhibit or reduce an uncomfortable increase in external or internal stimuli on the brain. When the baby is looked at by another who is strange, when its mother breaks away from the mutuality of gaze, or when interest moves too rapidly toward excitement—in other words, when there has been an "incomplete reduction of interest or joy"—the intervention of shame restores a previously comfortable state of affairs. For Tomkins, shame is inescapable "insofar as desire outruns fulfillment." Because there will always be barriers to desire, "a pluralism of desires must be matched by a pluralism of shame" (p. 155). Also in that volume of essays Nathanson contextualizes Tomkins's work in "The Timetable for Shame," pp. 11–16.

40. Lacan, "Mirror Stage," p. 4.

tional image in the mirror with the symbolic order governed by the law of the Father. For Elias the demand for self-control—though to some degree a constant by-product of social life everywhere—arises in historically variant forms and degrees. What is important for my interest in embarrassment, however, is that both sociohistorical and Lacanian conceptualizations of the demand for self-control fix it so firmly within the cultural domain that embarrassment becomes a site where historicist and psychoanalytic investments in the subject converge. In writing about the experience of bodily shame as a form of social discipline in early modern English culture, I have followed but also tried to reconcile this unruly set of somewhat divergent theoretical practices. Humoralism promotes an excessive interest in bodily fluids—"today . . . only 'normally' visible in children"—and their movement into and out of the body. The language of humoralism, thoroughly suffused by signifiers we assign to ethical discourse, establishes an internal hierarchy of fluids and functions within the body which is fully assimilable to external hierarchies of class and gender. Bakhtin identifies the contrast between the grotesque lower body's productions of fluids and the classical body's surface opacity as a politically active site for critical intervention. Elias offers a detailed coding of specific behavioral changes as advancing the thresholds of shame and embarrassment. And Lacan austerely challenges social codifications and the signifying chain to reproduce the history of lack-in-being.

In its particularity, transience, and insistent secularity, embarrassment is an affect well suited to the evidentiary requirements of the materialist historian of the body. It is a convenient, legible emotion because its cultural specificity may be taken as axiomatic and its behavioral content as arbitrary or even trivial. As Andrew Morrison has argued, compared to contempt, humiliation, and other forms of shame anxiety, "embarrassment is a less searing, less intense form of shame that is more readily acceptable to most people and that, therefore, may more readily be acknowledged in psychotherapy or analysis"[41]—or, I would add, in the textual detritus of the past.

Procedurally, the five chapters in this book move between and among a variety of textual materials, both chosen and found, wherever traces of humoral embarrassment might be uncovered or wherever what "went without saying" about humoral being-in-the-body

41. Morrison, *Shame*, p. 15.

might be glimpsed. These materials include medical writing in the vernacular, prose works, proverbs—all contextually directed toward the represented body in the drama, which is the center of my enterprise. That the represented body was, like the actor's actual body, a humoral entity is a silent, hence rarely thematized element of dramatic representations in gesture or discourse. But as the material body's fictional embodiment, what and how the actor's body signifies is always at issue. This is particularly true within the dramatic convention of the Elizabethan-Jacobean theater, which prescribed and accepted female impersonation by transvestite actors and hence acknowledged the indeterminate, variant relationship between two ambiguous and mutable social texts—between the actor's body, natural and social, and the specific attributes, natural and social, of his fictionalized being. Because of the cultural uniformity of bodily techniques we can also expect the body of character and actor alike to express and promulgate changes in the canons of bodily propriety.

The drama offers at least two other advantages for the materialist historian of the early modern body: the public playhouse was a relatively new cultural site, still engaged in negotiating the terms of its allowance and authority, and it promoted a new form of commercial enterprise, depending for signification on the self-conscious relationship between, and control over, practiced bodily behaviors and the professional mimesis of affect. From this point of view the actor's body offers to the spectator the contrast between fictional outer and insufficient inner which a mirrored image offers the baby, a body of behavioral completeness, significance, and desirability. The actor offers what Mauss calls "a prestigious imitation,"[42] offers the aesthetically successful and authoritative performance of behaviors that are themselves explicitly interpretative and canonical even when they imitate what would be transgressive or embarrassing in actual behavior. Above all, the actor can offer the image of an affective and physical control so masterful as to quell, if only for a time, the inner turbulence of his own humorality. The actor is in or out of a humor not of his own making but well within his affective command.

In the five chapters of this book, I isolate different internal and external functions of the humoral body as textually complex signifiers of embarrassment formations in early modern English culture. Without too much embarrassment, I "clearly and openly" evidence a

42. Mauss, "Techniques of the Body," p. 73.

childlike interest in bodily secretions. But because bodily functions work together physiologically and sociologically, the chapters tell a story of bodily embarrassments in a structure that is to some degree contingent. The book begins with a chapter devoted to urinary incontinence in women not because loss of bladder control was or is a minor form of embarrassment, leading either logically or historically to more tendentious forms of bodily discipline. Rather, it begins this way because the two comic scenes in Jonson's *Bartholomew Fair* and Middleton's *Chaste Maid in Cheapside* which depict women needing or failing to relieve themselves discreetly were *my* starting point. I discovered that references to urinary function to be found in English proverbs, emblems, and medical treatises construct the female body as effluent, overproductive, out of control. Critical silence about these two scenes became the origin of my wider interest in specific representations of bodily shame enacted onstage but later repressed by a critical tradition formed by the discursive disciplines of the civilizing process. Succeeding chapters were composed in an order prompted by my growing theoretical understanding of the internal procedures of the humoral body, in which all fluids were reducible to blood, and of the medical practices devolving from humoral theory. Thus Chapter 2 concerns bleeding both voluntary and involuntary; it argues that blood in the humoral body, differing from itself in purity and refinement, encodes cultural narratives of engenderment. The blood of Shakespeare's warriors, typically depicted as voluntarily shed or metaphorized as phlebotomy, differs from the involuntarily shed, hence shameful blood of woman. Chapter 3 takes on the alimentary purge, a central practice of humoral medicine with a paradoxical relation to the disciplinary mechanisms of the civilizing process. Purging recalls the deeply pleasurable ministrations of passive early experience, but it also threatens the bodily boundaries and self-mastery of the subject. And because the story of reproductive embarrassments in the humoral body is very complex, Chapters 4 and 5 divide between them the events from conception through birth to lactation and weaning.

Throughout, new readings of plays, though they are sometimes an indirect product of the argument, are not its express goal. Reading Elizabethan-Jacobean plays is rather the *means* to the end of discovering the signifying properties of the humoral body and the disciplinary protocols of its long-term transformation in culture. But the signifying properties of the humoral body, and humoral theory in general, do make a significant difference to the reading of early modern plays, for they introduce an insistent materialism into locutions once understood solely as figuration.

One embarrassment of my own is discoverable in the pages of this book—the all-too-prominent part Shakespeare's plays take in these chapters, especially Chapter 2. Since Shakespeare has become a far more massive presence in contemporary Anglo-American literary culture than he was as a practicing playwright, the predominance of his plays in any broadly based study introduces a distortion that must be acknowledged—as I freely do here. My own investment in Shakespeare's plays is such, however, that their presence was finally too insistent, their suggestiveness for my topic too great to be suppressed either on the mere ground of canonical embarrassment or any more substantial intellectual ground. In any case, the uniformity of humoralism's internal habitus, for which I have argued, finally makes the question of the authorship of specific plays treated here very much beside the point. My interest throughout lies in how all the texts of the early modern body inscribe the ideological effect of humoralism per se on the changing canons of bodily propriety, how such texts help us learn how embarrassment changed the reciprocal functioning of the humoral body and the humoral self within it.

Finally, the difficulty of siting as well as of seeing the bodies of which I write is not just a function of their distance in time, for the unobvious and far from simple Lacanian reason that we lack unmediated access to our own bodies as well as to others'. But despite, or perhaps because of, the theoretical richness of the background to my enterprise, the hermeneutic circle I follow to and from the seventeenth century turns out to be more elliptical than Vitruvian. The textualized bodies at its (off)center remain shadowed and inaccessible—as much dark interior as visible surface, the effect of powerful cultural fictions even to the thoroughly problematized selves that may be said to inhabit them.

CHAPTER ONE

LEAKY VESSELS

The Incontinent Women of City Comedy

The incontinence on which this chapter focuses is not the relatively comfortable subject of sexual incontinence in women but its much less comfortable analogue—bladder incontinence. In particular, I want to discuss the two odd occasions in Jacobean city comedy which represent women needing or failing to relieve themselves. The first occurs in Ben Jonson's *Bartholomew Fair* when the urgent need for a chamber pot brings Win Littlewit and Mrs. Overdo to Ursula's booth, the second in Thomas Middleton's *Chaste Maid in Cheapside* when the gossips at the Allwit christening wet the floor beneath their stools. Though both plays have received a goodly share of critical discussion over the years, neither of these episodes has provoked sustained comment. It is easy to understand why. Even now, when so much intellectual attention is directed toward the social formation of the historicized body and its literary representations, the cultural inhibitions that are part of the body's history have made sex easier to discuss than excretion. The bedroom is a discursive site as the bathroom or—to be less anachronistic—the chamber pot and the privy are not, because we are the silenced inheritors of what Keith Thomas has called "the cult of decorum."[1] Norbert Elias, acknowledg-

1. Keith Thomas, "The Place of Laughter in Tudor and Stuart England," *TLS*, 21 January 1977, p. 80.

ing that "in considering this process of civilization, we cannot avoid arousing feelings of discomfort and embarrassment," counters that "it is valuable to be aware of them."[2] However protected by the historical distance and impersonal mediation provided by a scholarly focus upon seventeenth-century comedy, in writing about women excreting I take the risk of evoking embarrassment or distaste.

But criticism should be wary of marginalizing the literary reproduction of any behavior, especially an everyday behavior mentioned so rarely in literary discourse, let alone represented onstage. To the charge that there is little in the physical needs of Win Littlewit or Dame Overdo to write about in the form of historical argument, I would point out the sheer gratuity of staging biological need as engendered joke in the first place. In spite of the recent television appearances of elderly but still attractive female stars delicately promoting the virtues of reinforced underclothing for adults (assumed to be mostly female) who want to get back "into the swim" of vigorous physical activity, the bladder incontinence at the source of Middleton's joke against the gossips is still protected by the taboo of silence.[3] Far from being beneath our critical notice, the two scenes in *Bartholomew Fair* and *A Chaste Maid in Cheapside* constitute important and by no means isolated instances of early modern English culture's complex articulation of gender—the weaker vessel as leaky vessel.

At these moments onstage two affective formations are at work. One involves that signifying practice we call "manners"; the other

2. Norbert Elias, *The History of Manners* (1939), vol. 1 of *The Civilizing Process*, trans. Edmund Jephcott (New York: Pantheon, 1978), p. 59.

3. A recent story in the *Washington Post* explores the ferocity of that silence in relation to the unavailing attempts by Johns Hopkins University Press to secure publicity for *Staying Dry: A Practical Guide to Bladder Control*, written by Kathryn L. Burgio, K. Lynette Pearce, and Angelo J. Lucco, two doctors and a nurse specializing in geriatric urology (Baltimore, 1990). None of the morning talk or news shows expressed willingness to feature the authors; none of the major book chains would feature the book until the press inserted a letter about the book in an Ann Landers column. At that point, requests for the book outpaced the press's ability to keep it in print. Urinary incontinence most affects the elderly, causing "humiliation and anxiety in many, many people," the *Post*'s article quotes Burgio as saying, but it also affects "women in their forties and fifties who have had several children" (*Washington Post*, 27 September 1990, p. C1). Recently Camille Paglia has broken the taboo, praising the efficiency of male urination and its "arc of transcendence" as a "genre of self-expression women will never master" because they, "like female dogs, are earthbound squatters." See *Sexual Personae: Art and Decadence from Nefertiti to Emily Dickinson* (New Haven: Yale University Press, 1990), p. 21. Such a binarism between urinating male as culture and urinating female as nature is, I will argue, both simplistic and ahistorical.

a culturally familiar discourse about the female body, an anxious symptomatological discourse to be found in a variety of other texts including Renaissance medical texts, iconography, and the proverbs of oral culture. This discourse inscribes women as leaky vessels by isolating one element of the female body's material expressiveness—its production of fluids—as excessive, hence either disturbing or shameful. It also characteristically links this liquid expressiveness to excessive verbal fluency. In both formations, the issue is women's bodily self-control or, more precisely, the representation of a particular kind of uncontrol as a function of gender.[4] This ascription of uncontrol is further naturalized by means of the complex classification of bodily fluids to which Galenic humoralism was committed both in theory and in practice. Thus the conventional Renaissance association of women and water is used not only to insinuate womanly unreliability but also to define the female body even when it is chaste, even when it is *virgo intacta*, as a crucial problematic in the social formations of capitalism—an instance of corporeal waste of the female body, representing, in Julia Kristeva's phrase, "the objective frailty of symbolic order."[5]

Natalie Zemon Davis has argued that the deepening subjection of women in the early modern period can be understood as a "streamlining" of the patriarchal family for the economic efficiency required by emerging capitalist modes of production.[6] Representations of the female body as a leaking vessel display that body as beyond the control of the female subject, and thus as threatening the acquisitive goals of the family and its maintenance of status and power. The crucial problematic was whether women as a group could be counted on to manage their behaviors in response to historically emergent demands of bodily self-rule. This book's starting point, proposed in the Introduction, is that the question of bodily control took on a new interest and urgency in early modern European culture, legible from the publication in 1530 and frequent reprintings thereafter of Erasmus's treatise

4. On the relationship between corporeal openness and garrulousness in women, see Peter Stallybrass, "Patriarchal Territories: The Body Enclosed," in *Rewriting the Renaissance: The Discourses of Sexual Difference in Early Modern Europe*, ed. Margaret W. Ferguson, Maureen Quilligan, and Nancy J. Vickers (Chicago: University of Chicago Press, 1986), pp. 123–42.

5. Julia Kristeva, *Powers of Horror: An Essay on Abjection*, trans. Leon S. Roudiez (New York: Columbia University Press, 1982), p. 70.

6. Natalie Zemon Davis, *Society and Culture in Early Modern France: Eight Essays* (Stanford: Stanford University Press, 1975), p. 126.

De civilitate morum puerilium. The bodily controls Erasmus begins to
enjoin upon upper-class boys more often concern table manners and
bodily carriage than the "natural" functions I concentrate on here.
Even so, the new injunctions against urinating or defecating in public,
for example, though frequently ignored in practice even by upper-
class males, begin to inscribe what Lacan calls "the laws of urinary
segregation"—laws employing gender norms to compel restraint and,
more important, to distinguish between the norms of restraint for
men and women.[7] The modesty that is an ethical norm for women
governs not only their own expression of excretory functions but also
what men may or may not do in the presence of women. Elias quotes
from German court regulations of 1570 calling those who would relieve themselves in front of ladies "rustics who have not been to court
or lived among refined and honorable people."[8]

The advance of the shame threshold affects discourses of the body
no less than behavior in ways that begin to clarify differences of both
class and gender. One proof of Erasmus's success in inscribing greater
shame in the boys he addresses is that, unlike later writers on manners, he does not seem reluctant to mention the behavior he is trying
to refashion.[9] This growing delicacy, especially as displayed by those
imitating without sufficient warrant the more refined behavior of
their social superiors, becomes a powerful signifier of class identification and newly drawn boundaries. In *The Winter's Tale*, for example,
Autolycus employs euphemism to establish a firm social distance between himself and Perdita's shepherd family. At first, the shepherds
have some difficulty accepting the downwardly mobile Autolycus's
word that he is "courtier cap-a-pe" (4.4.736), despite the hauteur with
which he asserts, "Seest thou not the air of the court in these enfold-
ings? Hath not my gait in it the measure of the court? Receives not thy
nose court-odor from me? Reflect I not on thy baseness court-
contempt?" (731–34). The evidence of his clothes is ambiguous since,
as the Old Shepherd notes to his more credulous son, "His garments
are rich, but he wears them not handsomely" (749–50). But the young
shepherd counters with evidence of refinement in bodily care: "A
great man, I'll warrant; I know by the picking on's teeth" (752–53).

7. Jacques Lacan, "The Agency of the Letter in the Unconscious, or Reason since
Freud," [1957] in *Ecrits: A Selection*, ed. and trans. Alan Sheridan (New York: Norton,
1977), p. 151.
8. Elias, *History of Manners*, p. 131.
9. Ibid., p. 58.

Finally Autolycus, looking for an excuse to get himself temporarily away from their company, pretends urinary need and invokes a familiar phrase: "Walk before toward the sea-side. . . . I will but *look upon the hedge* and follow you" (4.4.826–28, emphasis added). Several such expressions were available, any one of which would probably have served Autolycus's turn here. Morris Palmer Tilley cites as proverbial "to pluck a rose" and "to water the marigolds."[10] But the phrase works as a perlocutionary demonstration of rank, enacting more verbal refinement from Autolycus and arguably more of a desire for bodily privacy than would be expected in an itinerant peddler—or than the shepherds would have expected from a fellow rustic, a male member of their own class. In so elaborately signaling a desire for privacy in excretion, he is following the recommendation of the conduct books. One such book, published in 1619, declares:

> Let not thy privy members be
>   layd open to be view'd,
> It is most shameful and abhord,
>   detestable and rude.
> Retaine not urine nor the winde,
>   which doth thy body vex,
> So it be done with secresie,
>   let that not thee perplex.[11]

Autolycus mimics excretory refinement, represented both in language and in act, not only to excuse himself but to reinforce the social differences between himself and his companions. For later readers and editors of the play, however, for whom such strictures about excretory decency would be entirely archaic, Autolycus's urinary improvisation becomes a piece of "low" stage business worthy of notice mostly in order to protect Shakespeare from the charge of taking an undue pleasure in the scatological. As Eric Partridge has vigorously asserted, "Shakespeare was not a Rabelais: he took very little pleasure in the anatomical witticism and the functional joke unless they were either witty or sexual. Scatology he disdained, and non-sexual coprol-

10. See Morris Palmer Tilley, *A Dictionary of the Proverbs in England in the Sixteenth and Seventeenth Centuries* (Ann Arbor: University of Michigan Press, 1950). The proverbs in question are M 662, p. 444, and R 184, p. 576.

11. From Richard Weste, *The Schoole of Vertue* (London, 1619; STC 25265)2; rpt. as *The Booke of Demeanor*, ll. 141–48, in *Meals and Manners in Olden Time*, ed. Frederick J. Furnivall, EETS, no. 32 (London: Kegan Paul, Trench, Trubner, 1868), pp. 213–14; quoted in Elias, *History of Manners*, pp. 131–32.

ogy he almost entirely avoided; if one may essay a fine, yet aesthetically important distinction, Shakespeare may have had a dirty mind, yet he certainly had not a filthy mind."[12] Thus the Arden editor, glossing Autolycus's behavior here, dismisses the business as "merely a dramatic device (chiefly for the groundlings)."[13] Admittedly, if Autolycus had simply wanted to get away from the two rustics for a while, an excuse clearly might have been fashioned *otherwise*. What is at stake editorially is Shakespeare's part in his text's excretory humor. The editor's marginal comment serves to detach the playwright from pleasure in the joke and transforms the actor's physical business of pretending to piss into an act of authorial condescension to the "lowly" part of his audience, making *them* and not Shakespeare responsible for promoting an interest in bodily excretions.

Since the sign of the body natural is often a means of leveling social distinctions, it is slyly comic that Autolycus can remake the social management of the lower bodily stratum into a marker of *false* boundaries, the signifier of a counterfeit distinction. But the larger issue that Shakespeare evidences through Autolycus here is one of creating and managing social distance and intimacy, with excretory behavior as a generally available signifier of both class and gender. In the material realm of real practices, what Elias calls "the isolation of the natural functions from public life, and the corresponding regulation or molding of instinctual urges" are profoundly implicated in the overlapping structures of class and gender difference.[14] Thus, in *The Metamorphosis of Ajax* Sir John Harington enjoins his implied audience of great "housekeepers," all male, to adopt his new invention of the flushable water closet as a particular courtesy for great ladies, indeed, as a courtesy they should not hesitate to offer "boldly":

> If you would know whether you should show it to Ladies? Yea in any wise to all maner of Ladies, of the Court, of the country, of the City, great Ladies, lesser Ladies, learned ignorant, wise simple, fowle welfavoured, (painted unpainted) so they be Ladies, you may boldly prefer it to them. For your milkmayds, & country housewives, may walke to the woods to

12. Eric Partridge, *Shakespeare's Bawdy: A Literary and Psychological Essay and a Comprehensive Glossary* (London: Routledge and Kegan Paul, 1968), pp. 8–9.

13. J. H. Pafford, note to William Shakespeare, *The Winter's Tale*, ed. Pafford, Arden Shakespeare (London: Methuen, 1966), p. 133.

14. Elias, *History of Manners*, p. 139.

gather strawberies, &c. But greater states cannot do so; & therfore for them it is a commoditie more then I will speake of.[15]

In Harington's coy "&c.," euphemism—the discursive formation of shame—gathers force. Etcetera covers the country maids' retreat into the woods while exposing their reasons for going, opening a gap between the mentionable task and the unmentionable need. Etcetera may also work to excuse Harington's specification of gender here, from which I infer that other possible contrasts—between great lords and country husbandmen, for example, or between the two ranks apart from gender—would not carry enough rhetorical force in the social promotion of the water closet. Here for a moment there is almost a glimmer of excretory pathos. Not only do all men have greater freedom than all women in excretory behavior (for reasons we will begin to explore later), but lower-class women have greater freedom than women of higher station and whoever wishes to behave like them. Harington represents great ladies as trapped *in their houses* by the obligation to maintain their "greater states," which are constructed as both social and bodily. The degree of their discomfort, like the degree of their physical and social relief, is the "commoditie more then I will speak of." It seems—at least from Harington's point of view as an upper-class male—that to live "greatly" in the body is to be not more free but much less so. Though ladies necessarily have the same bodily needs as milkmaids and country housewives, they lack their freedom of bodily expression—or what *looks* to Harington like the expressive freedom of a state of nature implied in the festive cover of strawberry gathering. Indeed, the obligation of excretory privacy and the aristocratic disinclination to go into the woods "to gather strawberies, &c." becomes a litmus test of rank—"*So* they be ladies, you may boldly prefer it to them" (emphasis added).

By this cultural logic, by the laws of urinary segregation in a hierarchical society, great ladies and whoever wishes to imitate them have the greatest need to maintain their social position before the fact of bodily need and the greatest difficulty in doing so. It is precisely that difference—the greater danger for the elite woman of exposure and bodily degradation—that motivates the distinctions to be explored in

15. Sir John Harington, *A New Discourse of a Stale Subject, Called the Metamorphosis of Ajax*, ed. Elizabeth Story Donno (New York: Columbia University Press; London: Routledge and Kegan Paul, 1962), p. 219.

this chapter. The danger of such exposure underlies the notorious joke in *Twelfth Night* when Malvolio spells out an unmentionable word and commits a verbal trespass against Olivia by confounding the evident differences between her handwriting and her habits in urinating: "and thus makes she her great P's" (2.5.89). In this complex moment of redoubled humiliation, Olivia becomes the object of erotically unstable and ambiguous desires not only on Malvolio's part but on the part of anyone who finds an image of her bodiliness in the letters.[16]

In fact, there is a joke about the spectacle of women urinating here that—like the joke of Autolycus and the hedge—I will not hesitate to ruin by overreading. If considered closely, the joke has several social meanings far more specific than the idea of deflating by their bodiliness the pretensions of those born or aspiring to greatness. Such deflation, then as now, conventionally utilizes excretion to promote a leveling vision of the great at stool; Harington quotes "the old English proverbe that ends thus; *for Lords and Ladies do the same*."[17] Randle Cotgrave, defining the word *pisser*, for example, quotes the French proverb, "Les bonnes gens, pour cela, ne pisseront plus roide."[18] Yet matters of quality and quantity are precisely what are evoked, punningly, by Malvolio's slip. Risking the obvious, let us ask why Olivia is said to make *great* P's and why it is funny to hear Malvolio say so. Perhaps the joke is that for a social overreacher such as Malvolio no part of greatness is lowly; if quantity elides with quality when it comes to making water, the Lady Olivia would make great P's. Or perhaps the joke is that Malvolio's pretensions to indispensability and universal authority in household affairs should extend to such useless knowledge as this.

But the core of this joke, it seems to me, as with the joke of Autolycus and the shepherds, centers on issues of social and physical distance, of intimacy and intrusion. *Both* Olivia and Malvolio are subject

16. In a brief essay titled "Textual Properties," Jonathan Goldberg offers a reading of this moment from which I have both benefited and diverged. Though he mentions Lacan's laws of urinary segregation as the signs of a socially constructed, hence "fully arbitrary desire," he is more interested in how the letters that spell out "an unspeakable word for female genitalia" are castrating letters aimed at Malvolio: "He supplies the letters that cut him down to size." Goldberg's sensitivity to Malvolio's wound should not, however, blind us to Olivia's exposure here and its consequences. See "Textual Properties," *Shakespeare Quarterly*, 37 (1986), 213–17; the quotation appears on p. 217.

17. Harington, *Metamorphosis of Ajax*, p. 83.

18. Randle Cotgrave, *A Dictionarie of the French and English Tongues* (London, 1611; STC 5830; rpt. Menston, England: Scolar Press, 1968).

to critical exposure and a diminishing humiliation even though Olivia, here the innocent, unintended victim of Maria's emplotments, has no part in the scene at all. For this reason, the fact that Malvolio comes onto the scene of his humiliation having been observed "practicing behavior to his own shadow this half hour" (2.5.17–18) cannot be separated from the joke of the great P's and the narrative of possible difference enacted by Malvolio's puns. His criticism of Sir Toby's manners, company, and use of time introduces the larger questions of self-discipline and self-control basic to my continuing theme.

In an imagined future encounter with Sir Toby after his elevation to the place of Olivia's husband, Malvolio reveals himself as a willing disciple of Erasmus's most ferocious strictures about the exquisite control of deportment. Idealizing self-portraiture characterizes the steward as one who claims social superiority on the unfirm basis of manners alone. Malvolio presumes to correct the manners of those above him, indeed, to maintain distance between himself and Sir Toby by reversing their social positions. He constructs an Erasmian situation in which his new kinsman's behavior has become *his* embarrassment and thus his disciplinary obligation and opportunity: "I extend my hand to him thus, quenching my familiar smile with an austere regard of control" (65–66). Malvolio's claim to the mastery of self-presentation here turns the contest between him and the revelers into a contrast between the newer forms of self-possession enjoined upon the English gentleman and the increasingly archaic unconstraint of the elite. The liberty of that unconstraint has been summed up in Toby's exhortations to Sir Andrew to showcase his physical prowess, talents Toby knows to be largely imaginary. Signally for my purposes here, those imaginary talents include the vivid phallic display of urinary prowess as the capstone of male desirability and stylistic accomplishment: "Why does thou not go to church in a galliard, and come home in a coranto? My very walk should be a jig. I would not so much as *make water* but in a sink-a-pace" (1.3.127–31, italics mine). This is the unashamed phallic version of what it is to make great P's, the "arc of transcendence" here deconstructed by its association with Sir Andrew.

As Malvolio misreads the letter, his presumptive familiarity with Olivia's manner of producing bodily wastes, knowing *her* great P's, enacts a narrative revealing his compulsory inferiority of rank and perhaps a urinary encoding of Olivia's presumptuous arrogation of male prerogatives to rule her own household and specify her own objects of desire. Elias argues that the rules of hierarchical society allowed the great to expose their bodies before their inferiors without shame or self-consciousness precisely because the knowing gaze of their inferiors did not count socially: "It becomes a distasteful offence to show oneself exposed in any way before those of higher or equal rank; with inferiors it can even be a sign of benevolence."[19] For Malvolio to "know" Olivia in this way could come from not counting in her eyes, or even from having the duty of emptying her chamber pot and imitating that exquisite combination of intimacy, degradation, and privilege belonging to the body servants of the great, most famously the royal grooms of the stool.[20]

Perhaps in this connection, and for the sake of thoroughly parsing this joke, it is well to note that the household regulations for the male monarchs always specified which household officer bore responsibility for the king's waste products. The records are much more circumspect, however, when it comes to the officers of Elizabeth's privy chamber. As one modern chronicler of the household notes, Elizabeth never "formally appointed anyone to the post" equivalent to the Groom of the Stool.[21] Thus, though some of her ladies presumably had charge of disposing of Elizabeth's wastes and had a quasi-official interest in the state and functioning of the monarch's body natural, historians of Elizabeth's household are screened from the intimate view of her body's functions which they have of her male relatives'. Elizabeth, even more than Olivia, is the best exemplar of Harington's point about the expressive imprisonment of the bodies of "greater States."

Punishing Malvolio's presumption is of course the point of Maria's plot, being set in motion here. The joke of the letters spelling c-u-t, Malvolio's telling failure to speak the difference between "my lady's hand" and her vagina, is a carnivalesque joke rising up, Bakhtin would say, from the lower bodily stratum.[22] It exposes Malvolio as

19. Elias, *History of Manners*, p. 139.

20. Mark Girouard has brief comments about this privilege in *Life in the Elizabethan Country House* (New Haven: Yale University Press, 1978), pp. 57–58. See also David Starkey, "Intimacy and Innovation: The Rise of the Privy Chamber, 1485–1547," in *The English Court: From the Wars of the Roses to the Civil War*, ed. Starkey et al. (London: Longman, 1987), p. 78.

21. I am quoting here from Pam Wright, "A Change of Direction: The Ramifications of a Female Household, 1558–1603," in *The English Court*, p. 149.

22. Michael D. Bristol offers a brief carnivalesque reading of the agon between Malvolio and the revelers in *Carnival and Theater: Plebeian Culture and the Structure of Authority in Renaissance England* (London: Routledge, 1985), pp. 202–4.

blunderer and ensnares him verbally in two ways, involving him ei- ther in behavior that would be offensive and intrusive between social equals of the *same* gender or in behavior that identifies him as beneath social notice altogether. Either way he is hoist with his own Erasmian petard, indecent in precisely the ways he would be correct. But the joke confounding her letters and her genitals works just as vividly to expose Olivia. Sir Andrew Aguecheek's dim repetition of the letters— "her c's, her u's, and her t's: why that?" (2.5.89)—ensures our specific attention to the stylistically ambiguous matter of Olivia's bodiliness and her great P's as the rhetorical climax to Malvolio's desire. The leveling vision catches Olivia in the act and exposes her to the imagin- ary gaze and unstable desires of all Malvolio's listeners. Or it imagines Olivia and Malvolio together in an act of desire the precise nature of which is left excitingly unclear: "*Thus* makes she her great P's." It is even arguable that what opens up, briefly and contextually here, is the coprophilic material of the Elizabethan jestbooks.[23]

The joke's "lowness" effects a shift from one category of construct- ing women by class, which recognizes the social differences *between* women, to constructing women by gender, in which all such dif- ferences are subsumed in the body. This is the proverbial basis of the bed-trick, the material site of the reductive judgment that "Joan is as good as my lady in the dark."[24] No longer a unique individual known by that personal sign of scriptive identity, her handwriting, not even a member of the class of literate gentlewomen, Olivia is reduced to the lowly status of generic female by that specifically shameful female signifier—the "cut." The pun opens out contextually to transform the mediation of the letters into something very like a transgressive en- counter, Malvolio becoming a parody of Actaeon and Olivia of the naked Diana. But the voyeuristic thrill of *that* transgressive moment— already referred to by Orsino (1.1.20–22)—is here made erotically ambiguous by the trajectory of Malvolio's desire, his letter-by-letter sequencing from the genital to the excretory, from "cut" to "p's," from Diana bathing to Olivia peeing.

23. David O. Frantz contends that "the English show themselves particularly ob- sessed with the scatological, and they used it for a variety of effects from the bawdy and satiric to the obscene." See *"Festum Voluptatis": A Study of Renaissance Erotica* (Columbus: Ohio State University Press, 1989), p. 165.

24. For a helpful discussion of the competing classifications of women-as-the-same and women-as-different, see Stallybrass, "Patriarchal Territories," p. 133. The proverb is Tilley, *Dictionary of the Proverbs*, J 57, p. 347–48; he cites C50, "When candles be out all cats be gray," as parallel.

   That Malvolio should be trapped into an Actaeon-like transgressive
intrusion adds mythological motive to his punishment, but none of
the motives to punish Malvolio precisely settles the question of why
Olivia should suffer from such a high level of low exposure here. I
would argue that because the audience too is led to envision her "cut"
and her "great P's," the wider cultural motives to discipline unruly
women through degrading reminders of their bodiliness come into
view. If Toby and Maria lack sufficient motive thus to humiliate
Olivia, the play itself does not.[25] As Cesario has already asserted,
"What is yours to bestow is not yours to reserve" (1.5.188–89). Olivia's
declared withdrawal from the gaze of men into the confines of her
house and the enclosure of her veil—an enclosure already penetrated
by the importunate Cesario—is a presumptuous individualistic claim
not only to social but to bodily autonomy. But that claim is con-
tradicted by the "open" evidence of her great P's, which robs her of
her difference from the common fate, the common bodiliness of
woman. More than that, the presumptive fact of her bodily openness
is token of the inevitability of her eventual marriage, token of the
nature that brings her into neat alignment with Harington's country
maids. If the state of living greatly is what Olivia, walling herself off
from unwanted social intrusion, has claimed, Malvolio's "slip of the
tongue" takes it away from her. His pun strips her of the veil of
excretory privacy that going to the woods "to gather strawberies, &c."
affords Harington's country maids and transforms her, vividly if momentarily, into a carnivalesque figure knowable not by a hand and the
intellectual products of its writing but by her lower parts and the
waste products of "great" appetite. From this point of view, it does not
at all matter that Malvolio misrecognizes the letters, sees Olivia's mark
where she has not made one. As we shall find confirmed by sweating
Ursula, Jonson's pig-woman, the liquid letters of this humiliation belong to Olivia and to all women alike.

≈

   What is at stake here is a semiology of excretion in which an ostensibly natural behavior becomes thoroughly implicated in a complex

   25. The most powerful discussions of the punishment of Olivia are Stephen Greenblatt, "Fiction and Friction," in *Shakespearean Negotiations: The Circulation of Social Energy
in Renaissance England* (Berkeley: University of California Press, 1988), pp. 66–93; and
Jean E. Howard, "Crossdressing, the Theater, and Gender Struggle in Early Modern
England," *Shakespeare Quarterly* 39 (1988), 432–33.

structure of class and gender differences. The two examples of excretory behavior I have drawn from *The Winter's Tale* and *Twelfth Night*,
seen in the sociogenetic context provided by Elias, suggest its social
expressiveness and its relevance to larger questions of class and gender in city comedy. The taboo of silence, still existing to some degree
for us, existed to a much lesser degree for Erasmus primarily because
his treatise appears early in the formation of discursive norms for
bodily behavior.[26] But Elias's argument also implies that euphemisms
such as those employed and breached by Malvolio and Autolycus
assume greater instrumentality for people in more vulnerable or ambiguous subject positions—for people, that is, like women. In *Bartholomew Fair*, both Win Littlewit and Mrs. Overdo display much
greater reluctance to acknowledge their urgent bladders than did
Autolycus, perhaps because they really do need, as it were, to relieve
themselves, whereas Autolycus is only pretending a need in the body
in order to accomplish other social tasks. Finding herself among a
group of strangers at Ursula's booth, Dame Overdo must "entreat a
courtesy" of Captain Whit, but she cannot reply to his expansive offer
to "shpeak out" and "entreat a hundred" because—"with modesty" (4.
4.185–87)—the courtesy she requires can only be un-spoken.[27]

Win's reluctance is even more noticeable. Leaving Ursula's booth
with her husband, she resists his entreaty to see more of the fair
together, saying "I know not what to do. . . . For a thing, I am ash-
am'd to tell you, i'faith, and 'tis too far to go home" (3.6.113, 115–16).
Her evident desperation depends upon a recognized need for privacy
which cannot be met merely by turning away or—until their discovery
of Ursula's chamber pot—by any measure short of an actual return
home.[28] But Win reacts indignantly to the assumption that her embarrassment is caused by the presence onstage of Leatherhead, the
puppet-seller: "Hang him, base bobchin, I scorn him" (120). The
sensation of shame is a function of social structure. In hierarchical
societies, one does not feel the same bodily shame before inferiors as

26. Elias, *History of Manners*, p. 74.
27. I quote from the Revels editions of Ben Jonson, *Bartholomew Fair*, ed. E. A.
Horsman, and *The Alchemist*, ed. F. H. Mares (Cambridge, Mass: Harvard University
Press, 1960 and 1967).
28. One might extrapolate from this evidence that the pissing alleys we know to have
been numerous in London may have been frequented only or primarily by men.
Thanks are due here to Peter Blayney, not only for his rediscovery of Pissing Alley
behind the bookshops of Paternoster Row but for the benefit of countless conversations
on this lowly archaeological topic.

before equals or superiors. By such logic, Win has no reason to feel ashamed, has no social cause for verbal squeamishness if she, like Autolycus, feels superior or at least equal to her companions onstage.

But the vehemence of her response may tell us more than her word. Poor Win is experiencing a redundancy of shame, here the social shame of *feeling ashamed* to acknowledge urgent bodily need not to an inferior but merely in his presence. In this instance, the operative distinctions helping to constitute an embarrassment based on the laws of urinary segregation are those of gender and class and also those of urban or rural identification. Unlike Harington's country maids, the city wife has no woods to cover her retreat and prevent her exposure. She is trapped by the relentless copresence of the crowded metropolis, her sense of respectability, and the lower thresholds of offensiveness characteristic of urban life. If we accept what she says, then her husband's presence or even the otherwise unacknowledged presence of an audience has molded Win's confusion, has called forth a redundancy of euphemism: "I have very great what sha'call'um, John" (3.6.120–21).

If Win's problem is more cultural than physical, so too is its solution. Ursula's booth—the fair's central locus—is usually associated with the body as part of the play's apparent celebration of Carnival. Thus, in Jonathan Haynes's Bakhtinian representation of the booth's symbolic functions, "the material bodily principle is magnificently embodied in the enormous flesh of the pig-woman Ursula and in her booth, which caters to all the body's needs (eating, drinking, defecating, fornicating)."[29] Here, as so often, the call of culture is mistaken for the call of nature, and a generic body, like Leatherhead's puppets lacking sex or gender, stands in for concealed cultural norms that distinguish sharply between the bodily "needs" of men and women. No character in *Barthomolew Fair* is known to defecate offstage in Ursula's booth. And only female characters are shown to need and want Ursula's chamber pot—in actuality "the bottom of an old bottle" (4.4.203)—because, unlike Autolycus or any other male character in this period who needs to urinate, they cannot merely "look upon" the nearest stage property hedge but are tied by the invisible leading strings of culture to a concealed receptacle. Thus is Malvolio's verbal trespass constituted; "Thus makes she her great P's."

29. Jonathan Haynes, "Festivity and the Dramatic Economy of Jonson's *Bartholomew Fair*," *ELH* 51 (1984), 647.

As Haynes suggests, Jonson may well intend Ursula's booth to situate his festive advocacy of "the material bodily principle," and Ursula, by virtue of her office, may represent at one level a de-idealized version of the goddess Nature. Such a symbolic placement is itself fully conventional in binary Renaissance constructions of gender whereby man is associated with culture and woman with nature.[30] We ought to notice that Ursula describes herself as an archetypal representation of woman because, in standing over the hot fire, she becomes a vessel leaking and melting, to be known by her loss of corporeal being—loss of content, form, and integral identity—and marked like Olivia by the liquid letters she makes: "I shall e'en melt away to the first woman, a rib, again, I am afraid. I do water the ground in knots as I go, like a great garden-pot; you may follow me by the S's I make" (2.2.50–53). She and her booth are mutually identifying—in Overdo's words, "the very womb and bed of enormity! gross, as herself" (2.2.107–8). Yet, as proprietor of the booth and supplier of the chamber pot, Ursula crosses over the boundaries of gender to become the agent of culture, the instrument of patriarchy, for the cultural norms constraining Win Littlewit and Mrs. Overdo to seek out the booth as privy function to keep them there as prostitutes. That is, because the booth is the central locus of desire in the fair, it serves prevailing cultural requirements in transforming the women from subjects to objects. The chamber pot has become a bawd, the "jordan" a seller of flesh literalized in Jordan Knockem, the horsecorser. Perhaps Ursula herself senses some of the ideological contradictions in her function, for she objects to helping Mrs. Overdo to a jordan and tells Whit to find Captain Jordan instead: "I bring her! Hang her," she tells Whit furiously, "heart, must I find a common pot for every punk i'your purlieus? . . . Let her sell her hood, and buy a sponge" (4.4.198–201).

Behind Ursula's rejoinder is a specific linkage between whores and urine, which also surfaces in *The Alchemist* (2.1.43–45) when Surly imagines self-punishment to take the form of a whore pissing out his eyes. I discuss this image at some length in Chapter 3; here, let me note the logic of the connection only briefly. It was thought that whores used urination immediately after copulation both as a form of

---

30. See Ian Maclean, *The Renaissance Notion of Woman: A Study in the Fortunes of Scholasticism and Medical Science in European Intellectual Life* (Cambridge: Cambridge University Press, 1980), pp. 2–4 and passim.

contraception and as a preventative against venereal disease.[31] If business at the fair was good—and the attempted recruitment of Win and Mrs. Overdo certainly contributes to that impression—then the whores' demand for Ursula's chamber pot would have been great and her resistance reasonable enough. This semiotic connection between whores and the chamber pot suggests why the wives' desire to use the chamber pot is found to be so compromising and how a bodily behavior so commonplace among fairgoers then and now could become the groundplot of a final, humiliating exposure.

But as far as Win Littlewit's putative transformation from wife to whore is concerned, a wonderful irony is at work. In persuading the pregnant Win to pretend a "longing" to eat Bartholomew pig, John Littlewit had caused his wife to manifest one of the conventional weaknesses of women—the bizarrely irrational cravings of pregnancy, which had to be satisfied in order to prevent harm to mother and unborn baby.[32] If visiting the fair is an act of irrational appetite, the proctor will sanction and justify his weakness by displacing it onto his wife and, through her, women at large. It is Littlewit who acts most powerfully to make his wife into an emblem of female desire: "You may long to see, as well as to taste, Win: how did the 'pothecary's wife, Win, that long'd to see the anatomy, Win? Or the lady, Win, that desir'd to spit i'the great lawyer's mouth, after an eloquent pleading? I assure you they long'd, Win; good Win, go in, and long" (3.6.12–16). Similarly, it is Win who publicly confesses to having "very great what sha'call'um," but later the proctor seems to have it too. Ursula tells Whit that "an honest proctor and his wife are *at it*, within" (4.4.204–5, emphasis mine), thus forcing poor Mrs. Overdo to wait to use the bottle. But given the multiple functions of Ursula's booth, we should also notice here the multiple significations of her phrase, the sexual suggestion in "at it."

We are back, it would seem, in the unstable oscillations of Malvolio's erotic imagination, the libidinal vision of great P's. Like Malvolio's slip

31. See James T. Henke, *Gutter Life and Language in the Early "Street" Literature of England: A Glossary of Terms and Topics Chiefly of the Sixteenth and Seventeenth Centuries* (West Cornwall, Conn.: Locust Hill Press, 1988), sub *pissing after copulation*, p. 192; also E. J. Burford, *Bawds and Lodgings: A History of the London Bankside Brothels, c. 100–1675* (London: Owen, 1976), p. 173. Interestingly, in connection with *Bartholomew Fair*, which takes place at the fair in August, Henke also cites the phrase, "as wholesome as a whore in dog-days," as quasi-proverbial (p. 286).

32. Audrey Eccles, *Obstetrics and Gynaecology in Tudor and Stuart England* (Kent, Ohio: Kent State University Press, 1982), p. 64.

of the tongue, Ursula's pun makes physiological sense because Galenic humoralism proposed a structural homology among all forms of evacuation, including the bodily release of male and female "seed" in sexual climax. (Indeed, it is the Galenic image of female ejaculation of seed that makes phallogocentric sense of the upward displacement of genital desire in the lady longing to spit into the eloquent mouth of the great lawyer.) For Win and Mrs. Overdo to express literally unspeakable desires for the bodily release of urination is to bring them within the overall humoral logic of bodily repletion, a logic of the lower bodily stratum in which the sensory differences between excretion and copulation blur and lose distinction. It can hardly be coincidental that once Littlewit has abandoned his wife at Ursula's booth in order to see how his puppet show is going forward, other conventional uses of her and Mrs. Overdo can be culturally sanctioned—and made intelligible to a modern reader. As Ursula tells Knockem, "persuade this between you two, to become a bird o'the game, while I work the velvet woman within (as you call her)" (4.5.17–19).

How and why these two women find themselves at Ursula's booth, therefore, is just as revealing of gender norms as what happens to them afterward. The chamber pot is bawd indeed. It is not that Ursula confuses the two city wives with Ramping Alice or any of the other Bartholomew birds but rather that she and Knockem merely act upon the implication of the wives' presence, without male escort, at her booth. Just as Malvolio sees the image of his desire brought closer in the unlawful letters ending with P, so here unlawful access to otherwise inaccessible women is made possible by the odd but crucial mediation of the chamber pot: it discloses their vulnerability, announces an occasion of physical and social permeability, hints at the outermost horizon of their desires.[33]

But even beyond the linkage established by Jonson's play between the whore and the city wife who thus makes her great P's, there are other connections between bodily fluids and the contemporary constructions of woman. That women's bodies were moister than men's and cyclically controlled by that watery planet, the moon, was a given of contemporary scientific theory. Their bodies were notable for the production of liquids—breast milk, menstrual blood, tears, and great P's. Both popular and medical discourse, moreover, conceptualized all

33. See Stallybrass on the contrasting signs of the chaste woman—silence, the closed mouth—and the whore—"her linguistic 'fullness'" and her open mouth in "Patriarchal Territories," pp. 126–27.

these fluids as related forms of the same essential substance. Breast milk was the purified form of menstrual blood, "none other thing than blood made white."[34] It changed color according to function by means of a process that occurred in two veins—"occult passages"—which carried the fluid back and forth between the breast and the womb.[35] And to judge from the discursive evidence of one proverb—"Let her cry, she'll piss the less"—tears and urine also may have seemed interrelated in nature and function, flow from one orifice drawing off flow in another.[36]

But the proverb's permissive "*let* her cry" suggests another way of thinking about the matter of women's great pees—as occasions of patriarchal control and intervention, with the apparently desirable goal of making women "piss the less." Early modern culture was preoccupied with the quality and quantity of bodily evacuations as a crucial index of the body's solubility. Humoral medicine's nosology of evacuations constructed a complex symbology in which social differences were given objective verification and natural authority. In humoral medicine, urine was an evacuation of great epistemological potential. As with other signifying properties of the body, urine participates in a powerful hermeneutic circularity in which social distinctions govern both what is sought and what is found in the physical world. The attributes of sexual and other forms of difference were thought to be readily discernible in the body's liquids.

One of the things urine signified—and confirmed—was the nature of women. Thus most advocates of uroscopy were convinced that age and sex functioned materially in the taxonomy of urines along with other key determinants such as color, temperature, quantity, smell, taste, "substance," and "contents." In his 1623 treatise on urine, for example, John Fletcher cites recognized medical authority in insisting that "distinctione between men and womens urine is easily knowne by

34. Ambroise Paré, *The Workes of that Famous Chirurgion Ambroise Parey*, trans. Thomas Johnson (London, 1634; STC 19189), p. 947, quoted in Patricia Crawford, "Attitudes to Menstruation in Seventeenth-Century England," *Past and Present* 91 (1981), 51.

35. Eccles, *Obstetrics and Gynaecology*, p. 52.

36. Tilley, *Dictionary of the Proverbs*, G443, p. 237. Empirical interest in women's tears has not flagged, if the evidence of a 1987 Ann Landers column is any indication. Landers reprints a scientific report, submitted by a reader, that claims to prove a hormonal basis for women's teariness: "Research has shown that the hormone prolactin, which stimulates lactation, also stimulates the tear glands. Women have 60% more prolactin in their blood than men do. It is Frey's theory that weeping is the body's way of excreting substances produced by the body in response to stress." See *Washington Post*, 31 October 1987, p. D16.

often comparing [the urines] together. *Fernel.*"[37] From men of the ideal, sanguine temperament came the standard urines by which all others were to be measured: in color "palew [*sic*], light saffron"; "meane" or moderate in substance and quantity; "in contents} equall, white, light"; "not stinking"; and produced "in due time without} paine, heat, cold."[38] Most women, being of colder temperament, were supposed to have urines lighter in color and greater in quantity than those of healthy adult males. "The chiefe and principall reason alledged for this," notes James Hart rather skeptically in *The Anatomie of Urines* (1625), "is, because men are commonly of an hoter constitution then women, which is the cause that their urines are dyed of an higher colour; and moreover, that the contents in womens urines, in regard of their idle and sedentarie life, do often exceed mens in quantitie." Hart is not sure that sexual difference in urine is easily detectable since men's urine may come to resemble women's characteristic production "by reason of great quaffing, daintie fare, and abundance of ease and idleness."[39]

He does not, however, dispute women's propensity to great pees, because to do so would put in doubt all of Galenic humoralism: women's bodies were simply more liquid than men's. But no matter how logical and necessary (given the humoral facts of the case) "pissing much" may have been, it is also a signifier that confirms women's place in unfortunate social alignments. It makes them part of an otherwise diverse group of great pee-ers, marked by bodily attributes of social deficiency such as immaturity, unproductiveness, passivity, and uncontrol. Fletcher, classifying urines by quantity, writes about what "much signifieth"—"lacke of sufficient heat to attenuate and concoct the grosser parts so in winter, drunkards, sleepers, idle persons, wozmen and children contents are moe."[40]

The categorical complexity of traditional uroscopy is likely to amaze the modern reader who moves without preamble into its discursive precincts. It is hard for us to recognize how a bodily fluid with which we, too, are intimately (if less professionally) familiar can differ so vividly and complexly from itself and can seem so deeply infused with historical particularity and social significance. But the physicians

37. John Fletcher, *The Differences, Causes, and Judgements of Urine* (London, 1623; STC 11063), p. 8.
38. Ibid., p. 107.
39. James Hart, *The Anatomic of Urines* (London, 1625; STC 12887a), p. 45.
40. Fletcher, *Differences, Causes, and Judgements*, p. 57.

who read urines did not see themselves as fantasists. They were eager to distinguish their own practice in assessing the true signifying potential in urine from the grander claims of uromancers—those who read samples of urine to tell fortunes—or even from the practice of those empirics, women healers, and other lay practitioners who judged urines apart from other bodily signs and often diagnosed disease without examining the patient.[41] Physicians inspecting urines believed themselves engaged in the scientific recovery and classification of bodily signs that were objectively *there*. To the trained uroscopist, urines came in a rainbow of twenty or twenty-one colors ranging from several shades of white at the pale end of the spectrum through saffrons, reds, greens, blacks. These variations gave rise to conventional descriptions of great particularity and even beauty. We find urine "nygh as yelowe as saffron of the garden" or "reed as a brennynge cole," "redde as it were the lyver of a beast," "grene as wortes," "blacke & shinyng as a Ravens fether."[42]

But each color betokened differently for men, women, children, and the aged. Thus the red-gold urine, ideal in a man of sanguine temperament, signified an elevation of temperature in the colder, woman, whose urine was normally pale—an elevation that could be the physical effect of an emotional cause. The anonymous writer of *The Key to Unknowne Knowledge* (1599) was repeating commonplace wisdom in declaring that "urine of a woman as bright as Gold, signifieth that shee hath desire or lust to the companie of a man."[43] But such wisdom did not go unchallenged. James Hart ridiculed any reading of lust in a maid's urine compared to the more direct behavioral signs of amorous interest: "The *sanguine* and best complexioned (which by consequence should produce the best urines) are not alwayes the most amorous. Many as ill coloured drabs as ever any hath seene, have not sometimes bene behind the best complexioned Gentlewoman in the land in such a case."[44]

41. On the historical context for this controversy, see Harold J. Cook, *The Decline of the Old Medical Regime in Stuart London* (Ithaca: Cornell University Press, 1986), chap. 1. Heywood's *Wise Woman of Hogsdon* contains a scene of uromancy (2.1.7–21), in which the wise woman pretends to find in a country wife's urine the symptoms she draws from the woman's simple husband in conversation. See *The Dramatic Works of Thomas Heywood*, vol. 5 (London: Russell, 1964), p. 292. This scene is quoted and the play discussed by Jean E. Howard in "Scripts and/versus Playhouses: Ideological Production and the Renaissance Public Stage," *Renaissance Drama* n.s. 20 (1989), 41–47.

42. I quote from *The Seeing of Urines* (London, 1562; STC 22161), sigs. Aiv–Aiiir; but the colors are repeated virtually verbatim in the other vernacular treatises on urine.

43. [F. Kett], *The Key to Unknowne Knowledge* (London, 1599; STC 14946), sig. Miiiv.

44. Hart, *The Anatomie of Urines*, p. 63.

As Hart's sarcasm implies, the struggle to ascertain the nosological value of urine becomes, in effect, a discursive site for the deployment and interrogation of other socially useful discriminations. He was skeptical, for example, that men's urine differed decisively from women's because he seems to have been suspicious of the clarity of bodily signs in a society marked by gender disorder: "If I should instance also in our virgins, more manlike then many men, how were any able to contradict it? But if I should send to the cunningest pisse-prophet in this kingdome the urine of some *Hermaphrodite* or man-woman, what would or could they say? and to which of the sexes would they ascribe the urine?"[45] The problem for diagnosis, it would seem, lay not with the urine but with a dismaying confusion of attributes in the society in which the urine was produced and read as signifier.

In urine that was *known* to be a woman's and where deciphering sexual difference was not an issue, other kinds of crucial bodily indicators were sought—whether or not the woman was pregnant, for example, and what was the sex of her baby. Even the "manner of pissing" was read as a indicator of changes whose meaning may seem more social than physical. Among the virginity tests the humanist physician Laurent Joubert cites are several concerning a maiden's manner of pissing. He has little use for two such tests, in which the young woman is given "a little powdered lignum aloe to drink or to eat" or asked to smell the smoke of "some broken patience dock leaves," whereupon, if she "does not bepiss herself, she is not a virgin."[46] But he seems surer that defloration will in fact alter *for the worse* a young woman's manner of pissing and take away a mark of distinction he seems to value both on aesthetic grounds and for its similarity to the phallic expressiveness of male urination. He imagines a case in which an invasive test for virginity has the unfortunate effect of breaking a hymeneal membrane and thus lowering the value in marriage of an adolescent female whose social status is suddenly unclear:

> The virgin's pissing is more unfettered and clear than other women, because her womb pipe is still tight and narrow, all the way to the outside end, which makes her piss straight and far, in rather the same manner as

45. Ibid., p. 46.
46. Laurent Joubert, *Erreurs Populaires* (1579). I quote throughout from *Popular Errors*, trans. and ed. Gregory David de Rocher (Tuscaloosa: University of Alabama Press, 1989), here, pp. 210–11.

a man, whose urinary canal is very narrow. Thus, once her privities are widened, by whatever thing it might be, she will piss like a corrupted woman and will have lost *this beautiful mark of maidenhood*, all the while remaining a virgin, that is, not known by a man, to whom one will want to attribute her defloration and, consequently, force him to marry her or to dower her in accordance with her station.[47]

(Perhaps it is Malvolio's conviction of Olivia's virginity that leads to his estimation of her great P's—that beautiful mark of *his* aspiration.)

In terms of the history of women's bodies, however, female leakiness was not just a purely illusory construct of Galenic humoralism. It was a real physical condition more or less peculiar to women, the inevitable result of primitive obstetrical techniques and the reproductive practices of the upper and aspirant classes. Dorothy McLaren has persuasively demonstrated the correlation between the extremely high fertility rates among rich women and their abandonment of breast-feeding, arguing that "the choice for wives during their teeming years in preindustrial England was an infant in the womb or at the breast."[48] That this choice may have been dictated largely by class norms is less important to my argument than the possibility that women, whether suckling infants or suppressing the flow of milk after annual childbirth, must often have seemed ready to overflow at the breast or leak down below. In some circumstances, the two thresholds were interchangeable. Joubert devotes an entire chapter to the question of "whether it is true that a woman who has just delivered is able to piss milk" and decides that it is, "as is the case when the parturient woman does not nurse."[49] Early gynecologists believed that women who had never been pregnant could have milk in their breasts, that "marriageable virgins full of juice and seed" could have as much breast milk as wet nurses.[50]

The cultural association of women and liquids was so deeply inscribed that it required little empirical support, as we see in the case of the milk-laden virgins. Given the intractability of gynecological disease in the period and the incessant childbearing of an important female minority, evidence for an iconology of women as leaky vessels

47. Ibid., p. 216, emphasis added.
48. Dorothy McLaren, "Marital Fertility and Lactation, 1570–1720," in *Women in English Society, 1500–1800*, ed. Mary Prior (London: Methuen, 1985), p. 46.
49. Joubert, *Popular Errors*, p. 188.
50. See Eccles, *Obstetrics and Gynaecology*, p. 53, for several references to this belief. Here she is paraphrasing Ambroise Paré.

must have seemed undeniable. Obstetrical instruments did in fact leave women mangled after difficult or protracted labors, threatening them with urinary incontinence.[51] And even among women who gave birth more easily, the frequency of childbearing must have severely weakened control of the urinary musculature. Or as another of Tilley's proverbs puts it, "Like an old woman's breech, at no certainty."[52]

Because the embarrassments of the bodies of old women were proverbial, they were the more easily appropriated for the needs of narrative emplotment. In Reginald Scot's *Discoverie of Witchcraft*, an old witch who has transformed an unsuspecting young Englishman into an ass, is discovered when she has to stay behind him on a trip into town:

> After three yeares were passed over, in a morning betimes he went to towne before his dame; who upon some occasion (*of like to make water*) staied a little behind. In the meane time being neere to a church, he heard a little saccaring bell ring to the elevation of a morrowe masse, and not daring to go into the church . . . in great devotion he fell downe in the churchyard, upon the knees of his hinder legs, and did lift his fore-feet over his head, as the preest doth hold the sacrament at the elevation. Which prodigious sight when certeine merchants of Genua espied, and with woonder beheld . . . the merchants aforesaid made such meanes, as both the asse and the witch were attached by the judge.[53]

According to Scot, the old woman's body, needing to "make water" at the wrong time, has betrayed her witchcraft. Able to manipulate the male body of another, she nonetheless lacks sufficient control of her own.

With such anecdotes inscribing the insinuations of popular discourse, the neutrality of gynecological facts breaks down. Uncertainty in the lower parts bespeaks unreliability or even self-betrayal in the constructed woman; overproduction at one orifice bespeaks overproduction at the rest. The demonized womb, for example—fully animate, capable of movement, sensitive to smells—was "so greedy

51. Michael MacDonald cites one such case in *Mystical Bedlam: Madness, Anxiety, and Healing in Seventeenth-Century England* (Cambridge: Cambridge University Press, 1981), p. 273n.

52. Tilley, *Dictionary of the Proverbs*, W667, p. 744.

53. Reginald Scot, *The Discoverie of Witchcraft* (London: John Rodker, 1930), p. 54, emphasis added.

and likerish" for male seed, according to one midwifery manual, "that it doth euen come down to meet nature, sucking, and (as it were) snatching the same."[54] "A likerish tongue a likerish tail," says the proverb.[55] More important, in its liquorish behavior the greedy womb bears a metonymic resemblance to women at the gossips' meeting, a comic subgenre Linda Woodbridge has linked to prevalent anxieties about gender boundaries in early seventeenth-century England.[56] In the most striking example of the genre, John Skelton's "Tunning of Elynor Rumming" (written around 1517 but reprinted in 1609), gossips with naked paps and untrussed hair rush into the alewife's house to taste her latest brew, bringing their household goods to barter if they have no money. One of them gets so horribly drunk that "she pyst where she stood" (373) and, having overflowed at one end proceeds to flow at the other: "Then began she to wepe" (374). Another woman, whose paunch "was so puffed / And so with ale stuffed," barely escapes the same embarrassment: "Had she not hyed apace, / She had defoyled the place" (570–73). That such drinking women are also typically garrulous is obviously very much to the point: Skelton's Latin colophon invites women "marked with the dirty stain of filth" or "who have the sordid blemish of squalor" or "who are marked out by garrulous loquacity" to listen to his record of their deeds.[57]

The action in Skelton's poem is a particularly coarse example of a portentous metonymic chain: a woman who leaves her house is a woman who talks is a woman who drinks is a woman who leaks. Any point in the linkage may imply or abridge the rest. Thus, going abroad is itself a leak, even potentially a flood, as in John Northbrooke's argument against allowing city wives and widows to go to the theater: "They wander abroade . . . and runne from house to house, and at the last go after Satan. *Give the water no passage*, no not a little (sayth Syrach) neyther give a wanton woman libertie to go out abroade."[58] Talking is also leaking, of course, especially in the em-

54. *Complete Midwife's Practice Enlarged* (1659), quoted in Eccles, *Obstetrics and Gynaecology*, p. 29.

55. Tilley, *Dictionary of the Proverbs*, T395, p. 674.

56. Linda Woodbridge, *Women and the English Renaissance: Literature and the Nature of Womankind, 1540–1620* (Chicago: University of Chicago Press, 1984), pp. 224–39.

57. I quote here from John Skelton, *The Complete English Poems*, ed. John Scattergood (New Haven: Yale University Press, 1983). For the colophon, see p. 452.

58. John Northbrooke, *A Treatise*, ed. Arthur Freeman (London, [1577?]; STC 18670; rpt. New York: Garland, 1974), p. 68. I owe this reference to Boyd M. Berry.

blem literature. For Geoffrey Whitney, a leaky barrel emblematizes "the blab," a figure unidentified by gender. But in the fable portion of the emblem, the barrel itself—with water pouring from its many holes—is the one filled by the daughters of Danaus as a punishment for killing their husbands.[59] That these daughters are visually absent from the emblem may imply the conventional force of their association with the barrel or perhaps the suppressed patriarchal anxieties to which gossiping women give rise. Pour as they will, the daughters of Danaus cannot fill their barrel or stop it from leaking: "No paine will serve, to fill it to the toppe, / For, still at holes the same doth runne, and droppe" (5–6). On the facing leaf is Whitney's emblem of the proud Niobe, "Which, yet with teares, dothe seeme to waile, and mone" (6). In the second emblem, like the first, the iconography is only partial: the offending woman is visually absent. What seems to link them thematically for Whitney is the question of female insubordination and its patriarchal punishment—perpetual leaking.

What is all too obvious in the coarse physical detail of Skelton's poem is also present by implication in Whitney's emblems: the threat of female independence has been renegotiated as an issue of female self-control in a form—a leaky form—obviously related to talkativeness but far more shameful. It is the potential shamefulness of the association of women and water I want to emphasize, a shamefulness present even when the trope is apparently reversed or subverted. When it is reversed, the dangerous unreliability of women can be used to establish the dangerous changeability of water, especially the waters of the body. Othello tells Emilia that Desdemona was "false as water" (5.2.134).[60] In the context of marital infidelity and accusations of whorishness, however, Othello's phrase may be set beside another commonplace expression that "urine was the physician's strumpet." Like strumpets with false colors and fair exteriors, like strumpets who flattered their customers with false promises of pleasure, a fair-colored urine might flatter patient and uroscopist with the promise of health but really betoken disease and death. Color, says John Fletcher, is especially uncertain "of signification, as beeing subject to many alterations of light cause. . . . yea in one day every urine that a man maketh is unlike an other in colour, so that here especially the in-

59. Geoffrey Whitney, *Choice of Emblemes* (Leiden, 1586, STC 25438; rpt. Amsterdam: Da Capo Press, 1969), p. 12.
60. Tilley cites this line as proverbial, *Dictionary of the Proverbs*, W 86, p. 706.

Frustrà.

TH E Poëttes faine, that D A N A V S daughters deare,
Inioyned are to fill the fatall tonne:
Where, thowghe they toile, yet are they not the neare,
But as they powre, the water forthe dothe runne:
   No paine will ferue, to fill it to the toppe,
   For, ftill at holes the fame doth runne, and droppe.

Which reprehendes, three fortes of wretches vaine,
The blabbe, th'ingrate, and thofe that couet ftill,
As firft, the blabbe, no fecretts can retaine.
Th'ingrate, not knowes to vfe his frendes good will.
   The couetous man, thowghe he abounde with ftore
   Is not fuffif'de, but couetts more and more.

Superbiæ

Superbiæ vltio.

O F N I O B E, behoulde the ruthefull plighte,
Bicaufe fhee did difpife the powers deuine:
Her children all, weare flaine within her fighte,
And, while her felfe with tricklinge teares did pine,
Shee was transformde, into a marble ftone,
Which, yet with teares, dothe feeme to waile, and mone.

This tragedie, thoughe Poëtts firft did frame,
Yet maie it bee, to euerie one applide:
That mortall men, fhoulde thinke from whence they came,
And not prefume, nor puffe them vp with pride,
   Lefte that the Lorde, whoe haughty hartes doth hate, [ftate.
   Doth throwe them downe, when fure they thinke theyr

Fabula Niobes
Ouid. 6. Me-
tamorph.

De numero fi-
liorum, vide
Aul. Gellium
lib. 10. cap. 6.

Effe procul leti, cernant mea funera trifies;
Non fimilis toto mæror in orbe fuit.
Bis feptem natos peperi, bis pignora feptem:
Me miferam! Diuûm fuftulit ira mihi.

Dirigui demum lacrymis, & marmora manant.
Sic mihi mors dolor eft; fic mihi vita, dolor.
Difcite, mortales, quid fit turgefcere faftu,
Et quid fit magnos pofthabuiffe Deos.

Bapt. Gyral-
dus.

B 3   *In vi-*

Facing pages from Geoffrey Whitney, *A Choice of Emblemes* (Leiden, 1586).
By permission of the Folger Shakespeare Library.

famie, that urine is a lying strumpet, hath some appearance of truth."[61] (He goes on, of course, to try to save urine from its metaphoric contamination by woman by arguing that, despite its apparent changeability, urine remains a valuable and truthful diagnostic tool.)

The trope comparing women and water appears in a subverted form in the famous iconographic depiction of female virginity as a sieve that does not leak, an allusion to the vestal virgin Tuccia who carried water in a sieve from the Tiber to the Temple of Vesta in order to prove her virginity. Roy Strong has cataloged many examples of the motif in portraits of Queen Elizabeth, who carries a sieve to symbolize not only her physical virginity but also the connection between that virginity and her ability to rule. Strong identifies the series of sieve portraits as symbolic arguments against the Anjou match. In the three portraits of 1579 (one of which I reproduce here) the iconography of the sieve, the motto in Italian from Petrarch's *Triumph of Chastity* beneath Elizabeth's coat of arms, and the globe visible behind her right shoulder link the Queen's virgin triumph over love to her imperial mission.[62] Yet, clearly, the association of Elizabeth with Tuccia's sieve, even though it links the queen to another, ostensibly historical woman, serves to separate her sharply from womankind as a whole—and thus from the contradictions of a woman ruler. For women less politically motivated to maintain the virgin state, the iconographic representation of Elizabeth's self-command produces an unflattering implication: if not-leaking becomes something of a mythological miracle reserved for a long-gone Roman lady and the occasional virgin queen, then leaking remains the normal punitive condition for women, and melting mother Ursula remains their representational archetype: "You may follow me by the S's I make."

61. Fletcher, *The Differences, Causes, and Judgements*, p. 110. Robert Burton uses the same figure: "And for urine, that is the Physicians' strumpet, the most deceitful thing of all, as Forestus and some other Physicians have proved at large." See *The Anatomy of Melancholy*, ed. Floyd Dell and Paul Jordan-Smith (New York: Tudor, 1938) p. 560.

62. Roy C. Strong, *Gloriana: The Portraits of Queen Elizabeth* (London: Thames and Hudson, 1987), pp. 97–99. I am grateful to John King for pointing this reference out to me. Strong notes the sieve as an emblem of discernment, as in Whitney's emblem of a sieve in action under the motto, "Sic discerne." The accompanying verse makes clear this sieve's identification with the intellectual operations of patriarchy rather than with the bodily propensities of leaky women: "By which is ment, sith wicked men abounde, / That harde it is, the good from bad to trie: / The prudent sorte, shoulde have suche judgement sounde, / That still the good they should from bad descrie: / And sifte the good, and to discerne their deedes, / And weye the bad, noe better then the weedes (Whitney, *Choice of Emblemes*, p. 68).

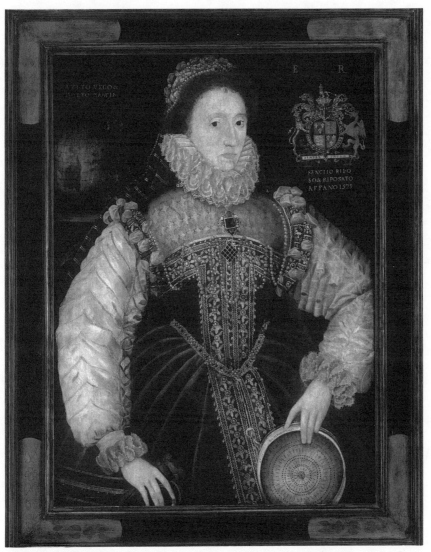

Portrait of Elizabeth I with a sieve, c. 1579. By permission of Mrs. Francis T. P. Plimpton.

꒰

Far more than even the leaking women of *Bartholomew Fair*, the female characters of *A Chaste Maid in Cheapside* reproduce a virtual symptomatology of woman, which insists on the female body's moisture, secretions, and productions as shameful tokens of uncontrol. Although this symptomatology is most striking in the christening scene in act 3, it is present from the very beginning of the play, when Mrs. Yellowhammer diagnoses her weeping daughter's languor as greensickness and prescribes a husband as the appropriate therapy:

> You had need to have somewhat to quicken
> Your green sickness—do you weep?—a husband!
> Had not such a piece of flesh been ordained,
> What had us wives been good for?—to make salads,
> Or else cry'd up and down for samphire.
>
> (1.1.4–8)

As R. B. Parker has pointed out, Mrs. Yellowhammer here associates sexually provocative foods such as highly seasoned salads with urinary function: samphire was considered to be both an appetite stimulant and a diuretic, provoking urine and an appetite for meat.[63] This early connection between sex and urination is repeated elsewhere in the play as part of a larger discursive link between urine and sexual incontinence.[64] But like Elias discussing the history of manners, Parker fails to see how deeply implicated this linkage may be with contemporary constructions of gender and anxieties about its boundaries. And he is not aware of the structural linkage between forms of evacuation in Galenic humoralism, which, as we have seen in the case of Win Littlewit and Mrs. Overdo at Ursula's chamber pot, blurs the lines between urination and copulation—and the appetites thereto.

In fact, though Parker is perhaps the play's most astute and sympathetic reader, he finds the urinary aspect of its discursive exploration of sexuality distasteful: it is "a criticism of eroticism pushed too far."[65] His discomfort is not surprising, since—if Elias is correct about the progressive lowering of the shame threshold—we are far less able

63. I quote throughout from *A Chaste Maid in Cheapside*, ed. R. B. Parker, Revels Plays (London: Methuen, 1969); for the note here, see p. 7n.
64. Parker, *A Chaste Maid*, p. lv.
65. Ibid.

even than Middleton's contemporaries to speak easily about excretory functions except in medical or scientific discourses. And we tend to segregate excretory discourse from erotic contexts as ferociously as we prosecute the laws of urinary segregation. Who can forget how central this very issue of "unisex public restrooms" was in the debate about the equal rights amendment, particularly among its female opponents. A provocative counterassertion of feminist demands was evident in a widely circulated poster showing the back view of two men in what is obviously a public restroom. But in between them, with her legs in a straddle parodying the male posture at urinals, stands a booted blonde in a fringed miniskirt. Contemporary contestants for power—in Lacanian terms, for possession of the phallus, concealed in this poster, which we are supposed to imagine this tall female invader now possesses—have met and mingled in the toilet. The urinal has become an object of desire, a symbol of contested privilege. We, having seen how the privy in *Bartholomew Fair* functions to subordinate women as sexual objects, may want to call this poster "Ursula's revenge."

But what also links this poster to representations of woman in *A Chaste Maid in Cheapside* is the symbolic use of the urinary function in discourses of power. In the early seventeenth century, this representation implied contests for control not of public territory—such as the restroom—but of the central domestic territory of the patriarchal family—the female body itself. In *A Chaste Maid*, this contest occurs most frequently as a function of competing explanations of behavior, as characters propose interpretations of motive and act that seem to be irreconcilable. These discursive collisions are most evident where the behavior of women is concerned. Thus, because Cheapside takes the physical frailty of women for granted, symptomatological explanations for female behavior—such as Mrs. Yellowhammer's response to Moll's tears—are readily available to articulate gender difference. But such conventions are radically destabilized by Cheapside's equally widespread acceptance of an economic determinism that opens the categories of class and gender to structural redefinition.

In the play, not surprisingly, bladder incontinence in particular is presented as an attribute of women of all ages, from the new Allwit baby, who is taken offstage in act 2 to get her bum wiped, to the drunken gossips who wet the floor in act 3 and discuss, among other things, a nineteen-year-old daughter who cannot be married because of "a secret fault," that she wets her bed (3.2.96). Her mother's willing-

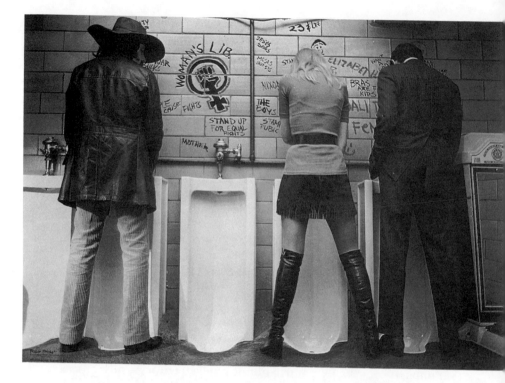

Testing the laws of urinary segregation. ERA poster, c. 1971. Library of Congress photo.

ness to reveal the shameful attribute is presented as a function of drink; as one gossip remarks cynically, wine can do what friendship cannot, cause women to talk freely as it causes women to leak.

The play's symptomatological discourse of women is perhaps most striking in the christening scene. There the gossips' enthusiastic eating and drinking finally chase their host from the room as their wet kisses chase Tim Yellowhammer, though not before one of the drunken gossips actually falls on him and requires a hoist up. The scene as a whole bears a strong resemblance in tone and action to Skelton's "Tunning of Elinor Rumming," except that instead of celebrating an alewife's latest brew, the gossips celebrate the safe delivery of the fecund Mrs. Allwit and christen a brand-new arrival to the sisterhood of woman. In fact the baby, "a large child," say the gossips, is presented as "but a little woman!" (3.2.14), rather than an infant, and

Middleton's broad comic play throughout the christening on the extraordinary facts of the baby's parentage serves to underscore the
asymmetry of gender and generation in a particularly striking way.
Though the gossips claim to see a resemblance between the baby and
Allwit, their inspection of the baby's features effects a metonymic
redistribution similar to what we observed in the subtext of the sieve
portrait. The gossips do not know what we do: that because the baby
has not been fathered by Allwit, only her resemblance to her mother
has a foundation in nature. And it is a resemblance that the gossips
link specifically to the two interchangeable thresholds of female appetite and vulnerability: the baby has her "mother's mouth up and
down, up and down!" (3.2.13). In this context the question of family
resemblance is thoroughly effaced by the constitutive force of gender.
The gossips really see in the baby a small version of themselves:

> A very spiny creature, but all heart;
> Well mettled, like the faithful, to endure
> Her tribulation here and raise up seed.
> (3.2.16–18)

The celebratory momentum of the christening itself produces an
even deeper sense of gender identity, because the gossips regress into
an infantile gluttony and incontinence, which bring them into the
tight circle of mother-daughter resemblance.

The christening in early modern Europe was an occasion that typically called for much eating and drinking, even when celebrated in
Lent, as this one is.[66] The signal feature of this christening, however,
is less the communal carnivalism than a demarcation of gender even
sharper than what we have seen in *Bartholomew Fair*, as the men band
together in vocal disgust at the women's gluttony, drunkenness, reek-
ing wet kisses, and finally incontinence. "They have drunk so hard in
plate," comments Allwit to his manservant, "that some of them had
need of other vessels" (3.2.171–72).

Allwit's male anxiety at the christening scene could not be clearer or
more representative of patriarchal feelings, even though they issue
from a man whose apparent desire to give over his rights to his wife's
body to the man who can keep them both in material comfort seems at
first glance to invert the patriarchal ethos. He stands apart as choric

66. Peter Burke, *Popular Culture in Early Modern Europe* (London: Temple Smith,
1978), pp. 191–99.

commentator while the nurse passes around comfits and wine. In his account of their gluttony, the women become sexually overpowering, grabbing at phallic sweetmeats with "long fingers that are wash'd / Some thrice a day in urine" (3.2.52–53), culling all the "long plums" and leaving nothing but "short wriggle–tail comfits, not worth mouthing" (3.2.63–64). The greedy mouth, furthermore, merges with the greedy womb, the women stuffing their pockets while they stuff their mouths: "Now we shall have such pocketing: see how / They lurch at the lower end!" (3.2.54–55). Allwit seems to see them in a sisterly collusion with his prolific wife, threatening to deprive him of a substance he defines as both material and sexual:

> No mar'l I heard a citizen complain once
> That his wife's belly only broke his back;
> Mine had been all in fitters seven years since,
> But for this worthy knight,
> That with a prop upholds my wife and me,
> And all my estate buried in Bucklersbury.
>
> (3.2.65–70)

For Allwit, the threat posed by a collective, hence Amazonian female appetite and female fertility is so catastrophic that it supplants the male rivalry, virtually normative in plays of the period, which Middleton's city comedies, with their obsessive feuding of merchant and gallant, usually lay bare. Indeed, what mitigates our sense of Allwit's gender anomalousness in giving up his wife's sexual services is that he so clearly defines them rather as sexual demands—costly ones. Her latest pregnancy is marked by a longing for "pickled cucumbers"—a sexually suggestive longing far more anxiety-provoking than anything other pregnant women of the stage, such as Win Littlewit or even the Duchess of Malfi, manifest. Allwit hopes the cucumbers will "hold [his] wife in pleasure / Till the knight come himself" (1.2.9–10). Mrs. Allwit's appetites can be satisfied only by dint of a sexual, financial, and psychological effort and expense that Allwit has craftily transferred to Sir Walter. It is Allwit, not his cuckolder, who congratulates himself on his escape from the alienated labor of sexual performance and the attendant anxieties of sexual possession:

> These torments stand I free of; I am as clear
> From jealousy of a wife as from the charge:

> O, two miraculous blessings! 'Tis the knight
> Hath took that labour all out of my hands:
> I may sit still and play; he's jealous for me,
> Watches her steps, sets spies; I live at ease,
> He has both the cost and torment.
>
> (1.2.48–54)

Here the enemy of middle-class conservation of wealth is women. "They never think of payment," complains Allwit (3.2.79) to the man who does offer payment for sexual privileges in the house, as they flee the room together. Here then, uniquely, cuckoldry becomes wittoldry. Erstwhile male rivals become partners in arms, banding together to conserve for themselves and the variously fathered offspring whom they feel obliged to support an economic and sexual substance that the appetite of woman and her conspicuous lack of self-control threaten to destroy.

In *A Chaste Maid in Cheapside*, however, the thematizing of female uncontrol through the discursive association of women and water, though even more striking than it is in *Bartholomew Fair*, is also more complicated because water symbolism and urinary references, while largely identified with women, are not exclusively so. The play's two most potent males, Sir Walter Whorehound and Touchwood Senior, especially, are linked with water symbolism in its male form—as semen. Thus in the play's dramatic economy, Sir Walter (pronounced "water") opposes his cousin Sir Oliver Kix, whose name means "dry stalk" and who will lose an inheritance to the watery Walter if his marriage remains infertile—or, in this dramatic idiom, dry.[67] We cannot be surprised, therefore, that water, when it is male water, has changed, now representing power, not leaking or loss of control. Male water, unlike female leaking, has economic value and under the right circumstances can even be shared in order to preserve or enlarge dynastic claims. Thus Sir Oliver seeks to cure his own dryness by ingesting medicinal water from Touchwood Senior, who promises that he "has got / Nine children by one water that he useth" (2.1.174–75). Of course he administers his "water" to the two Kixes separately—sending Sir Oliver off on a five-hour horseback ride after he has drunk the milky liquid and taking Lady Kix off to receive his more potent brand of liquid medicine in bed. The Kixes are so pleased with the effects of Touchwood's water—though presumably

---

67. On Sir Oliver's name, see Parker, *A Chaste Maid*, p. lv.

for different reasons—that at the end of the play, after Lady Kix has conceived, a delighted Sir Oliver exults in his newfound potency and in the victory of his "water"—conveniently hybridized—over that of his cousin: "The child is coming and the land comes after; / The news of this will make a poor Sir Walter" (5.3.14–15). He takes over for Master Allwit as the play's contented cuckold, inviting the Touchwoods to join their household.

This identification of water with male potency rather than simply with female leaking would appear to redefine the argument with which this chapter began, especially since Middleton seems interested in presenting male potency in so exaggerated a form that it starts to resemble the loss of self-control I have been associating with leaking women. The Touchwoods, for example, have impoverished themselves through overproduction:

> Life, every year a child, and some years two;
> Besides drinkings abroad, that's never reckon'd;
> This gear will not hold out.
>
> (2.1.15–17)

A virtual Priapus with an unquenchable thirst for such nondomestic "drinkings," Touchwood himself admits to having imperiled the harvests in nearby villages by taking so many girls out of service at haymaking time. For his part, Sir Walter worries that his unacknowledged offspring will marry, incestuously, the children of a future marriage. But Middleton creates a wonderfully comic context for his male fertility gods by linking the biological fact of male potency to the far more remarkable social facts of the play—that is, to the ingenious social and discursive arrangements by which male authority in Cheapside masks and serves its sexual drive and social ambitions. In these arrangements, since they focus so closely on the strategic containment of female appetite and reproduction and the strategic promotion of male potency, we return full circle to the social construction of women as shamefully leaky vessels with which we began.

Furthermore, as Mrs. Allwit's longing for pickled cucumbers suggests, the production of potent male water is often legitimated and rationalized as a function of female thirst. When this appetite is framed neutrally as a matter of female physiology, we are in the medical domain of the hungry womb "greedy and likerish" for the ingestion, as it were, of male seed and for the release of its own seed at climax. When this appetite is framed satirically, the womb's ingestion of male seed is indistinguishable from female appetite at other bodily thresholds. In one bawdy street ballad, for example, ale is used as a periphrasis for male seed.[68] The two extant versions of the ballad narrate one Watkin's seduction of a naïve young woman afraid she will "die a mayd." Her ignorance of what we still call the facts of life and her bibulous appetite for "ale" combine to produce a narrative at the nine-months' end of which a bastard has been born: "Good sir quoth she in smiling sort, / What doe you call this prety sporte / Or what is this you do to me? / Tis called Watkins ale quoth he." Word-play is built around the familiar pun of tale/tail; the ballads are full of coy equivocation about the delightful properties of "watkins ale." In her avid thirst for ale, the maiden seems to belong to the female society in "The Tunning of Elinor Rumming," except that here the transaction does not occur between female customers and an alewife. Instead, the alewife "Mother" Watkin disappears, to be replaced by a young man in the cask of whose body the potent "ale" is contained. In the manuscript version, the maid asks her lover in some detail about the properties of his ale:

> She said to watkin lovingly
> what ale is this which ronnes soe free
> tys watkings ale doe you not know
> tys now abroach and layd full low
>   yf watkings ale be such
>   I cannot drinke too much
>   I like so well the touch.

What I find remarkable here—amid the dreary conventionality of the maiden's naïveté, the ease of the seduction, and the inevitability of its outcome—is the ballad's evident phallic delight in the properties of the ale itself, a delight shared within the ballad by Watkin and the maiden both. In the broadside version Watkin advertises the ale as

68. "A Ditty Delightfull of Mother Watkins Ale" (London, c. 1590, STC 25107) and Bodleian MS Rawlinson Poet, 185, fol. 14v. The text of the broadside is reprinted in *Ancient Ballads and Broadsides*, ed. Henry Huth (London: Joseph Lilly, 1867), pp. 251–55; references also in *The Roxburghe Ballads*, ed. J. W. Ebsworth, vol. 7 (Hertford: Stephen Austin, 1893), p. xiv, and *The British Broadside Ballad and Its Music*, ed. Claude M. Simpson (New Brunswick, N.J.: Rutgers University Press, 1966), pp. 745–46. Natascha Würzbach includes references to this dialogue ballad in *The Rise of the English Street Ballad, 1550–1650*, trans. Gayna Wells (Cambridge: Cambridge University Press, 1990), pp. 70, 193, 194. The lines quoted from the manuscript ballad are from the transcription kindly made available to me by Peter Blayney, to whom I owe the original reference.

[60] THE BODY EMBARRASSED

"sweeter farre than Suger fine, / And pleasanter than Muskadine."
Two possible figurations of sexual intercourse seem to inhabit the
same textual field. In one reading of the ballads, sexual appetite is
mutual and mutually gratified; in the other, intercourse is a deceptive
transaction between a crafty seller and an unwary consumer whose
interest in the commodity being proffered is assumed. The joke depends on the maiden's ignorance of the *hidden* or long-term properties of the ale, permitting her to be duped into accepting pleasure in
the short term, which is gained at the expense of eventual shame.

The obvious humor and narrative shape are less useful to my purposes, however, than the self-delighted phallic hyperbole that hides
none too successfully behind its manipulation of the conventional
construction of female appetite as greedy at both ends. As the gossips
at the christening would have it: "Her mother's mouth up and down,
up and down." The seducer Watkin is merely a version of Touchwood, the seduced maiden a less skillful sister of Middleton's Country
Wench or her city cousin, Lady Kix. And once again, as with Touchwood or Sir Walter Whorehound, male repletion—here the condition
of being continually refillable with Watkin's ale—is emphatically contrasted to female openness. Female thirst—not male repletion—
causes the different fullness of pregnancy.

The extent to which such constructions help to maintain an existing
structure of gender differentiation is clearly visible. So too are the
ideological contradictions that any systematic articulation of gender
must seek to efface, which become particularly evident in Middleton's
characterization of Moll Yellowhammer and Lady Kix, the most sexually deprived of the women in Cheapside and hence the most labile
emotionally. As Burton describes that species of melancholy belonging to maids, nuns, and widows, "They are apt to loath, dislike, dis-
dain, to be weary of every object, &c. each thing almost is tedious to
them, they pine away, void of counsel, apt to weep and tremble."[69]
Full consideration of Lady Kix and Moll's circumstances, however,
exposes the discursive tyranny and incompleteness of any merely
gynecological interpretation of their behavior. Thus the "naturalness"
of Lady Kix's grief and frustration at her seven years of childlessness
is deconstructed by the presence of a strong economic incentive for
reproduction: "Think but upon the goodly lands and livings/That's
kept back through want on't," she tells her husband (2.1.150–51)—

69. Burton, *Anatomy of Melancholy*, p. 354.

"it" being, of course, Sir Oliver's "brevity," his phallic insufficiency. Her tears, then, are causally linked to her husband's dryness. But here the authority of gender to classify behavior—which is so compelling in the christening scene—is undercut by powerful competing economic and class determinants that bind the Kixes to each other and finally to a mutual reliance upon the potency of the Touchwood "water."

In the case of Moll Yellowhammer, Middleton is primarily interested in showing how social authority—here represented by the older generation—uses the discourse of nature oppressively to serve its own selfish ends. Thus the weeping Moll's emotional lability in the opening scene is immediately rationalized by her parents symptomatologically—as the telltale sign of maidenly greensickness. But their strong desire to supply the conventional remedy—a husband of their choice—only calls the interpretative completeness and objectivity of their diagnosis into question. Moll weeps not from greensickness, or at least not only from greensickness; she weeps more obviously from the effects of her mother's scolding and her parents' tyranny in the question of marital choice. By this logic, more tyranny will produce more water, more "leaking," and the constraints of culture will continue to be defined as inherent biological flaws in the nature of woman.

The exchange between the Yellowhammers about their daughter's behavior, furthermore, is also particularly revealing of the ideological tensions and contradictions occasioned by the asymmetry of gender. Mr. Yellowhammer scolds his wife for using socially pretentious diction to describe Moll's behavior just as she scolds their daughter for the ideologically aberrant behavior itself. "Errors?" he repeats. "Nay, the city cannot hold you, wife, / But you must needs fetch words from Westminster" (1.1.25–27). He identifies her language as the diction of a gadabout, a gossip, a woman who cannot be contained at home. His instruction in diction, intended to establish his authority and reassert the discursive boundaries of class, insists upon a patriarchal nomenclature for the faults of women and the presence of universal truth in the particular case:

> cracks in duty and obedience?
> Term'em e'en so, sweet wife.
> As there is no woman made without a flaw,
> Your purest lawns have frays and cambrics bracks.
> (1.1.33–36)

The Yellowhammers would proceed from symptom to cause, from the leak to the "crack," thence to the effective social remedy: "'Tis a husband solders up all cracks" (36). (The process may be particularly effective for a daughter whose dancing her mother has likened to that of "a plumber's daughter" [21].) But whereas the Yellowhammers clearly envision the therapy as mechanical—plugging the hole, mending the leaky pipe joint with the husbandly tool—we are bound to regard it as ideological. And the seemingly gratuitous authority lesson Yellowhammer has provided his wife reinforces the point. In this play, men discharge virtually all the responsibilities of culture, including the primary one—the containment of women.

In act 5, after trying unsuccessfully to elope by boat with Touchwood Junior, Moll pretends to sicken and die. Once again, her parents offer the diagnosis of nature to mask the constrictions of parental authority. "She has," her father asserts, "catch'd her bane o'th'water" (5.2.7). We supply the contextually subversive pun on the knight's name. The counterfeit illness itself, complete with a climactic swoon, is never offered up to diagnosis in the play, but it was fully diagnosable by current medical and popular thinking as suffocation of the mother—that is, a literal rising up of the cold, sexually deprived uterus toward the hotter organs, causing the sufferer to faint from the compression of heart and lungs.[70] Perhaps Middleton's audience recognized in Moll's counterfeit swoon not only a literary allusion but a gynecological symptom—the simulated fulfillment of her mother's diagnosis at the beginning of the play—since the swoon, like the tears, was symptomatic of hysterical sexual frustration. Only by imitating Juliet and undergoing a false funeral, does Moll escape her parents' discursive tyranny in a marriage to Touchwood Junior.

Yet Moll is a more obedient member of her culture, a more easily contained vessel, than her parents are able to recognize. Unlike Juliet, she has never initiated any part of her secret courtship, elopement, death, and resurrection but has taken direction from her resourceful lover and his powerful brother. In the discourse of this play, she merely makes a choice between kinds of male potency, refusing Sir Walter, her "bane o'th'water," for the more vital fluid of her lover, his "Watkins ale." Hers is a resurrection from drowning in the wrong water, but it is a resurrection ritualized and sanctioned by communal waters—the tears of the mostly female mourners. The reported

70. Eccles, *Obstetrics and Gynaecology*, p. 77.

deaths of the lovers "makes a hundred weeping eyes, sweet gossip," Lady Kix tells a companion at the funeral (5.4.22). The communal overflow, releasing the lovers from the Yellowhammers' restrictive containment, becomes the signal for the lovers to arise. Moll's tears have been transferred to the community and her sexual deprivation has been remedied by her husband's controlling potency. He says he has been momentarily rendered speechless by joy: "My joy wants utterance" (5.4.45). But phallocentric wordplay on *utter* defines his return to self-command as ejaculation—sex becoming discourse—and thus as sexual command. "Utter all"—that is, speak and ejaculate—"at night," his brother tells him (5.4.46). Just as Lady Kix's weeping has been controlled by Touchwood Senior's sexual power, so Moll's has been suppressed by the junior brother's.

Like the daughters of Danaus in Whitney's emblem, the leaky women of Middleton's Cheapside cannot by themselves keep their barrels full or their holes plugged. Attempting such impossible tasks becomes the self-imposed responsibility of the patriarchal order. In this play, moreover, the tasks themselves offer patriarchy the distinct advantage of promoting unusually stable male alliances—between Master Allwit and Sir Walter; between Touchwood Senior and the Kixes; between the Touchwood brothers themselves—to get the job done. Although the play seems to suggest that these male alliances are forged by necessity—a necessity occasioned by female unreliability and appetite—we can perceive in the construction of women as leaky vessels the powerful interests of patriarchal ideology. At the end, the leaky vessels of Cheapside have been contained, perhaps because they, unlike Win Littlewit or Mrs. Overdo, have not ventured into the free space of a fairground to follow mother Ursula and find the public chamber pot, Ursula's revenge.

LAUDABLE BLOOD

Bleeding, Difference,
and Humoral Embarrassment

The logic of cultural symbology requires, of course, that urine could never be the only semiotically vital fluid the early modern body produced or the only one to be fetishized. This and subsequent chapters attempt to describe the mostly obscured, even repressed relation between other body fluids and the early modern canons of embarrassment by deploying Bakhtin's contrast between the grotesque and classical bodily canons. In beginning with blood, I anticipate a skeptical question: what could be embarrassing about *bleeding*? It does not seem to belong logically to what Bakhtin calls the body's "gay matter"—dung, urine, sweat, and other bodily effluvia of the lower stratum.[1] Blood is not usually classified among the body's excreta (the category of bodily fluids most subject to ambivalent affect), since, unlike urine or sweat, it is supposed to remain contained within the body. In pre-Reformation religious symbologies, blood is precious and ritually efficacious.[2] Even in more secular vo-

---

1. Mikhail Bakhtin, *Rabelais and His World*, trans. Helene Iswolsky (Bloomington: Indiana University Press, 1984), pp. 334–35.
2. The popular beliefs attaching to blood in early modern Germany have been studied by R. Po-Chia Hsia as part of his discussion of the blood libel. See *The Myth of Ritual Murder: Jews and Magic in Reformation Germany* (New Haven: Yale University Press, 1988). He cites the following popular verse from Johann Weyer's *De praestigiis daemonum* (Frankfurt, 1586): "Sanguis mane in te, sicut fecit Christus in se. / Sanguis

cabularies, among them the several idioms of the Elizabethan-Jacobean stage, it is most often metonymy for important and laudable qualities such as mercy, sacrifice, or passion—both divine and human—or their tragic loss through violence and death. Thus Dr. Faustus, having signed in his "proper blood" the gift of his soul to Lucifer and finally facing damnation, has a vision of divine mercy: "See see where Christs bloud streames in the firmament" (5.2.1939).[3] And blood's power to blazon guilt—even more than the psychological enormity of the guilt itself—lies behind Macbeth's fear that "all great Neptune's ocean" will *not* "wash this blood / Clean from my hand" (2.2.57–58).

Logically, blood's symbolic weight and power would seem to derive from the obviousness of its importance to life itself, no matter which physiological paradigm holds sway. As Nancy Siraisi has commented, the "uniquely significant role ascribed to blood in Aristotle's work on animals," dividing animal creation into "blooded and bloodless types," remained influential in subsequent accounts of the physiology of blood.[4] The materialism so dominant in Renaissance thinking about behavior and the faculties of the soul allows blood's physical attributes to receive a high praise suffused with ethical implication. Blood, said the seventeenth-century iatrochemical physician George Thomson in a virulent attack on the practice of bloodletting, "is a most pure Sweet *Homogeneous, Balsamick, Vital Juice* . . . ordained to be the seat of Life, the principal matter for Sense, Motion, Nutrition, Accretion and Generation." As "the immediate instrument of the soul," its most important power was nutritive, "sweetly uniting all the parts of the Body for the conspiration of the good of the whole."[5]

But against this apparent immunity of blood to the early modern canons of embarrassment, let me immediately introduce the variable

---

mane in tua vena, sicut Christus in sua poena. / Sanguis mane fixus, sicut Christus quando fuit crucifixis," which he translates as follows: "Blood, stay in yourself, just as Christ in himself. / Blood, stay in your veins, just as Christ in his pain. / Blood, stay fixed, just as Christ was to his crucifix" (bk. 5, chap 4, pp. 311–12, quoted p. 145 n. 23).

3. I have used the text of *Dr. Faustus* from *The Complete Works of Christopher Marlowe*, ed. Fredson Bowers, vol. 2 (2nd ed.; Cambridge: Cambridge University Press, 1981).

4. Nancy G. Siraisi, *Medieval and Early Renaissance Medicine: An Introduction to Knowledge and Practice* (Chicago: University of Chicago Press, 1990), p. 105.

5. From the preface to Thomson's anti-Galenist, antibloodletting treatise, *Aimatiasis, or The True Way of Preserving the Bloud* (London, 1670; Wing T1021), p. 2. Although his ferocious attack on bloodletting and his defense of experimental chemistry make him a somewhat unorthodox figure, Thomson's praise of the blood is itself conventionally phrased.

of sexual difference—the gendered specter of female or womanly blood, the often demonized Other among the varieties of human blood, blood as bodily waste. With the reminder of menstrual blood, not only blood's relation to embarrassment but also its potential for ambivalent social coding begins to emerge. Blood was and is a far more powerful signifier than urine, but despite medical panegyric and the serious weight of Christian and other symbolisms, it is no less ambivalent or shame producing. Our own tragic experience of acquired immune deficiency syndrome and other blood-borne diseases indicates, too, that blood may be a bodily signifier of especially narrow historical specificity and affective power. Who before the recognition of AIDS in 1981 could have anticipated the cultural remystification of blood as the agent of a shame-laden fatal disease? Even in the far less charged arena of cultural histories of the early modern body, blood is suffused with ideological import. It is the bearer of a robustly hierarchized, elaborate semiology chiefly, though not solely, because in preindustrial English society where all the key structures of exchange and distribution of resources—whether material, symbolic, or libidinal—were still based on hereditary transmission, the key social attributes of blood could never be simply symbolic or metaphoric.[6] The importance accorded to a physical continuity located in the blood was one rationale for the culture's notorious obsession with female chastity, for example. Theological encodings and decodings of blood and bleeding, as English recusant history alone suggests, were decidedly unstable and, for the individual churchgoer or nonconforming nonchurchgoer, potentially even dangerous. Like other kinds of ideologically overdetermined signs, blood in early modern England was a discursive site of multiple, competing, even self-contradictory meanings and the relationship between blood and the individual body containing it was no less ideological than physiological. In one's blood were carried the decisive attributes of one's cultural identity.

This belief continued even after the empirical advances of the seventeenth century, Harvey's momentous proof of the circulation of the blood and the subsequent slow breakup of humoral Galenism. In his *Memoirs for the Natural History of Humane Blood* (1684), Sir Robert Boyle complained somewhat obliquely that the preoccupation of medical science with anatomy had taken attention away from physiology: "I

6. My preliminary thinking on these matters owes much to Leonard Tennenhouse, *Power on Display: The Politics of Shakespeare's Genres* (London: Methuen, 1986), pp. 20–36.

will not be so rash as to say, that to mind . . . the Solid parts of the Body, and overlook Enquiries into the Fluids, and especially the Blood, were little less improper in a Physician, than it would be in a Vintner to be very solicitous about the Structure of his Cask, and neglect the consideration of the Wine contain'd in it."[7] His own inquiry into the blood was intended to test—make that to debunk—the Galenic account of its composition, to make trial "whether the Humors, Phlegm, Gall, and Melancholy, be really contained in the Blood, as constituent Parts of it" or "whether some other substances may not with as much reason be admitted into the composition of the Blood." Operating within an ostensibly inductive paradigm, Boyle declared his object of study to be blood "not as 'tis form'd in the Vessels of a living Body, but as it is Extravasated." He further limited his experimental sampling to the blood of sound persons "that parted with it out of custom" in the normal course of prophylactic bloodlettings. And he reported with evident frustration a resulting problem of supply. Such limitation "was the main reason why I was so scantly furnished with Blood, that of sound persons being in the place I resided in, very difficult to be procur'd in quantity."[8]

Boyle sought to identify the physical attributes of blood. He investigated such topics as its taste and odor, its weight relative to water, and its inflammability when dried; he distilled blood serum and subjected it to various trials; he compared the properties of distilled blood and urine. But signally for the purposes of my argument, Boyle's list of topics for a thorough inquiry into the characteristics of blood—a project that his problems with an adequate blood supply prevented him from carrying out—includes the investigation of differences we now classify as socially constructed rather than materially "real." That is, having set aside Galenic humoralism as an adequate account of the internal structure of the blood, Boyle was determined to look elsewhere in the physical world for a system of differences. It seemed rational to him to start with external physical difference—visible difference—and hypothetically correlate it to difference within. Thus he proposed investigation of "the Difference between Humane Blood as 'tis found in sound Persons differingly constituted and circumstantiated, as men, women, (when menstruous, and when not), Children Moors, Negro's, &c" as well as "the Affinity and Difference between

7. Sir Robert Boyle, *Memoirs for the Natural History of Humane Blood* (London, 1684; Wing B3994), A2^v–A3^r.

8. Ibid., pp. 17, sig. A6^v, 96–97.

the Blood of men, and that of divers other Animals."[9] Returning to the classifications of Aristotle, Boyle would reexamine them anew.

To highlight Boyle's invention of these topics is not to accuse him of empirical naïveté, misplaced scientific zeal, or embryonic racism. That only the most trivial differences in blood chemistry exist within and among socially distinct groups could not have been detected or explained by any technology available to a seventeenth-century scientist, though that scientist could begin to formulate questions. The point, rather, is to show the determining potential of social difference even (or especially) for empirical inquiry, particularly in its foundational stages. Harvey's revolutionary demonstration earlier in the century of the circulatory movement of the blood, once accepted, encouraged fundamental reconsiderations of blood's constituent elements.[10] Boyle's *Memoirs* is an example. Because differences of age, gender, and race bear social meanings Boyle can only experience as natural, he turns to those differences to formulate scientific hypotheses.[11] Meanings attached to blood and bleeding as physical aspects of the body's structure and physiology could not be isolated from the inevitably hierarchical structures of social difference. Furthermore, Boyle's account of his trials of blood identifies many of the other variables and oppositions keying the textual relationship of bleeding to the canons of embarrassment—oppositions between blood within and outside the body, blood flowing and stopped, pure and waste, blood shed "out of custom" through phlebotomy and by other means, blood from persons sick and well, male and female, old and young. In the discursive operations of such variables the mechanisms of shame and embarrassment can begin to be read.

&

In these poststructuralist times it may almost go without saying that the meanings of blood as a signifier alter with specific discursive contexts. In the quasi-technical, incompletely formed early modern En-

9. Ibid., p. 14.
10. See Siraisi, *Medieval and Early Renaissance Medicine,* pp. 191–92.
11. My perception of the limits of Boyle's empiricism runs counter to the judgment voiced by Alfred White Franklin in "Clinical Medicine," his contribution to *Medicine in Seventeenth Century England,* ed. Allen G. Debus (Berkeley: University of California Press, 1974), pp. 113–45. "Paracelsus" he claims, "had been looking *for* something; for Boyle looking *at* things sufficed" (p. 127). But, as Ferdinand de Saussure and much of poststructuralist thought insists, how even a great scientist looks "*at* things" is subject to epistemic constraints.

glish medical discourses, the Galenic taxonomy of blood is confused and full of lexical as well as conceptual circularity—as perhaps befits an explanatory model nearing the end of its tenure. Blood was simultaneously a simple substance in the body and the compound containing it. Thus the French surgeon Ambroise Paré follows Galenic tradition in distinguishing between "the general name of blood, which is let out at the opening of a veine," and blood as the name for "an Humor of a certaine kind, distinguished by heate and warmnesse from the other Humors comprehended together with it, in the whole masse of the Blood." But besides blood, phlegm, bile (choler), and black bile (melancholy), the term *humor* also referred to a numerous subset of bodily substances, for a humor generally was "what thing so ever is Liquide and flowing in the body of living Creatures endued with Blood."[12] Contained in the neutrality of this definition is a significant distinction of kind, subdividing humors as either sustaining creatural life or inimical to it—"either natural, or against nature." Both kinds of humors, indeed all humors, were carried in the "whole mass" of the blood and determined whether and to what degree that blood was "laudable."[13]

Blood's lexical unwieldiness should not distract us from noticing a significant correlation between the scientific account of blood and the social hierarchies in which blood figures as a key signifier. Before Harvey early modern medicine followed Aristotle and Galen in viewing blood's production, composition, and movement within the body as conceptually dependent on a complex hierarchy of physical and spiritual attributes describable in ethically overloaded terms. Harvey demonstrated in 1628 that more blood flowed through the heart than could be produced as a result of digestion.[14] But before that (and for

12. Ambroise Paré, *The Workes of That Famous Chirurgion Ambrose Parey*, trans. Thomas Johnson (London, 1634; STC 19189), p. 12.

13. The adjective is a commonplace in the description of blood and other bodily fluids. See for instance, Helkiah Crooke, *Microcosmographia* (London, 1615; STC 6062.2), who thus describes the initial separation of aliment from excrement: "The thin and lawdable part of the Chylus (for the thicke excrements called *Alvinae foeces*, are forced into the great guts) together with that humour which is as it were a watery excrement, and was engendred in the concoction of the stomacke, is suckt away by certaine branches of the Gate-vein" (p. 134).

14. Gweneth Whitteridge summarizes this proposition as follows: "That the pulse of the heart transfers the blood incessantly from the vena cava into the arteries in so great a quantity that it cannot be provided by the food eaten and in such a way that the whole quantity passes through the heart in a short time." See her edition and translation of William Harvey's *De motu cordis*, entitled *An Anatomical Disputation concerning the Move-*

some time afterward), the body's production of blood was thought to be more or less directly related to consumption, and habits of consumption were related to a variety of factors, both social and physiological. Thus the bodies of the aged—since the aging process was thought of as a gradual drying out of the body over time and even after death—were thought to contain less blood than the bodies of younger adults. The sleepwalking Lady Macbeth's memory of Duncan's bloody corpse—"Who would have thought the old man to have had so much blood in him?" (5.1.39–40)—registers horrified surprise at the near-miraculous signs of vitality expended in the murdered king. Physician John Symcott, whose practice Lucinda Beier has investigated, would also have been surprised at Duncan's store of blood. Symcott caustically noted "what an adventure it is to take blood from an old withered man, whose fountains of blood-making may be justly suspected of weakness and some unsoundness."[15] Thus we would do well to consider the implications of Lady Macbeth's dismay over the quantity of Duncan's blood. Does spilling *less* blood make the spiller less guilty? Would killing a bloodless king be a less horrific crime?

Blood in varying states was considered to be the product of a series of three progressively refined transformations, or concoctions, of food and drink into bodily nutriment. The first concoction, which turned food into chyle, took place in the stomach: "All things which we eate or drink," says Paré, "are the materialls of blood . . . turned by the force of concoction [in the stomach] into a substance like to Almond Butter."[16] As a refinement upon food, Crooke notes, chyle was in the ideal both "laudable and well disposed." But it still contained "some unprofitable and excrementitious parts" and thus could never by itself constitute bodily nourishment: "This *Galen* seemeth to intimate when he sayth; *That nothing can perfectly nourish which hath not passed through all the concoctions.*"[17] The second concoction, sanguification, took place in the liver, where, Paré says, aliment "acquires the

---

ment of the Heart and Blood in Living Creatures (Oxford: Blackwell Scientific Publications, 1976), p. xvii. Her edition of Harvey's *Anatomical Lectures* or *Prelectiones anatomie universalis de musculis* (Edinburgh: E. and S. Livingstone, 1964), contains a concise and lucid summary of Galenic physiology—to which in 1616, the date of *Prelectiones*, Harvey was still committed. See pp. xxxviii–xxxix.

15. John Symcott, letter of 19 February 1641, quoted in Lucinda McCray Beier, *Sufferers and Healers: The Experience of Illness in Seventeenth-Century England* (London: Routledge and Kegan Paul, 1987), p. 109.

16. Paré, *Workes*, p. 12.

17. Crooke, *Microcosmographia*, p. 171.

absolute and perfect forme of blood."[18] This second stage of purification and refinement involved not only the transformation of chyle
into blood and the other humors but the infusion of chyle with "natural spirit." In sanguification, that is to say, inanimate chyle became
part of the living body and, as blood, was transported out of the liver
through the portal vein to the rest of the members.[19]

This understanding of sanguification implies the progressive separation of nutriment from excrement, the progressive differentiation
of bodily substances into materials of increasing purity or degradation: "With that blood at one and the same time and action all the
humors are made whether Alimentary or excrementitious." Phlegm,
for example, was blood "halfe concocted," which, says Paré, "may by
the force of native heat be changed into good and laudable blood."[20]
Organs of the lower belly (the area below the thoracic cavity) could be
classified according to whether and how they helped the liver in its
task of purification. Crooke mentions the spleen as "a great helpe to
the Liver" because it drew unto itself "the thicker part of the aliment,
not so fit to make pure blood." The spleen may be said "to purge and
defecate the blood, and to make it more pure and bright."[21] (The
final concoction, which further refined blood into seed, took place in
the spermatical vessels and becomes part of this argument later.)

Humoral theory, with its theoretical reliance upon the innate goodness of heat, classified the quality—the salutariness—of venous blood
by a hierarchy of attributes of color, consistency, temperature, movement, and refinement or lack of excrementitiousness. Laudable
blood, promoting the goal of bodily solubility, was thus thinner,
purer, redder, warmer, less sluggish than blood grosser in composition.[22] Such laudable blood not only nourished the body, but was
capable of transferring many of its positive attributes to kindred
organs. "From consideration of the colouring of each thing," writes
Harvey, "comes the knowledge of the degree of its kinship to blood, its
temperament and active movement."[23] Laudable venous blood was

18. Paré, *Workes*, p. 12.

19. On this rather complicated subject, see Gweneth Whitteridge's introduction to
Harvey, *Prelectiones*, p. xxxviii.

20. Paré, *Workes*, pp. 12, 13.

21. Crooke, *Microcosmographia*, p. 129.

22. For an account of solubility entering into the treatment even of wounds and
fractures to an initially healthy body, see Beier's account of surgeon Joseph Binn's
practice in *Sufferers and Healers*, pp. 60–61.

23. Harvey, *Prelectiones*, p. 23.

more "spiritous," less excrementitious than grosser blood. It was not, however, more spiritous than its ruddier counterpart in the arteries, which, before the public demonstrations of the great sixteenth-century anatomists, was thought to differ from venous blood not only in color and point of origin but also in composition. Some portion of venous blood—so went the theory—flowed to the heart, where, in addition to natural spirit, it received a second infusion of spirits transferred from the lungs to the heart and thence via the arteries to all parts of the body.[24] These were the so-called vital spirits or what Crooke, freely translating Galen, defined as "*a certaine exhalation of benigne or wel-disposed blood*" or "*a subtle and thinne body always moove-able, engendred of blood and vapour, and the vehicle or carriage of the Faculties of the soule.*"[25] The presence of the vital spirits gave arteries a clear privilege over veins with their load of humors and natural spirits. Thus Thomas Vicary, in his *Profitable Treatise of the Anatomie of Mans Body* noted that arteries "lye more deeper in the flesh then the Veines doo: for they cary and kepe in them more precious blood then doth the Veine."[26] Paré describes arterial blood as "more subtile, it runs forth as it were leaping, by reason of the vitall spirit contained together with it."[27]

As late as 1649 Harvey was still countering objections to his proof that the same blood circulates in the veins and arteries by seeking to reclassify natural and vital spirits from bodily fact—material carried in veins and arteries—to bodily metaphor:

> Though nothing is more uncertain and doubtful than the traditional teaching about the spirits, the majority of physicians appear to end in agreement with Hippocrates, who favoured a tripartite composition of our body, namely, the containing parts, the contents, and the driving factors. These last are interpreted as spirits. But if for driving factors spirits are to be understood, whatever in living bodies has force and drive would be styled spirit. . . . What, however, is specially relevant to my theme after all other meanings have been omitted from consideration as being tedious, is that the spirits escaping through the veins or

24. The arteries brought *spiritus* to the brain, where vital spirit was remade into the animal spirits (from *anima* or soul), which controlled nervous function and had a special role in vision. See Siraisi, *Medieval and Early Renaissance Medicine*, p. 108.

25. Crooke, *Microcosmographia*, pp. 173, 174.

26. Thomas Vicary, *Profitable Treatise of the Anatomie of Mans Body* (London, 1577; STC 24713; rpt. Amsterdam: Da Capo Press, 1973), sig. H3r–v.

27. Paré, *Workes*, p. 328.

arteries are no more separate from the blood than is a flame from its inflammable vapour. But in their different ways blood and spirit . . . mean one and the same thing. For, as wine with all its bouquet gone is no longer wine but a flat vinegary fluid, so also is blood without spirit no longer blood but the equivocal gore. As a stone hand or a hand that is dead is no longer a hand, so blood without the spirit of life is no longer blood, but is to be regarded as spoiled immediately it has been deprived of spirit.[28]

Whether refigured as bouquet, vapor, or the animating impulse, spirit in Harvey's somewhat defensive formulation retains its privilege as that which confers identity, integrity, and value on otherwise dead matter: blood "without the spirit of life" was "spoiled"; a hand that is dead, a hand in which no blood flows, is a stone hand. It is "no longer a hand" at all.

Harvey's great discovery of the circulation eventually broke down Galenic physiology, but it had no immediate effect on the practice of medicine, which still depended heavily on bloodletting, scarification, and cupping as major humoral therapies in the prevention and cure of disease. Renaissance medical writers of whatever persuasion and discourse were convinced of the relation of disease to the specific composition of the blood. "So great a power hath this liquid red matter to alter our conditions," says the iatrochemist Thomson with a professional devotion to blood verging on obsession, "that according as it is constituted in *Eumetry* and *Eucrasie*, our morality may be good or bad."[29] Thomson himself was violently opposed to bloodletting in any form, believing instead that diet or medicines sufficed for the restoration of the body chemistry and the promotion of solubility. More orthodox Galenists, however, believed the goal of the nonsurgical therapies of diet and "inward" physic to be maintenance of the "body's internal balance through evacuation"—including the evacuation of blood.[30]

28. William Harvey, "The Second Anatomical Essay to Jean Riolan," in *The Circulation of the Blood: Two Anatomical Essays by William Harvey*, ed. and trans. Kenneth J. Franklin (Oxford: Blackwell Scientific Publications, 1958), pp. 38–39.

29. Thomson, *Aimatiasis*, p. 1.

30. I take the quoted phrases here from Beier, *Sufferers and Healers*, p. 61. There is an extremely helpful introduction to the history and practice of phlebotomy from Galen to Vesalius in the introduction by John B. DeC. M. Saunders and Charles Donald O'Malley to their translation and edition of Andreas Vesalius, *The Bloodletting Letter of 1539* (New York: Henry Schuman, n.d.), pp. 5–36. But see also Siraisi, *Medieval and Renaissance Medicine*, pp. 136–41.

The key physical opposition here was between *"Fulnesse & Emptinesse,"* bodily states that Nicholas Gyer in *The English Phlebotomy* describes as having "between them selves a mutuall relation." The goal of diagnosis was to determine whether a given body was either too full or too empty of blood and, if its blood "offended," whether the offense lay in quantity, quality, or both. Internal imbalance of humors was always the culprit, variously cause or effect, but medicine made a distinction between two kinds of plethora. One was the *plenitudo ad vires* or "to the strength," when a patient knew him- or herself to be plethoric by a feeling of sluggishness. The second was *plenitudo ad vasa*, "to the vessels," when plethora presented symptomatically by broken blood vessels, as in nosebleeds or hemorrhoids. In a simple "repletion in qualitie," the vessels "conteine more good bloud and nourishment than the nature of the patient can wel rule or overcome." The repletion of disease "is when one humor alone aboundeth." All plethoric patients—whether suffering plethora *ad vires* or *ad vasa*—felt heavy, weary, drowsy, lumpish, or slothful in their members. Veins stretched, swellings appeared. In a state of plethora, the body could not use up all the blood it had produced in concoction, nor could it perfectly concoct all the food and drink it continued to take in. The resulting "discommodities" were many: "Moistnes thereby is too much increased, and naturall heate quenched." From the unconcocted food "proceede gross and undigested fumes," which annoy the nerves, trouble understanding and reason, even deprive the tongue of its office.[31] The plethoric body finally reached an internal state of what I would call virtual inanition, for its blood had lost its positive attributes of warmth, vigor, color and had become cold, clammy, slow moving, and full of gross excrementitious humors. Clearly such a body was far from "soluble."

Even so, when to let blood, how much to let, and where to open the vein were vexed questions, as Gyer explained: "It must not want art and judgement: For in it, consideration must be had of the inflicted wound: of the quantitie of the bloud: of choosing the aptest vaine: either to pull backe bloud, or to evacuate it quite: or to make it onely lesse in quantitie . . . whether the veine must be opened streight downe, or overthwart, of the same side of the bodie, or of the other."[32] Since the goal of phlebotomy was the restoration of an internal state

31. Nicholas Gyer, *The English Phlebotomy* (London, 1592; STC 12561), pp. 1, 7–8, 3, 10–11.
32. Ibid., pp. 25–26.

conceptualized as balance or homeostasis, moderation was inevitably the watchword of practice. The very old and the very young were not considered good candidates for bloodletting, or likely victims of plethora. Bloodletting was not customarily practiced on pregnant women, whose extra blood went to nourish the fetus (though Paré, an enthusiast of bloodletting, does suggest circumstances in which letting a pregnant woman's blood is advisable). Phlebotomy was not recommended in seasons of extremest heat and cold since opening and bleeding the body risked altering its internal caloric state. Prophylactic bloodletting in the springtime was thus routine for some, on the model of spring housecleaning, to rid their bodies of humors built up over the cold months when phlebotomy could not be indulged and the body's natural evacuations were slowed. Lady Margaret and Sir Thomas Hoby traveled to York regularly in the spring for doses of prophylactic physic, including bloodletting, and John Evelyn too "was frequently let blood."[33]

In some circumstances purging or bathing accompanied bleeding. In order to prepare blood to be let when it is "verie viscous, clammie, & grosse," Gyer advises a preparatory bath. If redirecting the humors was the phlebotomist's goal, the preferred course was bleeding by revulsion, or opening a vein to draw ill-humored or ill-tempered blood away from an affected part or inflammation toward the incision. Thus, for women whose monthly "courses" were stopped, surgeons prescribed the opening of an ankle vein to encourage the downward flow of blood. Revulsion was also recommended in cases of nosebleed or bleeding from the belly. Any one of several veins could be opened to relieve a more general case of repletion since, according to a Hippocratic aphorism noted by Gyer, the body was both *conspirabile*, "of a common and generall accorde together," and *confluxibile*, "alwaies running together." Theorists acknowledged that phlebotomy brought about "an exquisite evacuation of al the humors equally," even in cases where only one humor was the culprit.[34] The phlebotomist had to take care, therefore, neither to draw too much blood— allowing too many good humors to flow out with the bad—nor to cause too great and sudden a drop in the body's internal heat by a prolonged release of the heat-bearing blood.

For my purposes here, the cultural meanings of bodily plethora

33. See Beier, *Sufferers and Healers*, pp. 222, 171.
34. Gyer, *English Phlebotomy*, pp. 30, 53, 26.

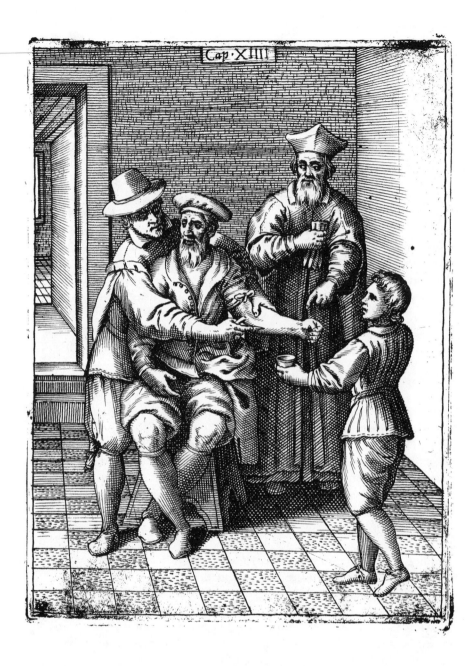

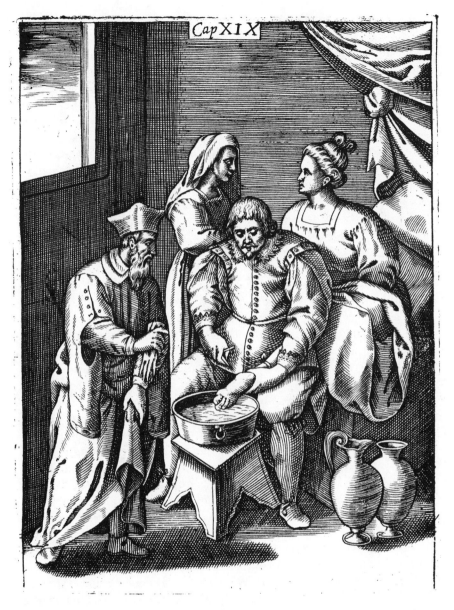

Bloodletting from a man's hand, to remedy plethora, and from a woman's left foot, to bring down her "courses." From Pietro Paolo Magni, *Discorsi di sanguinare* (Rome, 1626), pp. 26 and 40. By permission of the Folger Shakespeare Library.

[77]

have to be understood within the intellectual framework of precir-
culatory physiology, itself contained by and helping to reproduce the
ideological canons of patriarchal culture. As long as blood was
thought not to circulate continuously into and out of the heart and
lungs but to ebb and flow within a canalized body, blood participated
in a hierarchical signification of body parts based on ideologically
freighted notions of refinement and corruption, of relative distance
from more or less noble body parts, and simple binarisms such as
right/left, upper/lower. Blood took on and helped to impart attributes
of the parts with which it was associated. Blood issuing from the right
side of the body, for example, was to be regarded differently from
blood on the left. Blood's quality was a function, too, of the external
environment. The iatrochemist George Thomson argues that the
blood of persons living "in lofty places more remote from the
fæculent exhalations of the Earth" have more "rarified" blood and
circulation than those living near the lower surface of the globe.[35]

The idea of a body oppressed by the weight, volume, or poor quality of its own liquid contents—a body needing to be relieved of excess
or corrupt or excrementitious blood—has obvious ideological import
for the metaphor of the body politic and the material means of its
social reproduction. Of most concern to me here is the large-scale
correlation between the physical hierarchy of the blood in the discourse of nature and the social hierarchy of blood in the discourse of
culture. In particular, the structure of values in which blood participates, by which it is conceptualized, judged, and treated medically, is
conspicuously homologous to the structures of gender and other
forms of difference in early modern European culture. One familiar
reason for this homology is the momentum toward symmetry and
correspondence so notable in classical and Renaissance habits of
thought. Another, perhaps more important, is the result of a medical
discourse that produces such locutions as "laudable blood," because
habits of thought and discourse do not yet distinguish between the
ethical and physical domains. What I want to suggest is how the hierarchy of physiological values in the blood can be appropriated for the
canons of bodily propriety, so that bleeding is construed as an issue of
bodily voluntary and self-control. Bleeding thus comes to differ
from itself over the critical questions of purposiveness and agency,
becomes thoroughly traversed by questions of power and gender.

35. Thomson, *Aimatiasis*, p. 3.

As will become clearer hereafter, the emphasis of my argument differs from such accounts of classical and Renaissance physiology as Thomas Laqueur's history of classical thinking about sex, gender, and anatomy. For Laqueur, semiotically crucial differences in blood as sign become subordinated to a unitary (one sex/one flesh) conception of the human body: "In the blood, semen, milk, and other fluids of the one-sex body, there is no female and no sharp boundary between the sexes."[36] He rightly insists upon the "flux and corporeal openness" that Galenic humoralism attributed to human physiology and the fungibility of such bodily fluids as blood, mother's milk, and semen. Both men and women produced seed, the fluid essential for conception. More crucially for his argument, both men and women routinely underwent phlebotomy, as noted, in order to rid themselves of excess blood their bodies could not turn into nutriment or to remedy one of the many conditions—including nosebleeds, hemorrhoids, visible tumors, external ulcers, sore throats, and swollen glands—for which plethora was deemed to be responsible.

But the case of plethora as a common bodily event within the experiential domain of Galenic medicine is a notable limit-case of Laqueur's argument, for plethora differs from itself as soon as the variable of gender is introduced into its system of internal classification. Because of their colder, moister temperament, females were considered naturally plethoric; this was why they menstruated. Their bodies—and here the argument becomes very circular indeed—were naturally less soluble, since by virtue of its colder temperature their blood tended to be slower moving, clammier, grosser. Its natural attributes were also the attributes that, when magnified or increased, described disease. It follows—in the hierarchical logic peculiar to Galenic humoralism—that the finest female blood was less pure, less refined, less perfect than the finest male blood and, one infers, the more inclined to corruption.

I take these humoral axioms to imply that the blood of women as a category in nature was readily classifiable as superfluity or waste and that on the whole this was true no matter how soluble or evenly tempered a given individual woman might be either naturally or through the artificial evacuations induced by physic or surgery.

36. Thomas Laqueur, *Making Sex: Body and Gender from the Greeks to Freud* (Cambridge: Harvard University Press, 1990), p. 35; but see also his earlier discussion in "Orgasm, Generation, and the Politics of Reproductive Biology," *Representations* 14 (Spring 1986), 8–9.

Helkiah Crooke argues that women "have more bloud . . . and that is by reason of their colde Temperament which cannot discusse the reliques of the Aliment; adde hereto that the blood of women is colder and rawer then the bloud of men."[37] It was, in a word, less concocted. Laurent Joubert links the hierarchical difference between the blood of men and women to their different roles in reproduction. Women's blood

> is less refined and watery. Nature made it that way in order to provide nourishment for children, which women must normally carry for nine months. Children refine it further in their livers, which must not be left idle. The mother would be unable to generate the quantity of blood required if it did not remain imperfect. The father has less blood, but it is richer and more refined because of the semen that must come from it. He must furnish a more efficacious blood than the female.[38]

This lack of refinement in woman's blood is thus part of a providential biology; its inferiority is necessary to the overall workings of the re-productive plan. Because she must produce a greater quantity of blood in preparation for pregnancy, the *quality* of woman's blood suffers both as a result and, it would seem, as a matter of achieving gender complementarity: "The father has less blood, but it is richer and more refined." Moreover, compensating for the defects of its mother's imperfectly concocted blood gives the gestating baby's liver—"which must not be left idle"—something to do. Joubert's further suggestion that the father's blood must be "more efficacious" than the mother's implies his reliance upon the Aristotelian theory of the father's role in imparting form at conception, the mother's role in furnishing matter.

Menstruation was a special, though recurrent, instance of plethora. On one hand, it could be classified as one of the body's natural forms of evacuation, hence one means by which the female body sought to maintain and promote its "solubility." (Indeed, the value placed on solubility was one reason for the intense interest generated whenever the natural "courses" were stopped.) On the other hand, menstrual blood itself was always regarded as a form of excrement, blood that should not be retained by the nonpregnant woman. Crooke ponders

37. Crooke, *Microcosmographia*, p. 276.
38. Laurent Joubert, *Popular Errors*, trans. and ed. Gregory David de Rocher (Tusca-loosa: University of Alabama Press, 1989), p. 204.

the question of whether menstrual blood is produced in the second concoction—that is, at the same time as the rest of the blood—or in the third concoction, when blood underwent a further purification into seed. He temporizes:

> We say it is of both but in a diverse respect. It is an excrement of the second concoction, because the whole masse of bloud hath his first Generation in the Liver the seate of the second concoction, and from the Liver is powred as an overplus or redundancie into the trunke of the hollowveine [i.e., the vena cava]. It is an excrement of the third concoction, because it is as we sayd vomited away by the flesh when it is satisfied after the third concoction.[39]

Menstrual blood, we might infer, was doubly excremental, doubly superfluous. The difference in quality between male and female seed suggests why. The seed, says Thomas Vicary, "is made & gathered of the most best and purest drops of blood in all the body." But in men the seed is "hotte, white, & thicke" and would seem to leave no residue from concoction, whereas "womans sparme is thinner, colder, and feebler" and casts off its excrement in the form of menstrual blood.[40] But theories of the inferiority of female blood included the roles of both nature and culture. Thus, Crooke, weighing all the factors of women's temperament, concludes that "universally men are hotter then women, Males then Females, as well in regard of the Naturall Temper, as that which is acquired by diet and the course of life."[41] Women who lived idly did not use up their natural store of blood as readily as laborers, especially male laborers. Furthermore, even if menstrual blood in medical or scientific contexts could be regarded dispassionately as another form of bodily excrement, popular culture often followed Scripture in demonizing menstrual blood and the menstruating woman with a variety of taboos. Because menstrual blood was a form of plethora—even one recuperated into a narrative of biological providence—menstruation as a process took on an economy of impurity and waste, so that upper-class women who ate rich, moist foods were thought to flow more heavily than their lower-class counterparts.[42]

39. Crooke, *Microcosmographia*, p. 290.
40. Vicary, *Profitable Treatise of the Anatomie*, sig. M3ᵛ.
41. Crooke, *Microcosmographia*, p. 276.
42. Patricia Crawford, "Attitudes to Menstruation in Seventeenth-Century England," *Past and Present* 91 (1981), 70–72.

Thus women's purgative bleedings occurred monthly, but the issuings of men and women by means of phlebotomy were merely occasional responses to a diagnosis of nutritional repletion or the repletion symptomatic of disease. For Laqueur the distinction between
menstruation and phlebotomy does not affect the fundamental homology between male and female physiology: "What matters is losing
blood in relation to the fluid balance of the body, not the sex of the
subject or the orifice from which it is lost." His argument recognizes
no differences *that matter* between male and female blood: "Like reproductive organs, reproductive fluids turn out to be versions of each
other."[43] And it is true that his emphasis on homology as the central
component of the one-sex model of the human body does offer a
useful corrective to accounts of Renaissance conceptions of woman—
such as Ian Maclean's—which reduce gender differences to a rigid
and relatively simple set of binary oppositions.[44] Certainly, the hierarchical model by which woman's cold, moist body was an imperfect
version of the hot, dry, well-regulated man's requires analogy rather
than polarity to be the essential conceptual mode. But I would point
out that Laqueur's version of the physiology of sexual difference in
Renaissance culture fails to take sufficient account of the possibility of
simultaneous and contradictory ways of engendering sexual differences—or their material and discursive consequences. As long as hierarchical difference separates the generic attributes of male and
female blood, the perception of blood is capable of a profound—and
profoundly meaningful—engenderment. And with that engenderment, of course, comes an entire system of inherently unequal differences.

For my purposes here, the most important point about menstrual
bleeding is that, unlike the bleedings surgically administered to men
and women, menstruation is an involuntary and thus to some degree a
punitive process. Indeed, attitudes toward menstruation in the early
modern period often seem to betray an ironic double bind: whereas
the fact of menstruation could be used to demonstrate the natural
inferiority of women, the cessation or suppression of menses was also
blamed for all manner of physical and emotional maladies peculiar to

43. Laqueur, *Making Sex*, pp. 37, 38.
44. Ian Maclean, *The Renaissance Notion of Woman: A Study in the Fortunes of Scholasticism and Medical Science in European Intellectual Life* (Cambridge: Cambridge University
Press, 1980), passim.

the sex.[45] It seems to me, then, pace Laqueur, that physiological homology between the involuntary bleeding of the menstruating woman
and the opened vein of the phlebotomist's patient, whether male or
female, serves not to deny but to establish the difference between the
two processes as an issue of self-control. Monthly bleeding signifies as
a particularly charged instance of the female body's predisposition to
flow out, to leak. Menstruation comes to resemble the other varieties
of female incontinence—sexual, urinary, linguistic—that served as
powerful signs of woman's inability to control the workings of her own
body. It is not too much to argue that these historical signs of uncontrol bear implications for the ideology and politics of reproduction
that we live with still.

If I am right about inferences to be drawn from the meanings that
attach to menstrual bleeding, then the sign of phlebotomy is menstruation's cultural inversion. To its many adherents, "that exquisite
evacuation of al the humors equally," as Gyer called it, if properly
performed with the requisite "art and judgement" at the right time
and under the right conditions, represented precise application of
technical skill and theoretical know-how and the best hope for cure or
at least palliation of many bodily disorders.[46] It was, at least in theory,
a *controlled* opening and closing of the bodily container, a deliberate
invitation to that body to bleed where, when, and for how long the
phlebotomist and his patient chose. We cannot be surprised that phlebotomies often went disastrously wrong, causing soreness, infection,
amputations, and death, or that even when phlebotomies were tech-
nically successful, the patient succumbed anyway. To modern readers,
astonished at the lengths to which bleeding might go, it is harder to
account for reports of success, symptoms relieved and cures effected,
or to understand the subjective experience of those patients such as
John Evelyn who felt better after losing blood. The contingencies of
practice and the demonstrable risk involved in surgical bloodlettings
were disregarded as long as the underlying theory remained in place
and as long as patients continued to experience the psychological

45. See Audrey Eccles, *Obstetrics and Gynaecology in Tudor and Stuart England* (Kent,
Ohio: Kent State University Press, 1982), pp. 49–50. An earlier discussion is Hilda
Smith, "Gynecology and Ideology in Seventeenth-Century England," in *Liberating Wom-
en's History: Theoretical and Critical Essays*, ed. Berenice A. Carroll (Urbana: University of
Illinois Press, 1976), pp. 97–114.
46. Gyer, *English Phlebotomy*, pp. 25, 26.

benefit—the sensation of plethora relieved and bad blood evacuated—that followed upon loss of blood. Perhaps part of the mystique of phlebotomy as a branch of surgery, too, was that it was a form of treatment in which women medical practitioners never engaged, and thus, it may have come to epitomize the possibility of real, professional intervention against the physical woes of being-in-the-body.

In the articulation of social and bodily thresholds, the movement of blood *within* the body and the issuings of blood *from* the body play a crucial role. The corruption of blood, the differential purity of blood, the sexual difference of blood, the superfluity of blood, the age of blood—such phrases describe some of the potential conditions under which the blood of a single body or of many bodies was thought to differ physically from itself. But these conditions, believed to occur and to have significance in the natural world, cannot be separated for purposes of analysis and historical recovery from the effect of cultural values operative in early modern England. They also helped to constitute the metaphysical properties of blood on which so many kinds of social and material transmission depended. As conditions of *physical* difference, they logically encompass blood's physiological production, classification, nosological significance, and methods of treatment. As conditions of *social* difference, as we will see, they become the means of naturalizing various kinds of ideological production within the social body complex. More specifically, the control of blood and bleeding exemplified by the phlebotomist's art becomes a key determinant of agency and empowerment. In the dramatization of when, where, under what circumstances, and for whose benefit to bleed, the potential embarrassments of bleeding are realized.

ᔰ

The homologies between the internal structures of the blood and of society are given special visibility and ideological force onstage, where references to or appearances of blood are almost always narratively overdetermined, if not also semiotically overcoded. This is nowhere truer than in *The Merchant of Venice*, where resolution of the central crisis comes to hinge upon the privilege secured by a difference in blood. Shylock had asked Solanio and Salerio, his Venetian interlocutors and would-be tormentors, "If you prick us, do we not bleed?" (3.1.64). For the Jewish merchant, it is one in a series of more or less parallel rhetorical questions whose obviousness is intended to withstand contradiction. If pricked, the body of the Jew, like the body of the Christian, must display its common humanity by the blood flowing (if not yet, in these pre-Harveian times, circulating) in its veins and arteries. Indeed, it would have no power to do otherwise since, "fed with the same food, hurt with the same weapons, subject to the same diseases, heal'd by the same means" (60–62), the bodies of Jew and Christian alike participate in the same physical nature: "If you tickle us, do we not laugh? If you poison us, do we not die?" (65–66). In such an ethically overdetermined discourse, blood and bleeding function as the obvious, indisputable signifiers of natural law, the metonymies of what becomes here a physiology of insistent commonality. Furthermore, as the semiotic differences among the three paratactic questions about bleeding, tickling, and dying by poison imply, the signs of blood and bleeding carry an overload of cultural weight and resonance. Shylock's sly play with the near rhyme of "prick us" and "tickle us" barely conceals the significant differences of imagined intent and agency in the two kinds of stimuli, before the rhetorical and ironic climax of "if *you* poison *us*, do we not die?" The bodily signs bear a redundancy of self-evidentiality generated in part by the immense semiotic power of blood. For Shylock's rhetorical purposes bleeding is the sign of an essential undifference allowing him, slyly, to move onto the less stable ground of behavioral similarity: "And if you wrong us, shall we not revenge? If we are like you in the rest, we will resemble you in that" (66–68). To put it otherwise, the evident "naturalness" of bleeding and corporeality is used to limit and challenge the oppressive weight of ideological differences forming the social structure of Shylock's relations with Venice—differences finally symbolized in the self-sacrificial blood of Antonio which Shylock at the crucial moment is specifically forbidden to spill.[47] The essential difference in blood which Shylock denies as a obvious truth of nature (a truth Sir Robert Boyle might want to put to the test) is reinscribed as a truth of law at the moment when Portia reminds Shylock that, although Antonio's flesh is subject to the usurer's bond

47. In relation to Marlowe's stage Jew, G. K. Hunter has argued that "the whole Elizabethan frame of reference discouraged racialist thinking"; Jews differed from Christians "by faith (or lack of it) rather than race." See "The Theology of Marlowe's *The Jew of Malta,*" *Journal of the Warburg and Courtauld Institutes,* 27 (1964), 215–16. It could be argued, however, that Shylock's denial of difference in the blood is made to counter some contrary perception that is nothing if not "racialist."

and can be handed over to Shylock as "*thy* pound of flesh," Antonio's "Christian" blood is not. It is exempt from the traffic of flesh on the grounds, apparently, of its quotient of difference both from flesh and from non-Christian blood:

> If thou dost shed
> One drop of Christian blood, thy lands and goods
> Are by the laws of Venice confiscate
> Unto the state of Venice.
>
> (4.1.309–12)

A similarly inarguable, similarly essentializing deployment of blood as the signifier of material undifference is attempted by the King of France early in *All's Well That Ends Well*. But in this instance, blood's peculiar doubleness acts against the king's self-interest in his own blood. Blood is simultaneously an unevenly distributed signifier of rank and a physical entity common, according to Aristotle, to one half of animal creation. In the king's use of this complex sign, the contradiction lodged within it becomes clear. As the price of curing the ailing monarch of his "notorious" fistula, Helena specifies the free election of "what husband in thy power I will command" (2.1.194). From her horizon of choice she excepts only those of "the royal blood of France" (2.1. 196). Later, when Helena has announced her selection, the king rebukes Bertram for objecting to a match with "a poor physician's daughter" (2.3.115) by denying the grounds of difference between them:

> Strange is it that our bloods,
> Of color, weight, and heat, pour'd all together,
> Would quite confound distinction, yet stands off
> In differences so mighty.
>
> (2.3.118–21)

Like Shylock, the king seeks to validate the lack of essential difference in blood beyond any question by reference to medical discourse, proverbial utterance, and the familiar surgical practice of bloodletting. "There is no difference of bloods in a basin" was the proverbial counter to the assertion of social or ethical differences based merely on hereditary rank.[48] In the proverb blood retained distinction, "stood off," only when it moved within its bodily container. As Mary Douglas has suggested, because orifices symbolize the body's most vulnerable points, "matter issuing from them is marginal stuff of the most obvious kind. Spittle, blood, milk, urine, faeces or tears by simply issuing forth have traversed the boundary of the body."[49] But the king's recourse to the proverb in order to reprimand Bertram suggests that, at least for the purpose of effecting the royal will here, the meaningfulness of social differences was limited by the fact that the blood *failed* to stand off once it met and mingled with other "issues" in the surgeon's basin. Blood's social properties in other words were lost once it crossed the body's outer threshold and became no longer one's own. Extravasated, it became blood without a difference, or merely material blood mingling indistinguishably with the blood of any other subject of the phlebotomist's art. Extravasated, it became by definition bad blood, superfluous blood, or at the least, laudable blood issuing forth with bad humors, better spilled than retained. At that point, blood became what Harvey called "equivocal gore." It lost its spirit or driving force and became waste matter to be disposed of. Blood "without the spirit of life is no longer blood, but is to be regarded as spoiled immediately it has been deprived of spirit."[50]

Given Helena's success in effecting his cure when all other remedies had failed, the king's use of a medical idiom to correct Bertram here suggests his endorsement of the blood sign as a chemical solvent of social difference, as the semiotic destroyer of rank. But the king has at least tacitly accepted one form of distinction in blood which puts him in a position nearly as false as Bertram's and no less threatened: the distinction claimed for royal blood. Helena's readiness to except from her horizon of choice men of the royal blood may indeed signify what she claims it to be—her lack of "arrogance" (2.1.195). (Because Helena is completely uninterested in mingling bloods with anyone but Bertram, her deference to the royal blood seems to me more strategic

48. Morris Palmer Tilley, *A Dictionary of the Proverbs in England in the Sixteenth and Seventeenth Centuries* (Ann Arbor: University of Michigan Press, 1950), D335, p. 157. Tilley cites this passage from *All's Well* and the following from John Lyly's *Euphues and His England* as parallel texts: "You talk of your birth when I know there is no difference of bloods in a basin."

49. Mary Douglas, *Purity and Danger: An Analysis of the Concepts of Pollution and Taboo* (1966; rpt. London: Ark, 1984), p. 121.

50. Harvey, "Second Anatomical Essay to Jean Riolan," p. 38.

than real.) This exception does protect her from seeming in the king's eyes and perhaps ours to be a scheming marital overreacher, a figure of transgressive or socially destabilizing desires. For the audience, her qualifier may be meant, too, to make plausible even so desperate a king's willingness to agree to such an unorthodox method of payment for professional services. However uniquely skilled Helena may be and however threatening such unique skills may be in any woman, let alone in a female empiric, Helena shows herself to be a loyal subject by virtue of her acknowledgment of the material properties of royal lineage, its "real" foundation in "actual" blood. Nevertheless, for Helena to respect this difference is to throw any others severely into question. The difference she recognizes for royal blood as a scarce and precious resource, the firm social distinction she acknowledges between her commoner's blood and that of royal princes, has the effect of collapsing or at least effacing the differences between the "bloods" of other people—the difference Bertram would insist upon, for example, between the blood of the Count of Rossillion and that of a poor physician's daughter.

A similar complexity in the properties of blood and in the fragility of its power to confer distinction gives tragic force to the remarkable image of waste blood flowing into a sewage drain at the end of *The Changeling*. But in the tragedy, the same ambiguity of blood as the signifier of distinction takes an uncompromising form. If blood in a basin is to be regarded as waste blood, blood after it leaves the containment of the surgical basin for ultimate disposal was doubly waste. Beatrice-Joanna, carried bleeding onto the stage at the end of act 5, makes a metonymy of herself thus to her father with a self-judgment Frank Whigham aptly describes as "self-debasing, self-expelling":[51]

> Oh come not near me, sir, I shall defile you:
> I am that of your blood was taken from you
> For your better health; look no more upon't,
> But cast it to the ground regardlessly:
> Let the common sewer take it from distinction.
>
> (5.3.149–53)

51. Thomas Middleton and William Rowley, *The Changeling*, Revels edition, ed. N. W. Bawcutt (London: Methuen, 1958). My thinking on *The Changeling* in this regard is much indebted to Frank Whigham's essay "Reading Social Conflict in the Alimentary Tract: More on the Body in Renaissance Drama," *ELH* 55 (1988), 333–50; the phrase quoted appears on p. 340.

Beatrice-Joanna has decided that union with the baseborn DeFlores has defiled her, and she locates the pollution in blood specified as belonging to her father. It is an image denying Beatrice-Joanna any claim to self-ownership while sustaining her full culpability. By implication, she was never the self-authorizing container of her own blood but merely carried an originally pure portion of the patriarchal blood which has come to differ vilely from itself. We can find the theoretical groundplot for this inference in pre-Harveian physiology. In a canalized body, where blood flows but does not circulate, blood of greater and less purity moves unevenly, even irregularly to the parts. Thus, even as a divisible portion of the complex whole, Beatrice-Joanna was still capable of separate action and nature. She may be said to have failed, physically and morally, to sustain blood's nutritive mission. In George Thomson's phrase quoted earlier, this was "sweetly [to unite] all the parts of the Body for the conspiration of the good of the whole."[52]

In this physiological allegory of the patriarchal body, DeFlores plays a paradoxical role. The daughter's seducer and murderer, he also becomes the father's surgeon, practicing as it were upon the patriarchal body for its "better health." But *his* betrayal of Vermandero is almost completely effaced by hers: Beatrice-Joanna is not only the disease in the social body but a disease the bloodletting image identifies as plethora. In death she will become blood "taken" from the patriarchal body in order to purge it, to relieve it from a plethoric disease. In so doing she will lose the distinction she now finds so abhorrent and become even less than "equivocal gore." The social distinction—indeed, uniqueness—she has claimed from the very beginning of the play is denied here in a brutal image of extravasated blood. The blood drawn out into a basin flowed together with other blood; this blood has been poured into a common "sewer," a drain, where it will mix with all forms of filth and waste.

But the imagery of Beatrice-Joanna's extreme self-abnegation is founded, I would argue, not simply in the cultural practices of bloodletting, but also in the culturally sanctioned denigration of female blood in comparison to male blood. It is a function of the gendered properties of the discourse of blood that this image of the defiled heiress seeking extinction is an image of plethoric blood, blood in its lowest form, as waste. We have already seen the connection between

52. Thomson, *Aimatiasis*, p. 2.

femaleness and plethora, which explained menstruation and the inability of women's inefficient bodies to use up all the blood produced by concoction. This tendency was sometimes understood as aggravated by conditions of social privilege—by idleness, rich living, gluttony, appetitiveness. Here the implicit ethical judgment contained in the discourse of female nature is dramatically realized when the play's exemplar of female narcissism, having seen the justice of her punishment and exposure, seeks indistinction. Beatrice-Joanna has indulged a tendency to rebellion and disobedience which the imagery of plethoric blood connects with female bodiliness. In her recourse to the language of disease in the blood, Beatrice-Joanna justifies a patriarchal narrative naturalizing restrictiveness and endorsing principles of expulsion "for your better health."

&

What these examples suggest is how, in a hereditary culture, the sign of blood becomes a deeply contradictory site of multiple, competing, even self-contradictory discourses. The properties of blood as the metonymy of social differences—"of differences so mighty"—were not simply metaphoric or symbolic. As the plays' figurative turn to the semiotically overcoded discourse of internal medicine implies, in their embodiment and sequelae these differences were materially real. This is Sir Thomas Smith's point in the much-quoted passage from *De republica Anglorum* which seeks, on one hand, to limit the social authority of women but, on the other, to salvage hereditary transmission, even on the female side, by reminders of the culture's investment in the continuity of blood. In England women are not allowed to "medle with matters abroad, nor to beare office in a citie or common wealth no more than children and infantes *except it be in such cases as the authoritie is annexed to the bloud and progenie*, as the crowne, a dutchie, or an erledome for there *the blood is respected*, not the age nor the sexe."[53] On the other hand, as the French king's deconstructive rebuke to Bertram is intended to make clear, those social differences ceased to apply—became invisible—once respective "bloods" left the vessels of the bodies that housed them and were mingled in a surgeon's porringer. There is no difference of bloods in a basin.

53. Sir Thomas Smith, *De republica Anglorum*, ed. Mary Dewar (Cambridge: Cambridge University Press, 1982), p. 64. Also quoted by Tennenhouse in *Power on Display*, p. 21. The first set of italics is Tennenhouse's, the second is mine.

(What seems to be less clear to the king is that extravasated blood's loss of distinction brooks no exceptions, not even of the blood royal.)

Thus, I would argue that the play of signifiers in these three examples is more than a simple rhetorical opposition of social and medical discourses. It is more inflected than the king's crude references to the literal, material domains of medicine and physiology in order to deconstruct a more or less figurative discourse of blood as the metonymic signifier of rank and station. The king's perception that in medical or biological discourse social differences are set aside, fail to apply, or that blood loses difference and assumes mere materiality upon extravasation is commonplace and *to some degree* accurate. But that perception is also insufficiently attentive to the systemic hierarchizing of blood within medical and biological discourses, which, as we saw, fully articulates all the major tropes of cultural difference in early modern English culture. That is to say, in using proverb to authorize his reprimand, the king chooses to minimize the social difference between Bertram and Helena. Since he is obliged to respect her choice of partner, the proverb's erasure of distinction in bloods comes neatly to the purpose. But the king would be far harder pressed to deny the differences of purity, refinement, laudability that traditional scientific learning discovered in blood, which worked to naturalize the structure of gender and social difference on other than socially sanctioned grounds. In this respect, the fact that bloods mingle indistinguishably in a basin is irrelevant to the structural differences—between blood either of male and female or of any two individuals—with which medical science explained human physiology and upon which it based treatment.

It is crucial to my argument that bloodletting, as both sign and lived practice, reveals how blood could differ from itself in the material world of early modern England. More specifically for my preoccupation with the body embarrassed, phlebotomy is significant as a practice upon the body, an art of bodily culture, requiring professional skill and strategic application on the part of the surgeon and self-mastery on the part of the patient. If bloodletting can be understood as the cultural inversion of involuntary bleeding in any form, then the symbolic relation between the changes in canons of bodily propriety and the signs of blood and bleeding begin to emerge. Particularly on the stage—where the appearance of blood is almost always narratively overcoded—blood and bleeding become part of an insistent rhetoric of bodily conduct. The bleeding body signifies as a shameful token of uncontrol, as a failure of physical self-mastery particularly associated with woman in her monthly "courses."

In the organized visibility of dramatic representation, blood flowing from a wounded or dead body carries a potential narrative value that the hierarchies internal to humoral medicine make natural and available to gender coding. The male body, opened and bleeding, can assume the shameful attributes of the incontinent female body as both cause of and justification for its evident vulnerability and defeat. At such moments, the bleeding male's blood comes to differ, shamefully, from itself. This potentiality in the sign of bleeding takes on particular significance for the cultural history of the body in light of Bakhtin's distinction between the grotesque and classical bodily canons. We saw in Chapter 1 that woman is naturally grotesque—which is to say, open, permeable, effluent, leaky. Man is naturally whole, closed, opaque, self-contained. To be otherwise is both shameful and feminizing.

Transformation into female grotesqueness is precisely the fate, for example, from which Portia's identification of Antonio's blood as "Christian" spares Shylock's otherwise distinctly feminized victim, just as it is precisely the horrifying onstage display from which her legalistic distinction between flesh and blood spares *us*. Indeed, in a deeply encoded use of Bakhtinian bodily canons, the play's action suggests that Portia's bodily state and Antonio's are diacritically related. Portia has vowed to consummate her marriage to Bassanio only if Antonio's life is spared. It is Portia who, by interpreting the bond, specifies Antonio's blood as the core of his bodily security and privilege. If Shylock were to succeed in opening up Antonio's body, cutting off the pound of flesh nearest his heart, and letting his blood flow without stop, Portia's marriage would remain unconsummated. In effect, she has vowed that her virgin body will not shed its hymeneal blood unless Antonio's body has been sealed off from Shylock's predatory appetite and, of course, from Bassanio's use of it as collateral.

But we ought to notice the affective difference between the fates imagined or anticipated for the bodies of the two protagonists. The difference offers contrasting meanings for the loss of blood, for there is no shame in Portia's deflowering as there so clearly would be in Antonio's mutilation. He himself understands it as a form of castration:

I am a tainted wether of the flock,
Meetest for death; the weakest kind of fruit
Drops earliest to the ground, and so let me.
(4.1.114–16)

This reciprocity in the fates and bodily states of Portia and Antonio occurs because we accept the social and comic propriety of Portia's hymeneal bloodshed; indeed we are led to desire it and its sequelae, summed up in Gratiano's vow to "fear no other thing / So sore, as keeping safe Nerissa's ring" (5.1.306–7). We are also aware of the unstageability of deflowering as we could not necessarily be in the case of Antonio's mutilation and the excruciating embarrassment of his offering himself up so passively to the knife.

I am not suggesting any obvious equivalence between Portia's deflowering and Antonio's mutilation, between a form of bloodshed ritually celebrated and even perhaps desired and the bizarre and clearly fatal wound threatened for Antonio. Nor is the exchange of Portia's blood for Antonio's overtly thematized in the text of the play. But this economy of blood is encoded within the semiosis of Portia's ring and the vaginal threshold the ring represents. It is she who physically withholds herself from Bassanio pending the outcome of the trial in Venice even though she provisionally binds herself to him in marriage and bestows her ring upon him. Only when Antonio is prevented from losing any blood for Bassanio does Portia allow the full bestowal of her body, a blood-marked bestowal to which Gratiano's departing reminder of the "thing so sore" may crudely refer. Portia, that is to say, prevents Antonio from becoming a grotesque *and hence feminized* body in order to become a sexualized, hence fully grotesque female body herself. This is the sequel for the woman's body of her generically determined comic fate.

❧

The bleeding body that perhaps reveals the tropings of blood most fully is that of Shakespeare's Julius Caesar, in part because Caesar's corpse—that "bleeding piece of earth" (3.1.254)—undergoes a kind of exchange and display that is virtually unique for male tragic protagonists in the period. In the text of *Julius Caesar*, the *topos* of Caesar's body is not hidden. The Romans themselves, as we shall see in some detail, obsessively thematize it. The imagery of blood in the play, too, is so distinctly overcoded that, as Maurice Charney declared, the "central issue about the meaning of the play is raised by imagery of blood."[54]

In *Julius Caesar*, Bakhtin's two bodily canons are diacritically evoked as one way of articulating the crisis of difference that engages the Roman state.[55] Shakespeare's construction of the bodily canons differs from Bakhtin's, however, in possessing a metonymic specificity that transvalues what is essentially comic in Bakhtin's formulation into a tragic and also a religious idiom—into the bodily sign of the tragic grotesque. Recall that for Bakhtin the important fluids the grotesque body takes such pleasure in producing—dung, urine, sweat, and other bodily effluvia of the "lower stratum"—belong to a symbolic category he calls "gay matter."[56] In the high discourse of Shakespeare's Roman tragedy, however, the semiotically active fluid is blood and the essential bodily process is bleeding. Thus, I would agree with Charney that one way of phrasing the play's central political struggle until civil war breaks out after Caesar's funeral is to say that it occurs discursively as a struggle over kinds and meanings of blood and bleeding. But I would add that the discursive struggle is waged in increasingly gender-inflected terms. Both before and after the assassination, the conspirators use blood as a signifier that differentiates their bodies from Caesar's. They arrogate to themselves references to blood which belong to the symbolic order, and they justify their repudiation of Caesar by marking him discursively with the shameful stigmata of ambiguous gender, especially the sign of womanly blood. The assassination, then, discloses the shameful secret of Caesar's bodiliness. By stabbing and displaying his body, the conspirators cause the fallen patriarch to reveal an inability to stop bleeding which is one aspect of womanly incontinence. In the funeral oration, Antony's rhetorical task is thus not only to deconstruct the term *honourable*, which Brutus has appropriated for the conspirators, but to

54. Maurice Charney, *Shakespeare's Roman Plays: The Function of Imagery in the Drama* (Cambridge: Harvard University Press, 1961), p. 48.

55. See the influential discussion of the crisis of difference in René Girard, *Violence and the Sacred*, trans. Patrick Gregory (Baltimore: Johns Hopkins University Press, 1977), pp. 49–52. For relevant discussions of *Julius Caesar*, see the brief but suggestive comments of C. L. Barber and Richard Wheeler in *The Whole Journey: Shakespeare's Power of Development* (Berkeley: University of California Press, 1986), pp. 26, 36, and 236; and my book *The Idea of the City in the Age of Shakespeare* (Athens: University of Georgia Press, 1985), pp. 69–78.

56. Bakhtin, *Rabelais and His World*, pp. 334–35.

recuperate Caesar's body for his own political uses by redefining it—
even within the terms of its new engenderment as female—and re-
capturing for himself the meaning of Caesar's blood and Caesar's
bleeding.

The full relevance to Caesar of Bakhtin's distinctions may become
clear by means of comparisons to those Romans, in this play and the
other Roman tragedies, in whom shedding blood signifies self-control
or its lack. One such instance occurs in *Coriolanus*, in Volumnia's vehement response to Virgilia's horror at bloodshed:

> Away, you fool! it more becomes a man
> Than gilt his trophy. The breasts of Hecuba,
> When she did suckle Hector, look'd not lovelier
> Than Hector's forehead when it spit forth blood
> At Grecian sword, [contemning].
>
> (1.3.39–43)

Janet Adelman has seen in this striking image the deep linkage between feeding and phallic aggression in the play, which, through the
unspoken mediation of the infant's mouth, transforms the heroic
Hector "from feeding mouth to bleeding wound."[57]

But also at issue, I believe, is the barely suppressed anxiety, already
noticed in *The Merchant of Venice*, that in bleeding the male body
resembles the body of woman.[58] The physiological fungibility of
blood and milk becomes crucial here in two ways, for it provides the
symbolic linkage that Volumnia, aroused by Virgilia's feminine
squeamishness, must acknowledge in order to deny. Foreheads, like
breasts, can yield precious fluids. But in the patriarchal ethos for
which Volumnia speaks, male forehead can and apparently must be
differentiated from female breast by raising the question of self-
control, self-possession, voluntarism. Male bleeding is represented as
a "spitting forth," the combative verb serving to deny any causative

57. Janet Adelman, "'Anger's My Meat': Feeding, Dependency, and Aggression in
Coriolanus," in *Representing Shakespeare: New Psychoanalytic Essays*, ed. Murray M. Schwartz and Coppélia Kahn (Baltimore: Johns Hopkins University Press, 1980), p. 131.
58. Another instance of the bloody body as female is the murdered Duncan. See
Janet Adelman's essay "'Born of Woman': Fantasies of Maternal Power in *Macbeth*," in
Cannibals, Witches, and Divorce: Estranging the Renaissance, ed. Marjorie Garber (Baltimore: Johns Hopkins University Press, 1987), p. 95. That blood is the agent of gender
transformation is only implicit in Adelman's remarks, however, which focus instead on
Macduff's reference to Duncan's body as a "new Gorgon."

power to the Grecian swords and to endow the forehead itself with voluntary agency and passion. If struck, the seat of reason will bleed voluntarily from contempt rather than involuntarily as the effect of an enemy's external blow. ("If you prick us, do we not bleed?") Hecuba gives her milk to Hector, but Hector does not give his blood to Grecian swords. His would seem to be the kind of blood whose agency and power "more becomes a man," the kind of bleeding that differentiates manliness from motherhood.

It is true, as Caroline Walker Bynum has pointed out, that manliness could be assimilated to motherhood in late medieval religious discourse, particularly in the conventional iconography of Christ lactating blood.[59] Later, we will see the relevance of this image to the bleeding Caesar. Here it is important only to note that Christ's bleeding was necessarily perceived as a freely willed act and that Christ, unlike Hector, bleeds out of pity, not contempt. To bleed in contempt, then, is to reverse the imputation of woundedness and vulnerability, to deny permeability—or to displace one kind of bodily canon by another. Though an unwanted physical contact has occurred, the most negative implications of male bleeding can be effaced in narrative representation. A similar inference can be drawn when Martius himself appears, bleeding but seeking to define the physical process as both voluntary and therapeutic. To Titus Lartius's suggestion that he has lost too much blood to continue the battle against Aufidius, Martius responds by reconfiguring battle as work and blood as healthy sweat:

> My work hath yet not warm'd me. Fare you well.
> The blood I drop is rather physical
> Than dangerous to me.
>
> (1.5.17–19)

Martius effaces the evident fact of his permeability through the hyperbolic assertion of personal control in a therapeutic idiom. He has allowed to flow, he has *dropped* only excess blood. The protestation that his body is not yet "warm'd" implies that he could stand to release even more blood as a matter of promoting greater "solubility."

59. See Caroline Walker Bynum, *Jesus as Mother: Studies in the Spirituality of the High Middle Ages* (Berkeley: University of California Press, 1982), pp. 112–13; and Bynum, "The Body of Christ in the Later Middle Ages: A Reply to Leo Steinberg," *Renaissance Quarterly* 39 (1986), 403.

Bloodletting was in fact regarded as a therapy for excessive anger, as the following almanac verse suggests: "Blood letting cheereth sad minds, and anger pacifies, / And preserveth love from braine-sicke fantasies."[60] Hence Coriolanus's injury becomes phlebotomy. His adversaries, now his surgeons, administer health through an opening of the body which elides the difference between penetration and evacuation. Indeed, his surgeon adversaries may even assume something of the inferior status of a retainer or the eager purveyor of a desired service because, as Lucinda Beier points out, in the medical marketplace of seventeenth-century England, the patient—here the wounded but victorious warrior—was a consumer who "remained largely in charge of his or her own care."[61] Martius claims to be in charge even of his loss of blood. Such blood is voluntary in two senses: it is shed as a result of action freely undertaken, and it is shed virtually at will, "the blood *I* drop." When Martius later beseeches Cominius "by th'blood we have shed together" to return him to the fight (1.6.57), his invocatory phrase releases all the latent causal ambiguity of a verb that simultaneously signifies blood flowing from others and oneself, and blood being cast off, "shed" like surface exuviae or, more significant perhaps, like a plethora. To have excess blood to shed, therefore, does not create gender difference; what does is the possibility of shedding it at will. The male subject can regard such bloodshed therapeutically, as purgative, and can thus define it as enhancing rather than endangering somatic integrity and bodily solubility.

The psychic precariousness of this kind of assertion is clear in the refusal of Coriolanus to show the plebeians his wounds and beg their voices in his election. Janet Adelman is surely right to see this horror as rooted in his fear of dependency, a dependency we have seen imaged in the identification of feeding mouth and bleeding wound.[62] The play's language seems particularly severe in this regard, allowing for no saving categorical distinctions between new and old wounds, between flowing blood and healed-over scars. It is only logical then, that the imputation of dependency conjoins with the fact of compulsion: the autonomy Coriolanus has claimed in shedding blood in battle is threatened by his inability to forgo displaying his wounds.

The political implication of involuntary display is even clearer on those frequent occasions when Shakespeare associates freely flowing

60. *Richard Allestree's Almanac* (London, 1623; STC 407), sig. B6r.
61. Beier, *Sufferers and Healers*, p. 5.
62. Adelman, "'Anger's My Meat,'" pp. 114–15.

blood with the body of woman or with a bodily passivity linked to woman's subject position. In *Titus Andronicus*, Lavinia's bleeding body is likened to "a conduit with three issuing spouts" (2.4.29), one of them her mouth:

> Alas, a crimson river of warm blood,
> Like to a bubbling fountain stirr'd with wind,
> Doth rise and fall between thy rosed lips,
> Coming and going with thy honey breath.
>
> (2.4.22–25)

The fountain, Albert Tricomi reminds us, "is conventionally associated with the female sexual organs." In scriptural imagery, a stopped fountain symbolizes virginity and the flowing or bubbling fountain therefore represents "lost virginity."[63] But the language of Tricomi's interpretation, in service to a moral-allegorical critical practice, deemphasizes the physicality of what is represented so bloodily onstage. In a precise and wholly conventional metonymic replacement of mouth for vagina, the blood flowing from Lavinia's mutilated mouth stands for the vaginal wound that cannot be staged or represented, which has charged these images of warmth, movement, and breath with a peculiar eroticism and horror. The dramatic fungibility of mouth and vagina had a precise physiologic equivalence for members of a late sixteenth-century audience, who conceptualized their own blood as moving within a vascular system of linked canals, since vaginal or menstrual blood was thought to issue sometimes from other parts of the body—from breast or mouth.[64]

Furthermore, to the extent that images of fountains and rivers connote ceaseless, natural flow rather than sexual violence, they mask or subordinate the fact of bodily penetration. But blurring the idea of causality for Lavinia's woundedness does not work to reverse the imputation of vulnerability, to enhance Lavinia's agency, as was the case with Hector's forehead. On the contrary, to liken Lavinia's body to "a conduit with three *issuing* spouts" is to make her blood seem to issue from an absent, transcendent source, to make her blood seem hardly

---

63. Albert Tricomi, "The Mutilated Garden in *Titus Andronicus*," *Shakespeare Studies* 9 (1976), 94.

64. Crooke cites the case of an "ancient maide in Lincolnshire, who ever about the time she should have her Courses, for many daies together hath founde in her mouth in the morning when shee awaked, the quantity of foure or five ounces of blood more or lesse, and most part of it caked as it is in a Saser after blood-letting, and this continued with her for many yeares together" (*Microcosmographia*, p. 254).

her own. As a result, the blood flowing from Lavinia's mouth seems almost to become the sign of an immutable condition—the condition of womanhood—just as the sexual wound of defloration itself is symbolically a wound the female body cannot ever heal. But these meanings are ultimately inseparable from the more conventional meaning of vaginal blood as a sign of male mastery over the body of woman, or (as here) of male sexual violence.[65] In a chain of dramatic metonymies, Lavinia's inability to prevent her rape is equivalent to her inability to stop bleeding, is equivalent to her inability to speak her own bodily condition. The bleeding body of her sexual violation symbolizes—even as it results from—the political incapacity of the male Andronici, which may partly explain why Titus's own mutilation resembles hers, represents his overmastering by oedipally driven younger males. Even here, though, we ought to note that, unlike Lavinia, Titus mutilates himself, and therefore his wound—like Coriolanus's or Hector's—is at some level *willed*.

If we can see gender inflection in the symbolism of flowing blood, we can then see the dramatic role of blood in what I call the bodily canon of the tragic grotesque—a canon represented most obviously by the physical transformation and regendering of Julius Caesar. The gender inflectedness of flowing blood bears significantly upon the assassination of Caesar, for like Lavinia, Caesar cannot prevent his political victimization, cannot stop bleeding; when his body is displayed ceremonially, he depends on the voices of others to speak the meaning of his wounds. That these conditions combine to position Caesar as a woman in relation to the conspirators—with all the political disabilities attendant thereon—becomes clear both in the play's bodily discourse and in the presentational contrast of Caesar's wounds the self-wounding of Portia. It is a contrast precisely reversing the differences between Lavinia, on the one hand, and Coriolanus and Titus, on the other, a contrast underscoring the play's marked redistribution of gender attributes.

2▲

In the explicitly politicized idiom of *Julius Caesar*, the ideological potentiality of the bodily canons and their use value in the attribution

65. For a cogent discussion of the symbolism of vaginal blood and its relation as well to menstrual blood, see the now classic essay by Louis Adrian Montrose, "'Shaping Fantasies': Figurations of Gender and Power in Elizabethan Culture," in *Rewriting the Renaissance: The Discourses of Sexual Difference in Early Modern Europe*, ed. Margaret W. Ferguson, Maureen Quilligan, and Nancy J. Vickers (Chicago: University of Chicago Press, 1986), p. 333 n. 30.

of gender become especially apparent. For the conspirators, the most disturbing implication of Caesar's desire to be crowned is that it would replace differences with Difference. That is, it would replace a horizontal structure of highly individuated males within a traditionally self-authorizing class with a vertical structure that effaces all forms of patrician differentiation but that of not-being-Caesar. Furthermore, because the conspirators tend to present their own political integrity in somatic terms, their body images and Caesar's necessarily become functionally interrelated. If Caesar grows, the conspirators shrink; if Caesar reveals bodily weakness, the conspirators gain in strength; if Caesar is sick, the conspirators are whole. The process as it works here politically bears an obvious structural resemblance to social and medical constructions of gender—strong man; weak, even sick, woman. Not surprisingly, then, elements of Renaissance sexual binarism come increasingly into play, particularly that gendered equation by which men are associated with spirit and the symbolic order generally, women with matter.[66] To allow Caesar sway over themselves, Cassius implies, is thus symbolically to accede to a shameful feminization:

> Romans now
> Have thews and limbs like to their ancestors;
> But woe the while, our fathers' minds are dead,
> And we are govern'd with our mothers' spirits;
> Our yoke and sufferance show us womanish.
>
> (1.3.80–84)

Although the body of the father seems to be physically reproduced in the present, the *gender* of that body—says Cassius—has become shamefully and obviously ambiguous: "Our yoke and sufferance *show us* womanish."

The conspirators can remake themselves, it would seem, only by regendering Caesar, by displacing their own sense of gender indeterminacy onto the body of their adversary and renegotiating the differences between themselves and Caesar in the diacritical terms of the bodily canons. In this respect, how the conspirators come to regard Caesar's body contrasts sharply with the fear of Duncan's gender indeterminacy which Janet Adelman has noticed in Macbeth and other Scottish lords. She finds persuasive evidence that Duncan's an-

66. Maclean, *Renaissance Notion of Woman*, p. 2.

drogyny is "the object of enormous ambivalence" in his subjects because the perception of their king's femaleness "would rob his sons of his masculine protection and hence of their own masculinity." One reason Shakespeare does not stage Duncan's murder is to evoke the image of Duncan's bloodied body as blinding.[67] Caesar, by contrast, is *not* conspicuously gentle in character and, except for the physical reports of his frailty, is vulnerable neither physically nor emotionally. His murder can and, by this logic, *must* be staged and his corpse returned to the stage as the totemic object of the competing orations. Thus, what we hear is Cassius's defensive *attempt* to make Caesar seem the more womanly in order to assume a greater manliness in himself and the other conspirators. From this point of view, the much-noticed instability of Cassius's representation of Caesar in act 1, scene 2, is less a symptom of Cassius's own psychic fragility than it is the necessary construction of grotesqueness in Caesar, who, according to Cassius, is notably weak "as a sick girl" (1.2.128), yet prodigiously appetitive and swollen to immense proportions: "Upon what meat does this our Caesar feed / That he is grown so great?" (1.2.149–50). Caesar, we might infer, has become plethoric, in his own body as in the body politic. This contradiction between Caesar's physical inferiority to the other conspirators and his political domination of them bears an obvious resemblance to the chief political paradox of Elizabethan England—the queen herself. Elizabethan political theory, of course, managed the paradox by mystifying the queen's virginity and iconographically distinguishing her body from those of other women.[68]

In this play, this contradiction necessarily remains unresolved as Cassius's speech oscillates between literal narratives of Caesar's physical infirmities and explicitly figurative assignments of power, size, godhead:

> When could they say, till now, that talk'd of Rome,
> That her wide walks encompass'd but one man?
> Now is it Rome indeed and room enough,
> When there is in it but one only man.
>
>   (1.2.154–57)

67. Adelman, "'Born of Woman,'" p. 95.

68. See Montrose, "'Shaping Fantasies,'" pp. 49–50. On the cult of Elizabeth, see Roy C. Strong, *Gloriana: The Portraits of Queen Elizabeth* (London: Thames and Hudson, 1987); and Strong, *The Cult of Elizabeth* (London: Thames and Hudson, 1977).

The speech displays Cassius's need to find that Caesar imperils discursive as well as social boundaries. Caesar's transgression is articulated as one against the social body. By occupying more than his share of Rome, he offends against those norms of interpersonal behavior being promulgated with increasing efficiency throughout Europe in the sixteenth century.[69] The famous first scene has already shown that the right to urban space, to a place on the wide walks of Rome is a function of vested class interests. The plebeians' enthusiasm for Caesar offends against both time and place: indecorously they wear the "wrong" clothes, cull a holiday "out" of time and strew flowers when and where they do not belong.[70] For Cassius, such structural disruptions originate in Caesar's own lack of decorum, just as his rude refusal to "contain" himself bespeaks a threat to the exclusive community of gender. He would be "but one only man."

This imputation of bodily offense in Caesar, with all its consequences in the social formation, allows Cassius to place the apparent contradiction between Caesar's political size and strength, on one hand, and physical weakness, on the other, within the discursive logic of the bodily canons, to thematize his body in almost any manifestation as monstrously grotesque and structurally disruptive. Even the strange meteorological events on the eve of the assassination arise symbolically from Caesar's grotesque bodily uncontainment:

> Now could I, Casca, name to thee a man
> Most like this dreadful night,
> That thunders, lightens, opens graves, and roars
> As doth the lion in the Capitol—
> A man no mightier than thyself, or me,
> In personal action, yet prodigious grown,
> And fearful, as these strange eruptions are.
>
> (1.3.72–78)

Yet the imputation of bodily offense in Caesar allows Cassius and the other conspirators to maintain a sense of somatic integrity, primarily by distinguishing between their own physical self-control and Caesar's lack of it. Caesar is not the only Roman to manifest illness or handicap,

---

69. Norbert Elias, *The History of Manners*, vol. 1 of *The Civilizing Process*, trans. Edmund Jephcott (New York: Pantheon, 1978), pp. 53–55.

70. Richard Wilson, "'Is This a Holiday?' Shakespeare's Roman Carnival," *ELH* 54 (1987), 32.

but many of the play's references to Caesar's body before the assassination seek to interrogate his bodily condition in terms of self-
control. When Caesar chooses to swim the Tiber out of rivalry with
Cassius, his body fails him, as it does by contracting fever on cam-
paign in Spain, and as it will do in the marketplace when the plebeians
utter their "deal of stinking breath" (1.2.246–47). The aged conspirator Ligarius, by contrast, comes to Brutus's house to "discard [his]
sickness" (2.1.321) with the headkerchief that was its emblem. More
important, Brutus consistently frames the conspiracy itself in the canonical terms of the classical body, specifically what the body contains
or "bears." Brutus would be sure that the conspirators individually
"bear fire enough / To kindle cowards, and to steel with valor / The
melting spirits of women" (2.1.120–22). His is a reminder of the
difference in heat between male and female bodies and between more
and less manly men, the humoral difference between "real" men and
cold-blooded cowards and women. More than that, the heat of such
manliness is said to radiate outward to transform the minds and
bodies of the ambient citizenry. Given the humoral terms of everyday
bodily experience, the change Brutus hopes for is less figurative than
literal. In the charismatic bodies of such men, vital fluids are represented as having lost the stigma of mere or cold materiality in order to
become symbolic signifiers of patriarchal authority. Similarly, the assertion of somatic integrity in the conspiracy, imaged as a patriarchal
body of the whole, requires that oath taking be superfluous to the
common bodily seal of fellowship:

> Do not stain
> The even virtue of our enterprise,
> Nor th'insuppressive mettle of our spirits,
> To think that or our cause or our performance
> Did need an oath; when every drop of blood
> That every Roman bears, and nobly bears,
> Is guilty of a several bastardy,
> If he do break the smallest particle
> Of any promise that hath pass'd from him.
>   (2.1.132–40)

To break is to bleed shamefully, to be shamefully open, to be revealed
as bearing other than patriarchal blood. Patriarchal blood in such a
formulation is the blood one cannot bleed, the blood that cannot be

spilled without changing its nature. "In the spirit of men," says Brutus
with more than tautological force,

> there is no blood;
> O that we then could come by Caesar's spirit,
> And not dismember Caesar! But, alas,
> Caesar must bleed for it!
>
> (2.1.168–71)

Because the conspirators have defined Caesar's body as plethoric,
both in itself and as a member of the patriarchal whole, Brutus can
argue that "we shall be call'd purgers, not murderers" (180). To the
conspirators go all the phlebotomist's skill, self-mastery, and therapeutic praxis; to Caesar a passivity, uncontrol, and bodily wastefulness
gendered female.

Later in the same scene, Portia's self-wounding and voluntary self-
display corroborate the significance of bodily intactness as an ideological format of gender. Portia stakes her claim to knowledge of the
conspiracy by seeking to efface the physical difference that separates
her from her husband, difference that Brutus himself seems intent
upon marking. Since Shakespeare's text omits any prior reference to
Portia's illness (which Plutarch explains as a fever brought upon by
her self-wounding), Brutus's greeting of her is less explicable as a
reference to specific illness than as an invocation of difference:

> Portia! What mean you? wherefore rise you now?
> It is not for your health thus to commit
> Your weak condition to the raw cold morning.
>
> (2.1.234–36)

Her response—"Nor for yours neither"—by effectively denying difference in their conditions, undermines both hierarchy and gender as
causes for her exclusion. In fact Portia, appropriating the term *condition*, remarks upon Brutus's own bodily behaviors when contemplat-
ing the conspiracy—his sudden gestures, sighs, stares, head scratch-
ing, foot stamping. She attributes them to the involuntary, even
potentially transforming effects of "humor." It is an explanation, we
should note, which has the effect of opening to question Brutus's own
bodily state, even perhaps his own determinacy of gender. The
humor

> will not let you eat, nor talk, nor sleep;
> And could it work so much upon your shape
> As it hath much prevail'd on your condition,
> I should not know you Brutus.
>
> (2.1.252–55)

Portia's desire is to assimilate the bond of marriage with the bond of conspiracy, to have room in Rome rather than dwell in the suburbs of Brutus's good pleasure. She thus resorts to the only effective move by which woman's alterity could be blurred or modified, replacing the categorical restrictions of definition by gender—which, as Stallybrass says, construct women-as-the-same—with the privileges of definition by class or, even more narrowly, by family:[71]

> I grant I am a woman; but withal
> A woman that Lord Brutus took to wife.
> I grant I am a woman; but withal
> A woman well reputed, Cato's daughter.
> Think you I am no stronger than my sex,
> Being so father'd and so husbanded?
>
> (2.1.292–97)

Of course, in this claim to exceptional status, Portia (like Queen Elizabeth) affirms politically constraining gender norms for the rest of her sex. What she must distance herself from above all is woman's proverbial talkativeness, a condition culturally linked with the whores who dwelled in the suburbs and conventionally emblematized, as we saw in Chapter 1, by the leaking barrel. It was woman's normative condition to leak; Lavinia's bleeding body, as we have seen, constitutes the tragic representation of the trope. But Portia here, unable by talking to prove her ability to keep still, turns to self-mutilation. The gesture seems intended to imitate in little the suicides that Roman patriarchy valorized as the supreme expression of personal autonomy, which adumbrate her own and the other suicides at the end of the play.

Still, there is an apparent paradoxicalness in Portia's act—opening one's body to prove a capacity not to leak or break—which we may be able to decode and which is worth noting for its relevance to images of

71. See Peter Stallybrass, "Patriarchal Territories: The Body Enclosed," in *Rewriting the Renaissance,* p. 133.

Caesar before and after the assassination. In Plutarch's account, the scene of Portia's self-wounding is graphic, a little grotesque (thanks to the barber), and impressively bloody: "She took a little rasor suche as barbers occupie to pare mens nayles, and causing all her maydes and women to goe out of her chamber, gave her selfe a greate gashe withall in her thigh, that she was straight all of a goreblooode, and, incontinentlie after, a vehement fever tooke her, by reason of the payne of her wounde."[72] In the play, though the wound must somehow be physically demonstrable, Shakespeare chooses to present it only after the fact, far less bloodily than does Plutarch and without emphasizing the "incontinent" fever that Portia's pain brought on. Portia does not stand like mute Lavinia with blood flowing uncontrollably, and she does not require a male voice to signify her bodily condition: "I have made strong proof of my constancy, / Giving myself a voluntary wound / Here, in the thigh" (2.1.299–301). In this reading, Portia calls attention to this bodily site not to remind Brutus of her femaleness, her lack of the phallus, but rather to offer the wound paradoxically as substitute phallus. Hers is not the involuntary wound of the leaking female body but the honorifically gendered, purgative, *voluntary* wound of the male. It is the sign of a defiance that disallows automatic signification of woundedness, even here in the thigh, as castration and reconfigures self-punishment as honorifically male. Portia has bled not like Lavinia, with a wound that cannot heal, but like Coriolanus, like Hector.[73] She could even claim to have become her own surgeon, her own phlebotomist, for the wound she shows to her husband is not the vaginal wound of the signified woman, and the blood that has flowed is voluntary. The sign that she makes by her wound, like the voluntary opening of the phlebotomist's patient, is the cultural inversion of woman's monthly bleedings.

In her painful imitation of patriarchal bodily canons, Portia valorizes the conspirators' need to stigmatize Caesar's body discursively

72. "The Life of Marcus Brutus" in *Plutarch's Lives of the Noble Grecians and Romanes*, trans. Sir Thomas North (1579) reprinted in *Narrative and Dramatic Sources of Shakespeare*, ed. Geoffrey Bullough (London: Routledge and Kegan Paul; New York: Columbia University Press, 1964), 5:98.

73. I thus agree with Madelon Sprengnether that in Portia's self-wounding, manliness is equated with injury: "The sign of masculinity becomes the wound." See "Annihilating Intimacy in *Coriolanus*," in *Women in the Middle Ages and the Renaissance: Literary and Historical Perspectives*, ed. Mary Beth Rose (Syracuse: Syracuse University Press, 1986), p. 96. For an extended riff on possible (if improbable) sexual puns in this speech, see Frankie Rubinstein's entry for *thigh* in *A Dictionary of Shakespeare's Sexual Puns and Their Significance* (London: Macmillan, 1984), p. 273.

with the marks of difference, and by taking on maleness, she furthers the conspirators' ideological project of regendering Caesar. This project becomes most overt in Decius Brutus's interpretation of Calphurnia's dream, which, as David Kaula has argued, represents Caesar typologically as the redeemer Christ shedding blood for his people. Kaula is right, I think, to see the specific influence here of the medieval cult of the Holy Blood, which publicized miraculous stories of bleeding statues and paintings of Christ.[74] Caesar, as Decius Brutus anticipates, responds positively to this sacerdotal image of himself (perhaps even becoming a victim of witty anachronism on Shakespeare's part in his ignorance of basic Christian typology about the self-sacrificial nature of the Christ he is made to resemble here).

But even more significant in the exegesis is a detail that Kaula and other interpreters have passed over or evaded: that Decius Brutus specifically allegorizes Caesar as a lactating figure, a statue or fountain lactating blood:

> Your statue spouting blood in many pipes,
> In which so many smiling Romans bath'd,
> Signifies that from you great Rome shall *suck*
> Reviving blood, and that great men shall press
> For tinctures, stains, relics, and cognizance.
>   (2.2.85–89, emphasis mine)

Caroline Bynum has demonstrated that images and textual representations of a lactating Christ were familiar in late medieval Christian worship. The idea took variant forms. The body of the church, itself depicted symbolically as *ecclesia lactans*, was identified with the body of Christ, or Christ's nurturing flesh was identified with nurturing female flesh, or the bodily wound suffered at the Crucifixion was depicted near the breast in order to suggest a bleeding nipple. (All these images are related, furthermore, to the self-sacrificial emblem drawn from natural lore—the mother pelican, which, Christ-like, pecks her own breast to feed her young.) This iconography depends in the first place on medieval physiology, which, as we have seen, reduced all bodily fluids to blood. Just as medieval typology, for example, could assimilate the blood Christ shed on the cross with the blood shed at his circumcision and even with the monthly bleedings of

74. David Kaula, "'Let Us Be Sacrificers': Religious Motifs in *Julius Caesar*," *Shakespeare Studies* 14 (1981), 204.

women, so too could medieval Christianity, through the patristic analogy of spirit is to flesh as male is to female, see the humanized Christ
as having a female body. What Bynum's brilliant analysis allows us to
recognize is the distance between our frame of reference and that
of our forebears, who, far more than we, tended to perceive the female body as food and who "assumed considerable mixing of the
genders."[75]

But although late medieval Christians may not have seen any inde-
corum in the idea of a male deity giving suck from a flowing breast to
spiritually hungry worshipers, such may not be the case with modern
students of Shakespeare, who have avoided commenting on Decius
Brutus's crucial choice of verb here, or even with early modern Lon-
doners, whose cultural attitudes toward the female breast and breast-
feeding, as Dorothy McLaren has suggested, were changing.[76] It was
still possible, for instance, for King James in *Basilikon Doron* to recommend as one of a king's "fairest styles, to be called a loving nourish-
father to the Church."[77] Yet, the idea is left somatically indefinite, a
reference to maternal function apart from maternal anatomy. James
does not, like the lactating Christ, offer his body, even symbolically, as
food, nor was he depicted with a flowing breast. On the contrary, as
the breast became increasingly eroticized and as the suckling of infants or sick adults became the nearly exclusive province of lower-class
women, the image of the flowing breast was becoming more strictly
associated with woman.[78]

It is arguable, then, that part of the complex irony here in the
image of Caesar lies in its semiotic ambiguity in the matter of gender.
Caesar responds to an interpretation of the image which seems to
construe his body, like Christ's, as a magically powerful, ungendered,
symbolic source of nurturance; the image seems, in one possible construction, to offer the childless patrician a suitably powerful patri-

75. Bynum, "The Body of Christ," pp. 414–17, 429 plate 9, 421–22, 437. Bynum's
latest discussion of this theme appears in *Holy Feast and Holy Fast: The Religious Significance of Food to Medieval Women* (Berkeley: University of California Press, 1987), pp.
263–65.

76. Dorothy McLaren, "Marital Fertility and Lactation, 1570–1720" in *Women in
English Society, 1500–1800*, ed. Mary Prior (London: Methuen, 1985), pp. 27–28.

77. King James, *Political Works*, ed. Charles Howard McIlwaine (Cambridge: Harvard
University Press, 1918), p. 24; quoted also in Stephen Orgel, "Prospero's Wife," in
Rewriting the Renaissance, p. 59.

78. See Marina Warner, *Alone of All Her Sex: The Myth and the Cult of the Virgin Mary*
(New York: Knopf, 1976), p. 203, who argues for an increasingly class-specific semiosis
of nursing.

archal stylization. But it also gives expression to the conspirators'
more obscure need to re-mark Caesar's body with femaleness and to
cause his body—even if only discursively—to leak like a woman's.
Such bleeding, since it would signify the conspirators' overmastering
of Caesar, cannot truly resemble the freely willed eucharistic offering
of Christ or the patriarchal self-stylization of James. Yet this is exactly
how Decius Brutus interprets blood flow to Caesar here, flattering
him with an ambiguous, equivocal self-image in which there is a concealed irony: the image of god yields to an image of woman.

The ironic instability of Caesar's final haughty affirmation of patriarchal constancy and phallic power—"Hence! wilt thou lift up Olym-
pus?" (3.1.74)—is manifest in the feminizing effect of his bloody
death. For there is a precise and evocative resemblance between the
flowing body of Lavinia, with its "three issuing spouts," and the bleeding corpse of Caesar, its streaming wounds metaphorized as bodily
orifices, "weeping as fast as they stream forth thy blood" or "like
dumb mouths [that] ope their ruby lips / To beg the voice and utterance of my tongue" (3.1. 201, 260–61). Like a fountain—the fountain
Marcus Andronicus has seen in Lavinia's flowing wounds and that
Decius Brutus has made of Caesar's body in Calphurnia's dream—
Caesar's blood pools, allowing the conspirators to "stoop, then, and
wash" their hands in it. And its flow, at least symbolically, becomes
recurrent, as if it had now become the identifying condition of Caesar:

> How many times shall Caesar bleed in sport,
> That now on Pompey's basis [lies] along
> No worthier than the dust!
> (3.1.114–16)

These are no "voluntary wounds," nor do they speak for themselves. Indeed, Antony's recognition of this body's dependence on his
voice is at the center of his response to its newly feminized character,
as a "bleeding piece of earth" (3.1.254). For Antony cannot deny
Caesar's vulnerability, cannot, like Volumnia or Coriolanus or Portia,
transform the flow of this blood into a combative spitting forth, a sign
of maleness. On the contrary, both Brutus and Antony respond to the
bloody corpse and to the blood-marked conspirators in the eroticized
terms of male initiation ceremonies—the blooding of maiden hunt-
ers, maiden warriors. The closest canonical analogy is probably to

Prince Hal, who salutes his brother after the battle with "full bravely hast thou flesh'd / Thy maiden sword" (*1 Henry IV*, 5.4.130–31). Here Brutus urges his conspirators to "bathe our hands in Caesar's blood / Up to the elbows"—as if entering Caesar's body—"and besmear our swords" (3.1.106–7). Antony urges the conspirators to "fulfil your pleasure" (159) by killing him too.

Standing over the body of Caesar and speaking the meaning of his death, the conspirators seem momentarily to have resolved the crisis of difference for themselves in honorifically gendered terms. But they discover that to feminize Caesar by killing him is not to disable him, because, unlike any body's finite material existence, that body's discursivity is subject to seemingly endless renegotiation, and regendering. In a sense, to thematize Caesar's body, as they have done virtually from the beginning of the play, is already to have conceded the futility of actually killing him and the impossibility of controlling the semiotic uses to which his body and his blood can be put.[79]

Although the hostile construction of Caesar as female has helped to sustain the conspiracy, the terms of that construction are neither stable nor exclusionary. Caesar dead is no less obscurely or complexly gendered than Caesar alive, and his femaleness empowers Antony no less than themselves. Thus, it may be true, as Richard Wilson has recently argued, that the plebeians' riot after seeing Caesar's body and hearing Antony's oration may well result from "the exposure of Caesar's naked will." The signifier "will," which Wilson reads as "phallic pun," is repeated both as verbal auxiliary and as substantive twenty-seven times in thirty-odd lines (3.2.126–61).[80] Yet, even if Antony does seek discursively to reinvest the body with a portion of its original phallic power, he and Shakespeare make even more significant use of what I regard as its connotatively female affectivity. Even to receive Caesar's body from the conspirators as a token of political exchange and denial of hostile intent suggests Antony's acceptance of its use value as female and his own new patriarchal responsibilities to it.[81]

Dead, Caesar can be for Antony the perfect, mute Petrarchan object, demonstrably unable, like women generally, to control the work-

79. For a related discussion of the semiotic uses of Caesar's toga, see Alessandro Serpieri, "Reading the Signs: Towards a Semiotics of Shakespearean Drama," in *Alternative Shakespeares*, ed. John Drakakis (London: Methuen, 1985), p. 133.

80. Wilson, "'Is This a Holiday,'" p. 39.

81. On woman as object of exchange, see Gayle Rubin, "The Traffic in Women: Notes on the 'Political Economy' of Sex," in *Toward an Anthropology of Women*, ed. Rayna R. Reiter (New York: Monthly Review Press, 1975), pp. 157–210.

ings of his own body but thereby calling into being whatever powers of articulate closure his body's speaker possesses. Thus, the Petrarchan vocabulary Antony deploys in signifying Caesar's corpse, first in the capitol and later in the forum, accedes to the idea of femaleness as a source of Caesar's difference but refigures his body as a discursive site not of contempt or anxiety but of desire. Rather than deny Caesar's female vulnerability, he reifies it in the rents and tears of Caesar's mantle: "Look, in this place ran Cassius' dagger through; / See what a rent the envious Casca made" (3.2.174–75). In Antony's sentimental allegorical narrative, Caesar's blood responds to Brutus as to an unkind suitor, with a rather adolescent, even girlish naïveté. As Brutus

> pluck'd his cursed steel away,
> Mark how the blood of Caesar followed it,
> As rushing out of doors to be resolv'd
> If Brutus so unkindly knock'd or no;
> For Brutus, as you know, was Caesar's angel.
>   (3.2.177–81)

Particularly telling in this context, then, is Antony's use of the trope of putting a tongue into Caesar's wounds, a figure that seems to oppose mute femaleness to a phallicized image of speech. These wounds, are "poor, poor, dumb mouths," as tongueless and silent as Lavinia. Antony "bid[s] them speak for" him, ironically, as if to mark their affective power as constituted by female silence. But the wounds here are also bodily orifices, sites of potential interrogation, places to put tongues *in*. By fetishizing them to the crowd, Antony can eroticize "sweet" Caesar's female woundedness as the explicit motive of his rhetorical power, the source of his voice. It is he who *puts* the tongue in Caesar's wounds:

> For I have neither [wit], nor words, nor worth,
> Action, nor utterance, nor the power of speech
> To stir men's blood; I only speak right on.
> I tell you that which you yourselves do know,
> Show you sweet Caesar's wounds, poor, poor, dumb mouths,
> And bid them speak for me. But were I Brutus,
> And Brutus Antony, there were an Antony
> Would ruffle up your spirits, and put a tongue

> In every wound of Caesar, that should move
> The stones of Rome to rise and mutiny.
>
> (3.2.221–230)

The outbreak of civil mutiny in Rome can be seen, then, to result not so much from the disclosure of Caesar's "will"—his maleness—as from the disclosure of his wounds, his femaleness, and from the affective power these wounds have in flowing to transform Antony from part to whole, from Caesar's limb to motivated Orphic speaker, causing stones to rise up. Antony's oration cannot re-member Caesar or restore to his bleeding corpse the intact ideal maleness of the classical body. Instead, it takes up and redirects the political valences of the conspirator's own rhetoric of blood and bodily conduct, denying the conspirators exclusive rights to the Roman body politic. Plethoric womanly blood, however sublimated by Petrarchan discourse, has thus marked Caesar with the bodily sign of the tragic grotesque, but this marking has not achieved the conservative political results the conspirators had aimed for. Like all hegemonic efforts to limit signification and control the procedures of differentiation, the patriarchal attempt to limit and control the semiotics of Caesar's body was open to challenge. When Caesar was alive, his grotesqueness had served as justification for assassination. After he is dead, his grotesqueness diffuses throughout the body politic in the self-transgressions of civil war and turns that body, too, into a signifier of the tragic grotesque.

CHAPTER THREE

COVERING HIS ASS

The Scatological Imperatives of Comedy

Because formation of what I have called the internal habitus is historically and culturally specific, it follows that modes of bodily sentience and self-perception in early modern Europe must have differed profoundly from our own. Further support for this argument can be found in the centrality to early modern medical practice of the alimentary purge, administered in the form of emetics, laxatives, and enemas, which was experienced from time to time by nearly everyone from infancy on. The clinical importance of the purge was underwritten by humoral theory's emphasis on bodily solubility and by its conceptualization of the body as a canalized container. In humoralism, disease and organic dysfunction were explained as manifestations of corrupt bodily humors that had to be expelled. The efficacy of a particular purgative treatment was thus gauged not so much by whether the patient improved or recovered, as by the violence of its expulsive effect on the body.[1]

The possible cultural consequences of repeated violent evacuations on forms of sexual and social development may forever escape definitive analysis or recovery. But it seems reasonable to conclude that so

---

1. See Lucinda McCray Beier, "In Sickness and in Health: A Seventeenth-Century Family's Experience," in *Patients and Practitioners: Lay Perceptions of Medicine in Preindustrial Society*, ed. Roy Porter (Cambridge: Cambridge University Press, 1985), p. 119.

central a bodily practice would necessarily participate in the historical formation of the canons of bodily propriety being traced here. Thus, in this chapter I explore the possible effects of purging on one moment in the early history of the subject: the contest for physical autonomy every child wages with his/her primary care givers. In the physical practices of early modern England specifically (and by extension in those of early modern Europe generally), this contest may have become focused on the paths and sites of evacuation—the bodily thresholds of mouth and anus, mouth *as* anus—with a greater psychic intensity than we consider normal today. For whatever their physical or even therapeutic effects, emetics, laxative purges, and enemas constitute unmistakable interference with a child's growing experience of and mastery over his/her own ingestive, digestive, and excretory cycles.[2] For the most part, that interference would have been administered by women, who, as mothers, were the primary medical practitioners in their own homes or, as village "wise women," practiced medicine in their communities.[3] Then as now, mothers more than fathers handled the bodies of their children. And because this is so, as Julia Kristeva has argued, the maternal authority so early experienced as sphincteral training becomes integral to the subject's self-understanding of his/her own "clean and proper body."[4]

Few children in early modern Europe can have been subjected to the overscrupulous attention to every bodily event which the child Louis XIII suffered. His personal physician Jean Héroard not only measured the baby's food intake but customarily administered sup-

2. For a description of this developmental process, see D. W. Winnicott, "The Depressive Position in Normal Emotional Development," in *Collected Papers* (London: Tavistock, 1977), pp. 262–73; and James Clark Moloney, "Some Simple Cultural Factors in the Etiology of Schizophrenia," *Child Development* 22 (1951), 163–82. I owe the references in this context to Elizabeth Wirth Marvick, *Louis XIII: The Making of a King* (New Haven: Yale University Press, 1986), p. 13. I am assuming, at least for contemporary American child-rearing and pediatric practices, that better health and nutrition for children make the administration of enemas, rectal suppositories, and laxatives on the whole less frequent than was the case in early modern Europe. Moloney in particular argues for the importance of early patterns of rectal control or release to later sexual development, especially sexual neurosis, and makes an even larger claim that "sphincter control means living life on one's own terms, albeit anticipating, and thereby neutralizing, the commands of the mother" (p. 170).

3. See Hilda Smith, "Gynecology and Ideology in Seventeenth-Century England," in *Liberating Women's History: Theoretical and Critical Essays*, ed. Berenice A. Carroll (Urbana: University of Illinois Press, 1976), p. 108.

4. Julia Kristeva, *Powers of Horror: An Essay on Abjection*, trans. Leon S. Roudiez (New York: Columbia University Press, 1982), pp. 71–72.

positories to retain control over his bowel movements. The rectal protocols Héroard inflicted on the boy may not have been uncommon, however, since Héroard considered himself a conservative in prescribing purges, and he could not, in any case, have practiced a completely unorthodox medicine upon the little prince. Thus, though the decade-long struggle Louis waged for control of his body products and processes may seem protracted to modern students of childhood, it may not have been unusual in the period either in length or in the anal aggressiveness of its eventual formation.[5] The repeated bodily phenomenon of the purge, perhaps calling up unpleasant early memories of uncontrol and physical subjection, perhaps calling up pleasurable memories of genital/anal stimulation, would have been well known to many children and adults in early modern Europe and thus have helped to constitute normative forms of bodily self-experience. Such anal cathexes, I argue, are instrumental in the discourses of gender difference in early modern culture.

The many forms of purging and their bodily consequences are not themselves the subject of this chapter. Rather, I am interested in locating textual evidence of the internal habitus and the affect structures it helps to form. But I propose to find that textual evidence in the comic discourses of scatology and anality, bodily discourses regarded by modern criticism as too low for serious attention or as the object of only a prurient antiquarian, folkloric, or merely lexical interest.[6] To take scatology seriously—that is, without humor and as consequential—is to seek in it discursive traces of the early childhood experiences of uncontrol and anal cathexis, to see its formations as the external residue of unresolved struggles of infancy.

The symbolic contours of such early infantile experience are leg-

5. On this aspect of Héroard's care of the dauphin, see Marvick, *Louis XIII*, pp. 11–23. See also Marvick, "'Nature Versus Nurture': Patterns and Trends in Seventeenth-Century French Child-Rearing," in *The History of Childhood*, ed. Lloyd de Mause (New York: Psychohistory Press, 1974), where she contends that the "practice of syringe-administered enemas for children must have been widely diffused among the upper classes" (p. 273).

6. A notable exception to my generalization is to be found in John W. Velz's serious scholarly treatment of the medieval background of the scatological idiom in "Scatology and Moral Meaning in Two English Renaissance Plays," *South Central Review* 1 (Spring–Summer 1984), 4–21. I would point out, however, that Velz's interest in seeing scatology as moral troping puts him at a considerable distance from my own project here. I should note as another example of moral-aesthetic interrogation of the scatology of the play the work of William B. Toole, "The Aesthetics of Scatology in *Gammer Gurton's Needle*," *English Language Notes*, 10 (1972–73), 252–58.

ible in the scatological action and language of three early modern comedies—*Gammer Gurton's Needle, A Midsummer Night's Dream,* and *The Alchemist.* The scatology of these plays constitutes cultural documentation of genuine explanatory potential for recovering the affect structure of shame and delicacy as it is reproduced in very specific theatrical settings. The texts record a particular set of cultural transactions operating in and upon the intertwined psychic and bodily economies of theatrical audiences. In the case of *Gammer Gurton's Needle,* for example, the bodies most relevant to my argument belonged to Christ's College, Cambridge, undergraduates sometime in the late 1550s or early 1560s. The play's probable date is not unimportant to my argument, for some of the transactions I have in mind take on force and ideological momentum after 1530, the year in which Erasmus's powerfully formative treatise on good manners for boys was published. The rapid dissemination of Erasmus's canons of bodily propriety implies a new readiness to require a more exigent set of inner controls of the individual subject, to alter affect structures in service to emergent norms of civility and refinement.[7]

In *Gammer Gurton's Needle,* the issue of bodily autonomy and self-mastery is defined in exclusively male terms as an important outcome of engenderment, in particular as a matter of wresting control over one's body from a dominant older woman. Thus the two households organizing the social world of the play are both female headed. In both households the symbolic reciprocity of domestic and bodily thresholds as sites of social interference, exposure, and perilous change is evident. The needle was lost from Gammer's lap when she sat sewing in the light of the doorway, and it will be rediscovered lodged in Hodge's backside—but only after the dark interior space of neighboring households is cataloged, a cat is threatened with evisceration, and Dr. Rat, the vicar, has his head beaten with a door bar when trying to sneak into the back of Dame Chat's house through the "black hole" of a "privy way" (5.2.189, 187).[8]

Throughout the play, as Lindsay McFadyen has maintained, descriptions of the needle are "consistently phallic."[9] Such an identifica-

7. Norbert Elias, *The History of Manners,* trans. Edmund Jephcott (New York: Pantheon, 1978), pp. 53–59.

8. I quote here and throughout from Charles W. Whitworth's edition of *Gammer Gurton's Needle* in *Three Sixteenth-Century Comedies* (London: Ernest Benn; and New York: Norton, 1984).

9. N. Lindsay McFadyen, "What Was Really Lost in *Gammer Gurton's Needle?*" *Renaissance Papers, 1982,* ed. A. Leigh DeNeef and M. Thomas Hester (Southeastern Renaissance Conference, 1983), p. 11. McFadyen's argument runs counter to that of J. W.

tion justifies the village's consternation over the needle's loss, especially if, like McFadyen, we regard the play's fiction as virtually
transparent. Because the students were not adept female impersona-
tors, he argues, "it would be impossible for the audience to forget *the
real gender* of the actors playing Gammer Gurton or Dame Chat."[10]
We ought to resist such reification of gender. For adolescents, even
more than for anyone else, fixed and stable gender identity is less a
"reality" than a goal, an assertion of hierarchical difference constantly
to be maintained. Indeed, the very instability and arbitrariness of
gender construction makes sense of the fact that there seems to be
only *one* needle-phallus to go around. And for adolescents in the
academic audience watching other adolescents variously comfortable
in their fictional roles, the play's identification of phallus and needle
may yield a rather subversive, even unsettling semantic possibility.
Reversing the identification to ask not how the needle is like a phallus
but how the phallus may be like a needle, we discover that the proverbial phallus may be, like the proverbial needle, worthless, nonunique,
and too tiny to find.

However unhappy this possibility may be for the boy actors playing
Dame Chat and Gammer Gurton, it is nonetheless more damaging
(within the fiction) for Hodge, whose torn breeches Gammer was
mending. To Hodge, the loss occasions what seems to me an anxious
thematizing of narcissistic injury, a sense of genuine social and sexual
impairment. Hodge initially complains of bodily stain, which he specifically links to the frustrations of servile dependence. His desire for
retaliation is predictably anal:

> See, so cham arrayed with dabbling in the dirt—
> She that set me to ditching, ich would she had the squirt!
> Was never poor soul that such a life had
> Gog's bones, this vilthy glay has dressed me too bad!
> God's soul, see how this stuff tears!
>
> (1.2.1–5)

That Hodge articulates an oedipal desire to displace shameful uncontrol back onto its perceived source is not surprising. Yet here,

---

Robinson, who finds the suggestion that the needle and eel are phallic "somewhat
illogical" but does cite Henry Porter's *Two Angry Women of Abingdon*, where the phalli-
cism of the eel/needle is unequivocal. See Robinson, "The Art and Meaning of *Gammer
Gurton's Needle*," *Renaissance Drama* n.s. 14 (1983), 68.

10. McFadyen, "What Was Really Lost," p. 10, emphasis added.

though his anger takes on some gender inflection, the shamefulness of his bodily condition—particularly the state of his pants—is hypostatized as a function of class. To be a laborer like Hodge is to have clothes full of holes, is to be unable to keep one's body from being shamefully or offensively exposed to an audience of betters. This social fact, insofar as it has involuntary bodily markings, the needle cannot change: labor will always reopen holes in clothes Gammer will always work to repair. From this perspective, the sexual division of labor in the household appears rational and interdependent. The labor of both dependent male and dominant female is equally repetitive and nonprogressive, serving to situate both Gammer and Hodge in cyclical interdependence.

But once the needle is lost, Hodge realizes that the holes in his *other* pants, the ones he was to wear courting, have not been repaired. Issues of class are almost immediately overtaken by issues of gender and liminality. The routines of labor give way to directed heterosexual imperatives, as if to assert the primacy of gender as the basis of social organization and signification, especially for the male body sign of the open breech. Almost literally a floating signifier, the lost needle becomes to Hodge the talisman of gender difference and sexual maturation, becomes that which all the household's labor should function to preserve and utilize:

> Whereto served your hands and eyes but this your nee'le to keep?
> What devil had you else to do? Ye kept, ich wot, no sheep!
> Cham fain abroad to dig and delve in water, mire and clay,
> Sossing and possing in the dirt from day to day.
> A hundred things that be abroad, cham set to see them well,
> And four of you sit idle at home and cannot keep a nee'le!
>
> (1.4.23–28)

Hodge's realization of his phallic loss suggests the infantile rage and vulnerability of the male when maternal women retain control over male bodily thresholds and thus over access to contested arenas of social and sexual privilege. Small wonder that Hodge and the rest of the household so readily accept Diccon the Bedlam's suggestion that the precious needle is not lost but stolen—by Dame Chat, the community's other dominant woman.

In this play, then, household structures mirror and reify intrapsychic structures through the symbolic agency of the absent needle. The open breech is established as a male body sign of rusticity, immaturity, uncontrol, and anal subjection and is causally linked to female dominance. (Dr. Rat's broken head, wounds received at the hands of Dame Chat, will function later as an equivalent sign displaced to a higher social position and the upper bodily stratum.) In my view, the play's subsequent emphasis on coprophagy, anal raking, groping, farting, and penetration is evidence not of the "gleefulness" of its scatology (as if scatology were merely a high-spirited form of unthematic decor) but of the function of scatological discourse and behavior in the semiosis of gender.[11] It is precisely this aspect of the play that begins to explain its social meaningfulness to an audience composed largely of privileged but relatively powerless adolescent males in the company of their masters.

For Hodge, the crisis of gender formation is enacted not only through the loss of the signifying needle but also as a sequence of increasingly shameful bodily inscriptions that link bodily openness and dirt. His body is marked and thus soiled by increasingly privatized or personal forms of dirt, from relatively neutral field dirt in the second scene, to household dirt (including a cat's turd) picked up in his clothes when he wallows on the floor looking for the needle, to his own excreta released involuntarily in fear when Diccon pretends to conjure the devil as a way to find the needle: "By the mass, cham able no longer to hold it! / Too bad—ich must beray the hall!" (2.1.105–6).

The moment—which the play's most recent editor calls "gross"—is in fact critical to my larger argument. Note, first of all, that in the narrative economy of this play there is no such thing as waste. Hodge's failure of bodily control here requires him to change his clothes, though not his holes, requires him, that is, to put on the pants Gammer was mending when the needle was lost and thus prepares for the needle's discovery *in* those pants at the denouement.[12] And if the needle was never really lost, then the phallus and the sex-gender system it maintains—we are relieved to know retrospectively—was never really in danger!

11. "Gleeful" is Whitworth's term, *Three Sixteenth-Century Comedies*, p. xxxi, and he is quoted with approval by Douglas Duncan, "*Gammer Gurton's Needle* and the Concept of Humanist Parody," *Studies in English Literature*, 27 (1987), 188.

12. Whitworth agrees that "the grossness is not entirely gratuitous" because of its relevance to the denouement. See *Three Sixteenth-Century Comedies*, p. 26n. F. S. Boas was the first to commend the play's deftness of construction in *University Drama in the Tudor Age* (Oxford: Clarendon, 1914), p. 78.

But the needle's absence—from *before* the beginning until the very end of the play—identifies Hodge's private emergency as a structural crisis with implications for the whole community, since Hodge in his fear of shame and sexual impairment is willing to abrogate his bond of servitude to Gammer and transfer the labor of his body to the service of whoever finds the needle:

> Chill run, chill ride, chill dig, chill delve, chill toil, chill trudge,
>   shalt see.
> Chill hold, chill draw, chill pull, chill pinch, chill kneel on my
>   bare knee.
> Chill scrape, chill scratch, chill sift, chill seek, chill bow, chill bend,
>   chill sweat.
> Chill stop, chill stir, chill cap, chill kneel, chill creep on hands
>   and feet.
> Chill be thy bondman, Diccon, ich swear by sun and moon,
> And 'ch cannot somewhat to stop this gap, cham utterly undone.
>   (2.1.55–60)

Diccon's response to this unusually specific pledge of bodily devotion underscores the significance of stopping the bodily gap as an issue of power relations. For Diccon proceeds to enact a substitution critical to the play's symbolic economy, a substitution with special resonance in a university setting. Neither Hodge nor Gammer possesses any books, being unable to read them, but this illiteracy becomes privative only when Diccon pretends to invoke the mystical authority of Scripture as his own private means of containing and controlling Hodge. Unable to make Hodge swear by the book—that is, the Bible—to "be no blab" (2.1.67), Diccon constitutes his own breech as talismanic sign of Hodge's allegiance:

> I, Hodge, breechless,
> Swear to Diccon, rechless,
> By the cross that I shall kiss,
> To keep his counsel close
> And always me to dispose
> To work that his pleasure is.
>   *Here he kisseth Diccon's breech*[13]
>   (2.1.71–77)

13. In the tableau of the illiterate servant kissing the nether end of the Bedlam beggar instead of the Bible there is a wonderful carnivalization of religious ritual, the

The moment expresses more than, perhaps something other than, Diccon's contempt for Hodge because of the play's seriocomic endorsement of Hodge's necessity, its affirmation of the symbolism of stopping the bodily gap. In the twinned substitutions of the breech for the book and ass kissing for oath taking we can identify an early comic enactment of the metonymies of powerlessness and uncontrol which will become crucial to the reproduction of social position and gender in the later drama. Hodge kisses Diccon's backside as a *voluntary* act of submission on behalf of his heterosexual aspirations. Even in this predominantly male theatrical setting, the gesture seems to me homoerotic only insofar as homoeroticism can be identified as a kind of gender narcissism. For one with Hodge's sense of desperate sexual impairment, Diccon's unholey breech, like Diccon's assertion of generalized mastery, constitutes a fit object of desire.[14] But when Diccon begins to conjure the devil, Hodge's aspirations are imperiled yet again, this time by an *involuntary* bodily failure. In an action of symbolic downward displacement, Hodge's body itself confirms Diccon's fears about Hodge's ability to contain himself verbally. Poor Hodge can neither hold his ground nor avoid soiling himself out of fear: "Ich *must* beray the hall."

More important, this display of shameful uncontrol shows how a net of metonymies more conventionally identified with woman can also be used to reproduce hierarchies of class. In Chapter 1, I argued that conventional attribution of linguistic, genital, or urinary uncontrol to women serves to legitimate patriarchal strategies of enclosure and domination. Here, in order to reproduce difference on a male subject in the lower-class world of *Gammer Gurton's Needle*, shameful bodily openness has to occur in two ways—by way of the needle *and* by way of the fart. That is, as a problematic of gender, Hodge's shameful bodily openness is, as we have seen, linked to female dominance through the symbolic agency of the missing needle. As a problematic

---

precise suggestiveness of which is probably illegible to us without a clearer understanding of the play's date and occasion. Robinson does note the possibility that the villagers swore on breeches as a substitute for swearing on the "Breeches Bible," the 1560 Geneva Bible. He also argues that the scene primarily expresses Diccon's contempt for Hodge. See "Art and Meaning," pp. 62, 67.

14. Whether or not Diccon's breech *was* unholey is, I think, ambiguous. As Boas points out, neither contemporary accounts of ragged, unkempt Bedlam beggars nor Edgar's impersonation of poor Tom in *King Lear* seems to match this figure who speaks more or less standard English and whom the villagers accept and trust. See *University Drama*, p. 74. For the purposes of this argument, the icon of ragged Hodge kissing an equally ragged Diccon would have the effect of identifying gender anxiety as a subjective phenomenon.

of class, bodily openness is now blamed on Hodge himself. With the act of *soiling himself*, Hodge crudely but effectively naturalizes his subordinate class position. Perhaps he even enacts a crude equation: a needle is to Hodge what a book is to Hodge's audience—the means to avoid kissing somebody's ass and to keep one's body from physical or social shame. The villagers' shortage of needles is thus functionally related to their shortage of books, both shortages constituting a crisis of gender and power relations in which Diccon the Bedlam—a self-constituted authority from the outside world—has now intervened.

Just as important to my larger argument, then, are the implications of Hodge's metatheatrical notation of place here: "Ich must beray the *hall*." Despite their simplicity, the characters in *Gammer Gurton's Needle*, as often in farce, periodically acknowledge and address their audience, even attend to the physical reality of that audience in asking them to give room.[15] But here, Hodge's very bodiliness sets forth the semipermeable limits of mimesis. By noting the actual ground on which he stands as the place he is about to soil, the student actor as Hodge reifies the bodily tension between the requirements of narrative and the material constraint of the physical self. The moment acknowledges the difficulty of pretending to offend without actually doing so, of pretending shame in a fictional self without being actually ashamed on one's own. What is the excretory equivalent of stage blood, particularly in a play that has already made use of a cat's turd, produced (one supposes) by the college cat in her actual as opposed to theatrical capacity? The role the actor of Hodge has put on becomes as full of aporias as Hodge's clothes are full of holes, and the social determinacy of the body is showing through.

Furthermore, as the audience members recognize the limits of mimesis, contemplate the possible consequences of Hodge's bodily uncontrol, they are themselves drawn into a symbolic economy of laughter and shame made explicit by Diccon:

> Fie, shitten knave, and out upon thee!
> Above *all other louts*, fie on thee!
> Is not here a cleanly prank?
> But thy matter was no better,
> Nor thy presence here no sweeter;
> To fly I can thee thank!
>   (2.2.1–6, emphasis mine)

15. See, for example, 3.3.36.

What the young Cambridge men laugh at here, indeed, the narrative occasion for what they have laughed at from the very beginning of the play, is shameful bodily exposure—that which, as Michael Bristol has pointed out, constituted "the definitive category of laughing matter" in humanist theory.[16] Hodge's experience is indeed an exact instantiation of Stanley Cavell's definition of shame as "the specific discomfort produced by the sense of being looked at" and the response to shame as the desire to cover up "not your deed, but yourself."[17] Hodge's rage emanates from the fact that, properly speaking, he himself has not *done* anything to merit shame. And his shame is all the more pronounced because his body is being looked at where he himself has no possibility of ocular control.[18]

But, as the humanist physician Laurent Joubert argues in his *Traité du ris* (1579), unintentional exposure is the bodily state not only of the object of laughter but of the laugher as well. It is therefore helpful to my argument about the actor of Hodge and his audience that Joubert is far more interested in the physiological mechanisms of laughter than in its psychology (though that is a distinction he would not, in any case, have made). Laughter is for him a bodily phenomenon that one ought to find astonishing "if one examines it closely": "Indeed, who could not be amazed upon seeing in an instant the entire body thrown into motion and shaking with an indescribable stir for the pleasure of the soul . . . were we not already so used to it—so much so that one scarcely takes notice?" He devotes an entire chapter of the *Treatise on Laughter* to the question "whence it comes that one pisses, shits, and sweats by dint of laughing," and he begins—remarkably enough—by instructing his readers about the location, structure, and function of the sphincter muscles and the voluntary control we ordinarily have over them. In laughter, however, our will to bodily control is overcome by a violent solicitation from the body below:

16. Michael D. Bristol, *Carnival and Theater: Plebeian Culture and the Structure of Authority in Renaissance England* (London: Routledge, 1985), p. 135: "The buttocks are 'out of place' in a social situation. Nevertheless, they are objects of desire and in any case their existence is 'common knowledge.'"

17. See Stanley Cavell,"The Avoidance of Love: A Reading of *King Lear*" (1969), reprinted in *Disowning Knowledge in Six Plays of Shakespeare* (Cambridge: Cambridge University Press, 1987), p. 49.

18. For an extended meditation on the exposed buttock and our inability to see it as a specific of shame, see Eve Kosofsky Sedgwick, "A Poem Is Being Written," *Representations* 17 (Winter 1987), 126. See also Anthony Giddens's discussion "Front Regions, Back Regions," in *The Constitution of Society: Outline of the Theory of Structuration* (Cambridge: Polity Press, 1984), pp. 56, 122–29.

It is, then, likely, that when these muscles press a long time and with much violence, soliciting the bowels and the bladder to give up their contents (as it happens in laughter), if there is a quantity of liquid matter, all escapes us indecorously. For the agitation and jouncing is so strong that the sphincters are unable to resist, especially when after a long duration they become loose and weak, like the rest of the body, losing all strength.[19]

As the undergraduates in the audience of *Gammer Gurton's Needle* laughed at the nearness of Hodge's shameful lapse of bodily control, perhaps they were moved through laughter closer to the dangerous experience of their own bodily shame—as a structure of memory or as a momentary perception of bodiliness—and thus to a recognition of the social vulnerability of the bodily self. But given the crisis of gender formation which Hodge's bodily emergency signifies, such laughter is probably not a simple token of festivity, of benevolent communal self-recognition and psychological release.[20] As Joubert's account of the physiology of laughter makes clear, laughter operates indiscriminately but predictably on the body of the laugher, without regard for the social coordinates of age, rank, and especially gender by which hierarchical difference is constructed. Laughter here threatens to destabilize not only the structure of differences between Hodge and his audience but the hierarchical differences of rank and station within the audience as well because it threatens the bodily control that is construed in *Gammer Gurton's Needle* as a central attribute of male privilege. In such an economy of laughter and shame, covering one's ass is more than a narrative preoccupation for the rustic villagers; it becomes, almost literally, a mandate for the hall.

In the matter of voluntary physical self-mastery, Joubert's emphasis as a physician upon the physical consequences of laughter conjoins with Hodge's experience of the obstacles to heterosexual adulthood and returns this discussion to the question of formative bodily experience with which I began. From this point of view, Hodge's experience of shameful bodily openness is not to be regarded as the isolated comic predicament of an individually constructed male subject but

19. Laurent Joubert, *Treatise on Laughter*, trans. and ed. Gregory David de Rocher (University: University of Alabama Press, 1980), pp. 16, 59, 60.
20. See Bristol, *Carnival and Theater*, pp. 130–39, for a linked discussion of Erasmus and Joubert on laughter; I agree with Bristol on the antihierarchical function of laughter but would argue, here at least, for anxiety about threatened difference as a result.

rather as a regressive fantasy in which ambiguities of gender formation become encoded and hierarchized as a question of personal
bodily discipline. Thus attention to scatological discourse may well be
essential to recuperating the play's interactions with its immediate
audience because in this play scatology is the instrument of fantasy,
the common language of bodily memory.

ᴥ

Scatology, in *Gammer Gurton's Needle*, then, mediates between the
somatic control required by patriarchal culture and the antithetical
desire maintained in part by such bodily practices as the purge. It is a
dialectic of holding in or letting go, of self-mastery or release. With
the advent of the cult of Elizabeth, that dialectic of contradictory male
desires comes to focus upon the equally contradictory figure of the
queen, mother and virgin, woman and prince.[21] The structure of
regressive bodily memory encoded in *Gammer Gurton's Needle* is re-
enacted and circumscribed explicitly *as fantasy* in *A Midsummer Night's
Dream* and *The Alchemist*. Both plays displace Hodge's anxiety about
bodily boundaries and shameful genital exposure with a narcissistic
fantasy of erotic privilege and uniqueness. Bottom and Dapper stand
in for Hodge; Titania and Doll Common take over for Gammer.
Experience in the body here is an aspirant's fantasy of selection
and metamorphosis at the hands of a powerful female figure—
recognizably a version of the queen.

To look to the body in *A Midsummer Night's Dream* as a material
signifier of social allegory is to see the central scenes between Titania
and Bottom take on the aspect of an elaborately encoded scatological
joke. As in *Gammer Gurton's Needle*, scatology provides a narrative
content for the "fantasy of infantile narcissism and dependency"
which Louis Adrian Montrose and others have seen in Bottom's relation to Titania.[22] Scatology is encoded, first of all, in Bottom's name.
If the weaver, like the other mechanicals, is named by a metonymy of
his craft ("bottom" being the core of a weaver's skein), metamorphosis

21. Louis Adrian Montrose, "'Shaping Fantasies': Figurations of Gender and Power
in Elizabethan Culture," in *Rewriting the Renaissance: The Discourses of Sexual Difference in
Early Modern Europe*, ed. Margaret W. Ferguson, Maureen Quilligan, and Nancy J.
Vickers (Chicago: University of Chicago Press, 1986), p. 67.
22. Ibid., p. 35. My reading of the Bottom-Titania interaction corresponds in the
main to his brief discussion of the scene, except that I want to insist upon the relevance
to it of bodily practices specific to early modern culture and their psychic consequences.

activates the name's latent somatic pun.[23] It activates scatological possibilities as well, most of them derived from the trope of the speaking
ass—the motif of *proktos lalon* identified by E. R. Curtius as part of
"coarse" European folk humor from the Middle Ages on.[24]

Charges of coarseness aside, two things about this trope are of
special relevance here. One is its connection to misogyny. In one of
Curtius's examples of the motif, an outspoken old woman who doubts
the miraculous properties of the body of Saint Gangolf is punished by
a case of unrelenting flatulence: "During the rest of her life the woman could not speak a word on Friday but that it was followed by a
detonation."[25] A voluntary act of verbal transgression is disciplined,
shamefully, by involuntary transgression from below. By farting
against her will, the old lady's body enters the history of shame, takes
on the iterable identity of the textual. There is a similar connection
between scatology and misogyny in the bodily embarrassments Puck
delights in visiting upon old women. His mischief isolates the interchangeable thresholds of female appetite and vulnerability—making
an old gossip spill ale "on her wither'd dewlap," and "the wisest aunt,
telling the saddest tale," fall on her bum and, I believe, into a proverbial response to embarrassment: coughing to cover a fart.[26] Here

23. The *OED* does not support a lexical use of *bottom* as buttocks before the end of
the nineteenth century, but Eric Partridge in *Shakespeare's Bawdy: A Literary and Psychological Essay and a Comprehensive Glossary* (London: Routledge and Kegan Paul, 1968)
does cite analogous sexual wordplay on "sweet bottom-grass" in *Venus and Adonis* (v.
236). In contemporary American usage, of course, there is a pun on bottom/ass which is
not present in Elizabethan locutions. The *OED*'s first citation of *ass* as a dialect spelling
of *arse* is mid-nineteenth century. Shakespeare is playing on the word *bottom*, whether
specifically in its meaning as the posterior or more generally as signifying the lowest
part, the basis of anything, whether a social or a human body. The likelihood of somatic
troping on Bottom's name is increased, too, by the obvious somatic allusion in names
for the other mechanicals—Starveling, Snout, and Flute, whom Harold F. Brooks
characterizes as "a lackbeard with a fluty treble" in the Arden edition (London: Methuen, 1979), Dramatis Personae n. 12.
24. Ernst R. Curtius, *European Literature in the Latin Middle Ages*, trans. Willard Trask
(Princeton: Princeton University Press, 1953), p. 435. I owe this reference to Michael
Bristol.
25. Ibid.
26. See Morris Palmer Tilley, *A Dictionary of the Proverbs in England in the Sixteenth and
Seventeenth Centuries* (Ann Arbor: University of Michigan Press, 1950), F 64, p. 202.
James T. Henke also identifies "cough in the breech" as a cant phrase for a fart, in
*Gutter Life and Language in the Early "Street" Literature of England: A Glossary of Terms and
Topics Chiefly of the Sixteenth and Seventeenth Centuries* (West Cornwall, Conn.: Locust Hill
Press, 1988), p. 66. But neither Partridge in *Shakespeare's Bawdy* nor Frankie Rubinstein
in *A Dictionary of Shakespeare's Sexual Puns and Their Significance* (London: Macmillan,
1984) cites this in Shakespeare. Puck's image of the old gossip is linked to the female
attributes of gluttony and drunkenness, particularly at the gossips' meeting.

again is the comic specter of incontinent women and the gluttonous world of the gossips' meeting.

In other instances of the *proktos lalon* trope, however—perhaps when it is given a masculine inflection—the meaning of the speaking ass is inverted to become a signifier of remarkable bodily control, the nether source of a bodily music. Both Joubert in the *Treatise on Laughter* and the English physician Edward Jorden in his *Disease Called the Suffocation of the Mother* cite Saint Augustine, among others, as the source of this meaning for the trope. "Some let farts that do not smell," says Joubert, asserting the power of some rational souls over the bodies they inhabit, "as many as they want and of diverse sounds, so much so that they seem to sing from their arse." Jorden refers to "*Adrian Tournebus* [who] saw a rogue that gayned much money by shewing this feate."[27]

My point is not that Bottom—even as acted by the famous clown Will Kemp—was recognizably a version of the trope of *proktos lalon*. The point is rather that thematic traces of this scatological material constitute an embedded layer of meaning in the powerfully over-determined image of the ass-headed man taking his ease in the bower of the fairy queen. I have already tried to show how, in Hodge's scene with Diccon, Hodge's incontinence naturalizes his subordinate position in both gender and class relations. His body is shamefully open, hence feminized, because he is the victim of female domination; his body is shamefully open, hence ungoverned by the rational will, because he is a lower-class rustic. Hodge's heterosexual desire does not, however, take him outside the aspirations or boundaries of his class, nor does the mise-en-scène of *Gammer Gurton's Needle* venture beyond the boundaries of the rustic village.

But as Leonard Tennenhouse has suggested, *A Midsummer Night's Dream* dares to stage interhierarchical events in a complex social body just as it dares to imagine the dissolution of social boundaries in the forbidden mating of a queen with the grotesque body of the populace, represented by Bottom.[28] I believe the somatic pun on Bottom's name gives the metamorphosis an even more ambivalent social tonality than Tennenhouse implies because Bottom's relation to Titania parodies not only a transgressive social fantasy but a dangerous famil-

27. Joubert, *Treatise on Laughter*, p. 70; Edward Jorden, *A Briefe Discourse of a Disease Called the Suffocation of the Mother* (London, 1603; STC 14790; rpt. Amsterdam: Da Capo Press, 1971), p. 12.

28. Leonard Tennenhouse, *Power on Display: The Politics of Shakespeare's Genres* (London: Methuen, 1986), pp. 42–43.

ial one as well. Cultural discomfort with the powers of maternity is suggested at the very beginning of the play by Theseus's expository reference to his conquest of Amazonia and appropriation through marriage of its queen. A further part of the representational strategy of patriarchy here is to use Bottom's elevation as the basis for a parodic representation of maternal affection and nurture. We know that Bottom's metamorphosis is motivated by Oberon's desire to punish Titania for keeping the changeling boy in memory of his mother. As Montrose suggests, "What Oberon accomplishes by substituting Bottom for the boy is to break Titania's solemn vow."[29] But the substitution also constructs a parodic image of adult female sexuality in which the differences between heterosexual intercourse and the anal cathexes of maternal nurture become blurred.

Shakespeare's trope for the sudden elevation of a bumptious mechanical to be the intimate of a queen is an inversion of upper and lower bodily strata—the replacement of top by Bottom. Such a trope is fully consonant with the Bakhtinian paradigm of the grotesque body, emphasizing the parts and functioning of the lower stratum—both reproductive and excretory. But the somatic trope suggests, as well, an identification of lower-class bodily behaviors with the bodily behaviors of children. Shakespeare would seem to be endorsing as a matter of class differentiation Elias's argument that "the distance in behavior and whole psychical structure between children and adults increases in the course of the civilizing process."[30] Here, instead, the "distance in behavior and whole psychical structure between children and adults" reproduces the social hierarchy, so that the mechanicals—"every mother's son" (1.2.78)—seem to represent an early stage of psychosocial development, the patriarchal Theseus its maturity.

Metamorphosis from man to ass and whole to lower body part thus returns Bottom to infancy or confirms his ascriptive social position in a symbolic infancy that the somatic trope identifies as a dominantly anal stage, focused on retentive-eliminative modes of expression.

29. Montrose, "'Shaping Fantasies,'" p. 41.

30. Elias, *The History of Manners*, p. xiii. Without endorsing Elias's assertion as a sociogenetic truth, I cite it here as one kind of theoretical explanation for Shakespeare's infantilization of the mechanicals. Elias's thinking on this matter resembles that of some cultural anthropologists who, according to Mary Douglas, assume "that primitive cultures correspond to infantile stages in the development of the human mind" and who thus interpret rituals in such cultures "as if they express the same preoccupations which fill the mind of psychopaths or infants." See *Purity and Danger: An Analysis of the Concepts of Pollution and Taboo* (1966; rpt. London: Ark, 1984), p. 115.

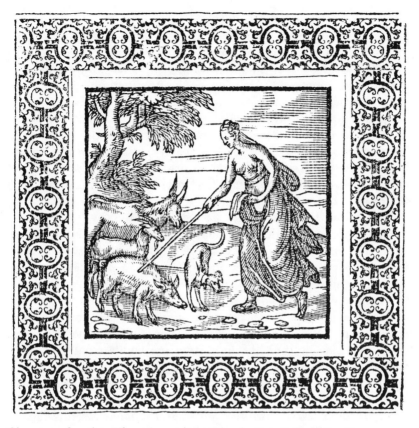

Circe transforming Ulysses' men into animals. Detail, from Geoffrey Whitney, *A Choice of Emblemes* (Leiden, 1586), p. 82. By permission of the Folger Shakespeare Library.

Scatology functions here, then, to naturalize Bottom's regressive behavior as both baby and lover, son and paramour—the charged admixture of roles produced by Elizabeth's eroticizing of courtier-sovereign relations. From Bottom's point of view as the bewildered object of such devotion, Titania's response to the intruder in her bower throughout the scenes between them seems hopelessly contradictory in tenor. Although she professes an instant and complete love for him as ass, a love for him *as is*, she seems intent upon enacting changes in him, exacting changes from him. The first of these, replicating Oberon's operations on her, is to appropriate Bottom through an alteration of affect: "Out of this wood do not *desire* to go" (3.1.152). Other changes, however, seem anally cathected, seeking to impose a stricter external discipline upon his bodily boundaries and orifices with the effect, intended or not, of infantilizing him. Her dotage is his regression. As if following upon the implication of the somatic pun in his name, Titania's instructions for his care seem designed to quiet the upper bodily stratum and to stimulate the lower. Though ostensibly in love with his song, she commands her fairies to "tie up my lover's tongue, bring him silently" (3.1.201), as if mistrusting his ability to keep from singing or—more to the point—from emitting what Stanley Wells calls his "involuntary" asinine brays.[31] A victim of his own presumptuousness, Bottom, like the old lady in Curtius's fable, threatens an incontinence of noise.

Even more important, Titania would refine upon his bodiliness: "And I will *purge thy mortal grossness* so, / That thou shalt like an aery spirit go" (3.1.160–61). The emphasis here is mine, for the phrase has attracted almost no attention from editors, as if Titania's intentions and methods at this moment were perfectly transparent. To the contrary, her language may well represent an instance of overdetermined meaning crucial to the scene at large but occluded for modern readers of the play by their distance from the bodily culture of early modern Europe. As the fact of editorial silence implies, the linked signifiers are easily assimilated to a figurative reading of Titania's intention as solely ethical and tutelary, since they point to what are for us signifieds of ethical practice and moral judgment. Thus "grossness" is a signifier for dullness, stupidity, want of instruction or for coarseness and want of refinement in habits, ideas, and speech.[32] As qualified by "mortal," grossness emphasizes Bottom's corporality and materiality in contrast to Titania's immortality. (Any more precise ontological distinction between the two beings, such as the bodilessness of fairies, collides comically with the facticity and corporality of drama.) The transferential meaning of "purge," signifying a process of moral or spiritual purification, also belongs to ethical or specifically religious discourses in Shakespearean as well as general usage. By concentrating on the abstraction in her speech, we can understand

31. In the Penguin edition (Harmondsworth, England, 1970), note to 3.1.196, p. 144.

32. The *OED* cites this line under *grossness*, "3a. Thickness, density, materiality, solidity." But see also "4. Coarseness, want of fineness or refinement: a. of food, feeding, or material substances."

Titania to announce a generalized intention to improve Bottom with education or adornment, to "purge" away the coarseness of his manners or the monstrousness of his physique.

But the humoral theory on which the practice of purging was based does not allow for sharp distinctions between the ethical and physical domains, between abstract and concrete signification in its technical vocabulary.[33] Its characteristic idiom—of *qualities, humors, temperaments*—had a firm, systematic function of physical reference which ostensibly figurative usages in the Shakespearean corpus do not dislodge. Thus Orsino's praise—"O, when mine eyes did see Olivia first, / Methought she purg'd the air of pestilence" (*Twelfth Night*, 1.1.18–19)—endows Olivia with a power against airborne infection in which physical and psychological operations commingle. A perhaps clearer instance of the commingling of physical and ethical occurs in *Richard II* when the king asks Bolingbroke and Mowbray to "purge this choler without letting blood," adding facetiously, "our doctors say this is no month to bleed" (1.1.153, 157). Richard employs the commonplace trope of combat as phlebotomy, of bloodshed as bloodletting discussed in Chapter 2. He seeks, ineffectually but nonetheless literally, to expel the choler of his feuding barons with the instrumentality of the royal word. Or we can look to another instance, closer in spirit to that of Bottom and Titania, in *Love's Labor's Lost*, when Costard replies to the promise of his freedom after being "bound". "True, true," he tells Armado, "and now you will be my purgation and let me loose" (3.1.126–27). To clear Costard from wrongdoing, an ethical procedure, is also to effect a physical change in him from bondage to freedom, a change whose significance he plays upon with the scatological pun. Similarly, Falstaff, at the end of *1 Henry IV*, contemplates the prospect of reward and reformation with a pun on moral and physical purgation: "If I do grow great, I'll grow less, for I'll purge and leave sack, and live cleanly as a nobleman should do" (5.4.163–65). His plan for physical reform, to take laxatives and reduce, cannot be separated from a plan for moral reform, as his play

33. For a discussion of the metaphysical underpinnings of Galenism, see Lester S. King, "The Transformation of Galenism," in *Medicine in Seventeenth Century England*, ed. Allen G. Debus (Berkeley: University of California Press, 1974), pp. 7–31. But see also an analogous case of the physical becoming ethical, or vice versa, in Georges Vigarello's discussion of "uprightness" and the courtly prescriptions about posture in "The Upward Training of the Body from the Age of Chivalry to Courtly Civility," in *Fragments for a History of the Human Body: Part Two*, ed. Michel Feher, *Zone*, 4 (1989), 149–96.

upon the quasi-religious paradoxes of "great" and "less" confirms. Both plans constitute modes of living "cleanly"—too cleanly, in fact, for Falstaff's unregenerate, unpurgeable brand of mortal grossness. The closest equivalent to the kind of purge Titania may intend for Bottom comes not elsewhere in Shakespeare, however, but in Rabelais's *Gargantua*: when the young giant's tutor Ponocrates asks a physician to "consider if it would be possible to set Gargantua on a better road, Theodore purged the youth in due form with black hellebore, and with this drug cured his brain of its corrupt and perverse habits."[34] The move from a scholastic to a humanistic education is facilitated or ensured by the strong purgative.

Titania's plans to "purge" Bottom of mortal grossness seem to me equally poised between, or inclusive of, ethical and physical reference, just as her interest in his physical state seems poised between the erotic and the maternal. Like an overcontrolling mother focused upon the body processes of her infant, Titania prescribes a *literal* purge, the alimentary purge from inside out. She commands that Bottom be fed a diet consisting entirely of fruits distinctly laxative in effect: "Feed him with apricocks and dewberries, / With purple grapes, green figs, and mulberries" (166–67). In part the menu impresses by its seasonal impossibility, early and late fruits being offered together at midsummer. But as Dale Randall has pointed out in connection with the dung-ripened apricots Bosola gives to the Duchess of Malfi, exotic fruit in general and apricots in particular were thought to be aphrodisiacs for men and women. This association, he says, explains why the Capulet cooks preparing for Juliet's bridal banquet "call for dates and quinces in the pastry" (4.4.2), why the pregnant Mrs. Elbow's craving for stewed prunes leads her to a brothel in *Measure for Measure*.[35] One could add to these examples of the sexual stimulation of fruit Lucio's decision to "dine and sup with water and bran" in order to control libido: "One fruitful meal," on the contrary, "would set me to't" (*Measure*, 4.3.153, 154).

What goes unspoken in these conventional associations of fruit with sexual appetite is the erotic effect of laxation, the erotic promise of the purge, particularly perhaps for Elizabethans accustomed from infancy to this form of bodily culture. Freud's account of the erot-

---

34. François Rabelais, *Gargantua and Pantagruel*, trans. J. M. Cohen (Harmondsworth, England: Penguin, 1955), pp. 86–87.

35. Dale B. J. Randall, "Physical Symbols in *The Duchess of Malfi*," *Renaissance Drama* n.s. 18 (1987), 179–89. He does cite this passage in *Dream* without discussing it (p. 183).

ogenic overloading of the lower bodily stratum may be useful here: "The peripheral stimulation of certain specialized parts (genitals, mouth, anus, urethra) which may be called erotogenic zones, furnishes important contributions to the production of sexual excitement."[36] This is precisely the suggestive ambiguity of an Elizabethan herbal's warning about ripe apricots that "they loose the belly, & engender *noughtie* humors."[37]

There is, moreover, an established connection between purging and sexual activity in the seasonal recommendations of popular medicine. The relation between sexual intercourse and excretion had scientific legitimation in the attention paid by humoral theory to the production and expression of all bodily fluids and in its theoretical assumption of their fungibility. In medical literature sexual release was regarded functionally as a form of evacuation, as an emission of bodily fluids necessary for health but requiring regulation and moderation. "Venus omitted," says Burton in *The Anatomy of Melancholy*, produces the same harmful effects as dysfunction in any other form of evacuation, such as the unhealthful suppression of menstrual periods, the abrupt stopping of a nosebleed, or the "detention of hemrods." Too much venery, Burton says, is "bad . . . *because it infrigidates & dries up the body, consumes the spirits.*"[38]

Humoral theory's broad definition presupposes and helps to sustain a preoccupation with evacuation throughout early modern culture generally and within the life cycle of the individual subject. Evacuation had not only a daily rhythm but a seasonal one as well. In popular medicine of English almanacs in this period, the short formulaic verses heading the monthly calendar pages contain common

36. Sigmund Freud, "Character and Anal Erotism" (1908), in the *Standard Edition of the Complete Psychological Works*, trans. James Strachey (London: Hogarth Press, 1959), 9:170–71. He wants to differentiate the formation or repression of anal erotism by reference to a theory of the "anal erotic character." My concern is to situate a cultural rather than characterological impulse to anal eroticism within the bodily and discursive practices of early modern Europe.

37. This is a quotation from Dioscurides in the Dutchman Rembert Dodoen's *Niewe Herball, or The Historie of Plants*, trans. Henry Lyte (London, 1578; STC 6984), p. 710, emphasis added, also quoted by Randall, "Physical Symbols," p. 179. I infer a possible pun here, even if unintended or unconscious, because of the semantic ambiguities forming around *nought/naught* and *noughtie/naughtie* in the period. The *OED*, interestingly, cites another instance in Lyte's translation for *nought*, "injurious *to*, bad *for*, a thing or person" (B 3, adj.), but the senses of doing wrong or acting immorally are always close at hand.

38. Robert Burton, *The Anatomy of Melancholy*, ed. Floyd Dell and Paul Jordan-Smith (New York: Tudor, 1938), pp. 204, 203, 205.

forms of dietary, medical, and sexual advice specific to each season and geared to an implied male reader. This advice always includes recommendations for those times of year best and worst for bathing, bleeding, purging, and venery—bodily events homologized as forms of "like evacuation."[39] Though gentle purgatives might be taken at any time, the porous body of humoral theory was vulnerable in the climatic extremes of the year, the months of greatest heat and cold, when the expenditure or release of bodily fluids was thought very inadvisable. Burton cites the case of a man who "married a young wife in a hot summer, *and so dried himself with chamber-work, that he became in short space from melancholy mad.*"[40]

More important, however, to the associations of sexual intercourse and the purge is the suggestion latent in almanac verse that purging, bathing, bleeding, and venery were not only functionally alike but alike as forms of bodily pleasure. Thomas Bretnor's 1615 almanac for the dangerously hot month of August advises, "Bid farewell Physicke, Wine & women shun, / least wo is me (thou criest) I am undone." Leaving physic, he implies, is like leaving wine and women—a farewell to sensual pleasure on all counts. George Dauncy's July verse singles out "venereous, great feeders," and August identifies "the lustfull and Phisicke takers" as seekers of undifferentiated pleasures and warns them from their pleasure in eating, purging, or copulating in the heat. There is an even broader hint of the erotic pleasure of the purge in Dauncy's verse for May, a kind of medical May song:

> Now art thou bid by gentle May,
>   Purge, vomit, bath and bleed:
> Leave bed, walke fieldes in morne, use meanes
>   Of Health to sowe the seede.

39. I quote here from "Observations in May" in *Rams Little Dodeon* (London, 1606; STC 6988), p. 17, but the thinking is commonplace. On the matter of bathing, Alain Corbin has demonstrated that in France until well into the nineteenth century "plunging into water involved a calculated risk. It was important that the duration, frequency, and temperature of baths be adapted to sex, age, temperament, state of health, and season. Baths were thought to exert a profound effect on the whole organism, because they were not an everyday event." Not surprisingly, given the humoral association of women and water, bathing for women was surrounded by all sorts of prohibitions, constraints, and moral judgments. See *The Foul and the Fragrant: Odor and the French Social Imagination* (Cambridge: Harvard University Press, 1986), p. 178.

40. Burton, *Anatomy of Melancholy*, p. 205.

The consequences of ignoring such advice were potentially disastrous. Witness the threat to a man's hopes for issue contained in the
July verse of Thomas Bretnor's 1615 almanac:

> Strike not a vein, nor do no phisicke take
>   unlesse thou wilt a breach in nature make:
> Nor middle not with wine nor wanton toyes
>   least thou deprive thy selfe of hoped joyes.

One almanac's September recommendations bear a close resemblance to Titania's diet for Bottom:

> Eate ripe fruites moderately,
> Take Medicines needfully,
> Figges, Grapes, and Spicery,
> Refresh the members dry.[41]

Though such fruit may "loosen the belly," according to this verse, it
will also, much more important, moisten a body dried up by August
heat and restore its sexual vigor. Fruit may be functioning here, implicitly if not explicitly, as a gentle aphrodisiac.

It is thus helpful to note that the anthropologist J. B. Loudon reports the common use in some African tribal cultures of powerful
purgatives as aphrodisiacs, a practice he likens to the British sailor's
slang formula for the structure of sexual experience as "a shit, a
shave, and a shove ashore."[42] Today we associate any sexual use of the
laxative purge with the practice of anal intercourse among male ho-
mosexuals. In Elizabethan erotic discourses, however, references to
buggery are not exclusively homosexual. Although anal eroticism in
Elizabethan sexual discourse remains exclusively within the stylistic
domain of male sexuality, there seems to be no reason to regard the
anally erotic stimulation of the laxative purge as either homoerotic or
a sensation sought out by a minority of males. But the purge in early

41. Almanac verse is more or less standard from edition to edition of the same
almanac as well as in different almanacs throughout the period. Quoted here are the
almanacs of Thomas Bretnor (London, 1615; STC 420), George Dauncy (London,
1614; STC 435.5), and Richard Allestree (London, 1623; STC 407.6).

42. J. B. Loudon, "On Body Products," in *The Anthropology of the Body*, ed. John
Blacking (London: Academic Press, 1971), pp. 173 and 176n.

modern culture, even apart from its possible use in specifically sexual practice, was prescribed to assuage anxiety and depression, or to relieve the oppression of melancholy humors. Burton accounts "costiveness, and keeping in of our ordinary excrements" as main causes of melancholy.[43] After taking syrup of roses for an ague, the Puritan diarist Ralph Josselin notes that it "wrought very kindly with me, gave me 9 stools brought away much choler."[44] Henri IV, unlike Héroard, his son's physician, was a firm advocate of the therapeutic value of frequent enemas and powerful purgatives. Perhaps, like Loudon's Africans, the aggressively heterosexual monarch found them erotically stimulating or used them to treat his frequent bouts of depression. Henri's son, as Elizabeth Marvick has demonstrated, in reaction to Héroard's early and frequent use of suppositories on him, would request an enema or would refuse to accept one when prescribed as a strategy in his protracted struggle with his adult governors for bodily and psychic autonomy.[45]

Belief in the value of even violent or prolonged evacuations, though by no means universal or indiscriminate, was widespread. Burton does warn against the overzealousness of physicians who "prescribe too much Physick, and tire out [patients'] bodies with continual potions." He creates the impression that some melancholics or their doctors were virtually dependent, physically or psychologically, on the administration of purges: "Aëtius will have them by all means therefore to give some respite to nature, *to leave off now and then*."[46] The purge, downward or upward, was the bodily route to psychic wellbeing, to an elevation of spirit.

But this homology among the pleasures of the lower bodily stratum does not occur only in medical or quasi-medical discourse, and outside those semiotically safe discourses, it gives rise to considerable anxiety. A curious feature of the seasonal recommendations of almanac verse is how matter-of-factly they specify the several forms of erotic activities. The therapeutic sanctions that underlie the practice of purging redefine the functionality of coition and offer sexual ac-

43. Burton, *Anatomy of Melancholy*, p. 203.
44. Ralph Josselin quoted by Beier, "In Sickness and in Health," p. 117.
45. See Marvick, *Louis XIII*, pp. 80–81, for an account of Henri IV's sexual recklessness, periodic depressions, and advocacy of violent evacuations; on Louis's struggles with Héroard over the issue of enemas and bowel training in general, see pp. 12–13, 20–23, 30, 65–66.
46. Burton, *Anatomy of Melancholy*, p. 391, emphasis added. On the belief in violent evacuation, see Beier, "In Sickness and in Health," p. 112.

tivity a protection from ethical judgment. By the same token, however, it could be argued that the moral and psychic transgressiveness of sex has the potential for contaminating with a dangerous eroticism the therapeutic bodily activities with which it is functionally linked. Thus Sir John Harington in the *Metamorphosis of Ajax* compares the allure of the privy to that of the brothel and the erotic satisfactions of the stool to the "sweet sinne of lecherie" with its "sowre sawce" of repentance and disease:

> This surpassing pleasure [of sex] . . . I have heard confessed before a most honourable person, by a man of middle age, strong constitution, and well practised in this occupation, to have bred no more delectation to him (after the first heate of his youth was past) then to go to a good easie close stoole, when he hath had a lust thereto (for that was his verie phrase). Which being confessed by him, and confirmed by many; makes me take this advantage thereof in the beginning of this discourse, to preferre this house I mind to speake of, before those which they so much frequent; neither let any disdaine the comparison.[47]

The theoretical assimilation of defecation and sexual intercourse in medical discourse does not mitigate Harington's odd, defensive over-emphasis, discernible in the speaker's assurances of the heterosexual vigor and social rectitude of his informant (one resembling himself), the confessional honesty of that informant's avowal "before a most honourable person," and the dialogic citation of another's "verie phrase." Harington seems somewhat surprised by his informant's use of the word *lust*, his simple identification of sexual desire with the excretory impulse. He insists, nonetheless, that recognition of the erotic satisfactions of the close stool is widespread, "confirmed by many," if ordinarily in a more covert fashion. Perhaps such confirmation is allowable only after the rigorous truth of another's "confession."

Some or all of these possibilities could register here as Titania's purpose to purge Bottom's mortal grossness. My own division of that purpose into conceptual subcategories labeled erotic, medical, ethical, or psychotherapeutic does not at all reflect the less differentiated Elizabethan taxonomy of bodily culture. Rather, my categories are

---

47. Sir John Harington, *A New Discourse of a Stale Subject, Called the Metamorphosis of Ajax*, ed. Elizabeth Story Donno (New York: Columbia University Press; London: Routledge and Kegan Paul, 1962), p. 84.

meant to suggest the possible complexity of signification and response in Titania's phrase. It is she, after all, who reminds Oberon of
the "distemperature" and the dangerous alteration of the seasons
their quarrel has caused (2.1.106–7), the unhealthy miasma whose
effects might be remedied for an individual by the proper course of
purgatives. Titania's identification with the moon might also link her
with purgatives since of the "foure naturall vertues" in astrological
medicine, "The vertue expulsive is governed of Luna."[48] But the idea
of the purge has the general effect, I think, of identifying Titania's
mastery and Bottom's passivity with the structure of early childhood
experience of the body, especially infantile experience of maternal
stimulation.

The significance of the scene as a structure of memory and bodily
recall may explain why the atmosphere of erotic promise created by
Titania's sudden infatuation seems far more recognizable to the audience than to Bottom, caught up in bewilderment and narcissistic
self-involvement. Whatever else that audience could in fact perceive
as Titania's erotic program when her fairies lead Bottom offstage to
her bower, we do know that she intends to purge him in some fashion,
to feed him, and to put him to sleep. The resulting affect formation, I
would argue, is complex and ambivalent, depending in part on multiple and overlapping possibilities in the audience of the heightened
identification and introjection that was one of the consequences of
playgoing.[49] For the male subject, the promise of erotic pleasure
through passivity could well have generated profound anxiety about
self-mastery and bodily boundaries. I find such an anxiety in *The
Metamorphosis of Ajax*. For Harington, the satisfaction of the stool is
constructed as an individually chosen form of sexual pleasure, as a
matter of preference. This is what Harington's informant "confesses"
his "lust" for. The mastery over one's own bodily processes in defecation, so crucial to the infant's sense of well-being, is compared and
ultimately preferred in terms of erotic gratification to sexual intercourse. Similarly, the recommendations of almanac verse presuppose
the exercise of volition in bodily culture, the possibility of regulating
appetites and purging—and the appetite *for* purging—according to a
rational, seasonally adjusted praxis. Though regularly cautioned to

48. I quote from the almanac of Thomas Buckmaster or Buckminster (London:
1571; STC 422.5), sig. A3ᵛ, but the thinking is commonplace.
49. See Steven Mullaney, *The Place of the Stage: License, Play, and Power in Renaissance
England* (Chicago: University of Chicago Press, 1988), p. 101.

consult a doctor, particularly at times of year only marginally safe for purging, bathing, or bleeding, the men addressed by almanac verse were nonetheless free to choose the manner and timing of their own purgations and presumably to self-administer them.

Such experiences would be quite different from Bottom's here, which involves having one's bodily processes taken over, voluntarily or involuntarily, by a powerful other. Thus, it may be significant for the production of male anxiety that Titania's instructions for Bottom's diet and nurture also include vaguely phallic threats of stealing "honey-bags from the humble-bees" and cropping "their waxen thighs" (3.1.169–70).[50] Such intentions may explain why Bottom's conversation with Titania's fairies touches upon the sexual immaturity of unripe peascods and the bodily events of bleeding and weeping, as if Bottom's sense of his own bodily boundaries were being endangered, or why when Titania's thoughts, at the same moment, project melancholy onto a weeping moon "lamenting some enforced chastity" (200), the reference to rape seems strangely ungendered. Bottom, whom the fairies are both to "wait upon" and to "lead," to serve and to control, is himself a sexual victim, his body in thrall to Titania and possibly subject to the massive interventions of the purge.

Titania's treatment of Bottom contains a full measure of what for the narcissistic infant constitutes paradoxical messages of love and discipline, affection and mistrust, or in my earlier terms of opposition, bodily retention and release. But the scene also makes clear that Bottom's narcissism is manifest only because of Titania's constitutive desire and maternal complicity—a maternal complicity represented as anally cathected and assimilated to the narcissism of contemporary court culture. If his lordly deportment turns Bottom into a comic version of Freud's His Majesty the Baby, Titania's interest in assigning her fairies to supervise the orifices of His Majesty Bottom is itself a possible encoding of the obsessive rituals involving the narcissistic body of the monarch. Recall that the Groom of the Stool who served the male monarchs was required by household rules "to give attendance upon the king's Highness when he goeth to make water in his Bedchamber." Though Elizabeth "never formally appointed anyone

50. Sometimes it is difficult to know how far to press sexual innuendo in Shakespeare. Partridge, however, glosses "honey" as "the sweets of sexual pleasure," *Shakespeare's Bawdy*, p. 128; and Frankie Rubinstein, citing the French *chatrer*, more specifically identifies taking honey away from beehives with castration. She cites equivocation among Cassius, Brutus, and Antony on "honeyless" and "stingless" Hybla bees in *Julius Caesar*, 5.1.35. See *A Dictionary of Shakespeare's Sexual Puns*, p. 128.

to the post," according to Pam Wright, some of her ladies presumably performed the same function for Elizabeth and had a quasi-official interest in the state and functioning of the monarch's body natural. James I's Groom of the Stool reported to Salisbury in 1610 that "his Majesty has been a little loose since his coming to Royston, but not in the extremity, and he does not lose his meat, so I hope he is past the worst."[51] We have already seen the similar prominence of anal cathexes in Héroard's care of Louis XIII. Bottom's royal infantilism, then, can be seen as his unconscious or at least spontaneous response to the regressive allure of matriarchal domination—the allure of being "every mother's son" by mother's remedies.

Fully to recognize Bottom as infant to mother Titania may well entail recalling one's own early subjection to maternal power and the complex affect of bodily pleasure, rage, shame, and helplessness it produces. But there is also the possibility of an even more complex and equally ambivalent response to the dramatic icon of Titania and Bottom, which comes from recognizing not only the passive infant but also the powerful maternal agent. We have been told that Oberon subjects Titania to dotage in order to humiliate and expose her to his gaze *and ours*. But what is missing from these scenes between Bottom and Titania is precisely the experience of shame in them, in Stanley Cavell's phrase, "the specific discomfort produced by the sense of being looked at."[52] The inhibition of shame, it might seem, is another function of Oberon's love juice, but such an inhibition is itself potentially shameful to any observer whose powers of introjection are activated. As Anthony Giddens has noted, "to be embarrassed for someone reveals a certain complicity with the conduct, a sympathy for someone who has been unnecessarily exposed."[53] Any identification with Titania here risks becoming implicated in the embarrassing self-witness of maternal shame: Titania is doting on an infantile monster, a braying, narcissistic creature oblivious to her magnificence and condescension. The threat is not only to her dignity but to her own autonomy as an adult, for her dotage seems to define this quasi-

51. On the Groom of the Stool, see David Starkey, "Intimacy and Innovation: The Rise of the Privy Chamber, 1485–1547," p. 78; Pam Wright, "A Change of Direction: The Ramifications of a Female Household, 1558–1603," p. 149; and for the report on James's "looseness," Neil Cuddy, "The Revival of the Entourage: The Bedchamber of James I, 1603–1625," p. 186—all in *The English Court: From the Wars of the Roses to the Civil War*, ed. David Starkey et al. (London: Longman, 1987).

52. Cavell, "The Avoidance of Love," p. 49.

53. Giddens, *Constitution of Society*, pp. 55–56.

maternal form of erotic love as itself regressive, even presocial: mother and child locked into a self-sufficient dyad in the mutual satisfaction of feeding and being fed. The moment turns into a culturally empowered misrecognition of and distantiation from the mother-child dyad, exposing the anal cathexis of early bodily experience and imposing a kind of memorial shame on it.

The asocial exclusiveness of the mother-child dyad partially explains Bottom and Titania's obliviousness to the presence of the four sleeping lovers onstage with them in act 4, scene 1. Nor are they aware of the real conditions of power in which they are enmeshed, since they cannot see Oberon, whose supervisory power—gazing down upon a stage of sleeping bodies—demonstrates his husbandly role as master of Titania's body and his princely role in arranging erotic alliances and social promotions. Furthermore, if Titania's intentions to purge Bottom register as designed to stimulate him sexually, to heighten his ardor and ability to perform, the purge as administered by mother has become indistinguishable from the aphrodisiacal purge of the courtesan. For women, the affective power of motherhood in this parodic form is perhaps just as ambiguous and anxiety provoking as the appeal of bodily passivity was for men.

Bottom's languor at his appearance with Titania in act 4, scene 1, his passivity and apparent bodily contentment at being scratched, petted, and adorned, may well suggest the postcoital. We are free to assume that in the interval since their first encounter in act 3, scene 1, the monstrous mating has occurred—an action manifestly unstageable but not unimaginable. But given the pregenital infantilism into which he has lapsed and the earlier references to purgatives, given Titania's dominance and maternal attentiveness to filling his ears with music and his mouth with food, the scene is also suggestive of postpurgative release—and thus of the kind of unstageable action we began to anticipate when Hodge abruptly left the stage in *Gammer Gurton's Needle*.

Clearly, it is difficult to distinguish somatic from social fantasy in this scene. It seems to contain a promise that, just as somatic release is the required response to maternal discipline, so regression is the way to promotion and passivity is a form of control. But that message of regressive pleasure is embedded in an ironizing, disciplinary context produced at one level by Titania's threatening domination and at another level by our residual awareness of Oberon's punitive stratagems. Titania's devotion, however maternal and thus in one sense unanswerable, is also grounded in an intended imposition of shame, in misrecognition and manipulation, in her own unconscious physical submission to Oberon's magical skill. But Oberon's presence in act 4, scene 1, may also serve to contain the fantasy's eroticism and the possibility of sustained engagement with its premises by men in the audience. Oddly enough, it may have been preferable to imagine that Titania would purge Bottom rather than mate with him, that she could have performed the offices of mother-nurse rather than mother-mistress. Even Oberon, though jealous of both Theseus and the changeling boy, seems to be less jealous of this latest object of Titania's affection. Titania's dotage on Bottom is, after all, the result of Oberon's deliberate intervention in her cognitive and affective processes, not, as in the case of the boy, the result of a parturition displacing him in her affections or, as in the case of Theseus, of an attraction to his adult double. The fairy king's apparent lack of jealousy is thus a function of Bottom's low station; the mechanicals are not only infantilized in their relations with their superiors but desexualized as well. Oberon's complaisance thus supports whatever resistance we may feel to imagining that the monstrous union has occurred.

In fact, no interpretative choice needs to be made in *A Midsummer Night's Dream* between kinds of erotic experience—between intercourse and purging. In the psychological formations of Elizabethan culture, they may well have been, or been felt or somehow counted as, the same. Thus, to acknowledge the possibility of the purge as an alternative to intercourse between Bottom and Titania is to recognize a narrative aporia; it is to give this moment of indeterminacy cultural significance and a narrative rationale. The moment may be a clear instance, furthermore, in which a dramatic text gestures toward and thereby recognizes its own distance from what Harry Berger has called the detextualized signifying practices of the body.[54] Such an inference is supported by what seems to be Bottom's repression of his experience in the woods, his imprecision of recall or utterance— "Methought I was—and methought I had" (4.1.207–8)—and his relocation of that experience into the psychological domain of the dream and past the reach of discursive explanation or the iterability of text. This may provide Bottom a psychologically efficient way of retaining the powerful affect of the erotic memory and an insistence on its

54. Harry Berger, Jr., "Bodies and Texts," *Representations* 17 (1987), 152.

meaningfulness while regaining the bodily control and sense of somatic boundary so decisively lost to Titania. His psychic stratagem—
if that is what it is—brings him close to Harington, whose point in
arguing defensively for the erotic satisfactions of the stool is precisely
the efficiency and safety, the greater satisfaction, of the solitary
purge—that is, of doing without the offices of woman altogether.

ॐ

I am aware that so desublimated a reading of the scenes between
Titania and Bottom may provoke repugnance. My best ally in answer-
ing such resistance is Ben Jonson, whose satirical rendering of the
Bottom-Titania relationship in Dapper and his "aunt," the Queen of
Fairy, focuses precisely on its anal coding—that is, on Dapper's fate to
be gagged, locked, and forgotten in the privy rather than have a
much-anticipated reunion with his doting relative. Admittedly, in
much of the language of *The Alchemist* there is an aggressive anality
with little demonstrable connection to *A Midsummer Night's Dream*,
which would seem to erode my ability to make Dapper's experience in
the privy contextual evidence for what I want to call Bottom's purge.
Anality has, after all, been identified as peculiar to Jonson's psycho-
genetic makeup and no part of Shakespeare's.[55]

But it is an important part of my project here to remove anality and
scatology—the bad boys of bodily discourse—from the semantic constraints imposed by particular constructions of authorial personality.
As Michel Foucault has argued, "The author is . . . a certain functional principle by which, in our culture, one limits, excludes, and
chooses; in short, by which one impedes the free circulation, the free
manipulation, the free composition, decomposition, and recomposi-
tion of fiction."[56] From this point of view, to attach anality to Jonson
as a psychological component of the author function is to deny
scatological and anal discourse a wider cultural significance and to
protect Shakespeare from anal contamination. I have been arguing,
instead, for the presence of anal cathexis in certain fictional and lived

55. Edmund Wilson, "Morose Ben Jonson" (1928), rpt. in *Ben Jonson: A Collection of
Critical Essays*, ed. Jonas Barish (Englewood Cliffs, N.J.: Prentice-Hall, 1963), 63–69.
See also David Riggs's account of Jonson's early "anal eroticism" and adult adaptive
mechanisms in *Ben Jonson: A Life* (Cambridge: Harvard University Press, 1989), pp. 3,
31–32.
56. Michel Foucault, "What Is an Author?" rpt. in *Contemporary Literary Criticism:
Literary and Cultural Studies*, ed. Robert Con Davis and Ronald Schleifer (London:
Longman, 1989), p. 274.

practices of Elizabethan culture because early bodily experiences such as regularly administered purges must have been psychologically formative. I do not deny the variability of early bodily experiences either among individuals or distributed among groups in the social formation. But the meaning any individual gives to his or her own bodily self-perception and experience—what I have called the internal habitus—is itself a matter of more or less conventional selection from the somatic discourses available at any moment in the *longue durée* of culture. To recognize as much is to give scatology, and any other kind of somatic discourse, a signifying potential in the strategies of gender and class differentiation—the strategies by which a particular body's physical attributes, functions, and behaviors participate in and reproduce conventional social meanings.[57]

The association of anal cathexis with shameful pleasure and somatic anxiety which we have seen in *Gammer Gurton's Needle* and *A Midsummer Night's Dream* is even more strikingly evident in the scatological invective of the opening of *The Alchemist*. Here, the genital exposure that to the rustic laborer Hodge seemed to impede passage to heterosexual adulthood takes on an even more complex semiosis. As so often with somatic behaviors, what genital exposure signifies depends on whether the condition can be construed as voluntary or involuntary. In Joubert's treatise on laughter, involuntary exposure is regarded as the essential state of the comic object, an introjection of humiliation and weakness bringing laughter from others and embarrassment for oneself in its wake. The more unusual and more ambiguous state of *voluntary* exposure, however, which Joubert does not discuss, seems able to support and signify notably aggressive projections of humiliation and shame. Clearly, the question of who defines as voluntary or involuntary any particular moment of bodily or psychic exposure is crucial in instantiating power relations. Making any such claim about one's own exposed body is contingent upon control over the gaze of others and a convincing appearance of bodily self-command. Subtle's expressions of contempt for Face are predicated upon a claim to superior self-possession even in the midst of a quarrel—a self-possession demonstrated through control over his lower body and its products as signifiers: "Thy worst. I fart at thee" (1.1.1).[58]

57. For theoretical guidance I am much indebted here to Giddens, *Constitution of Society*, esp. pp. 36, 50–55.
58. I quote here and throughout from Ben Jonson, *The Alchemist*, ed. F. H. Mares, Revels Plays (Cambridge: Harvard University Press, 1967).

Curtius's motif of the *proktos lalon* reappears here, but in this contest between males, the ass's "speech" is not represented as involuntary offense, as the embarrassing, feminizing attribute of public incontinence. On the contrary, Subtle must construe such a fart as deliberate and aggressive, signifying control, aim, the effectuality of will, and the social dominance implied by turning one's back.[59] Embarrassment shifts away from the possessor of the *proktos lalon* and toward the shamed opponent: "I fart *at* thee." After Face's threat to "strip" him naked, that is, to expose him involuntarily, Subtle again attempts to deflect the inscription of shame with an even coarser reply: "What to do? Lick figs / Out at my —— " (3–4).[60] He reconstitutes his body not as the object of Face's fury, but rather as an object of base, anally cathected desire, trying to reverse the customary trajectory of shame at a moment of otherwise involuntary genital exposure.

I contend that this quarrel demonstrates the negative homosocial potential of scatological language and gesture, the vocabulary of male intimacy and acknowledged interdependency gone sour.[61] The dialectical strategy of the quarrel depends upon a detailed narrative reconstruction of the emphatic, offensive, and finally regressive bodiliness of the other as the basis for claims of personal superiority. Each seeks to appropriate the patriarchal role of mind in order to subordinate the other as mere body, the signifier of uncontrol. In the emphatically urban mise-en-scène of *The Alchemist*, this strategy of stripping the other naked, physically and psychically, assumes cultural specificity and resonance in light of Margaret Pelling's work on psychosomatic anxiety about bodily appearance. She links the emergence of this anxiety in early Jacobean London in part to the epidemic spread of disfiguring venereal disease. More generally, however, she finds material evidence for "a climate of acute social competition" in the "remarkably thorough" distribution "over the whole City within the Walls" of barber-surgeons, who provided a full range of personal

59. This specifically offensive consequence of showing one's back (backside) is suggested by the meaning Francis Grose, the eighteenth-century antiquarian, records for *fart catcher*: "A valet or footman, from his walking behind his master or mistress." See *A Classical Dictionary of the Vulgar Tongue*, ed. Eric Partridge (London: Routledge and Kegan Paul, 1963), p. 140.

60. F. H. Mares assumes that in Subtle's threat to "gum your silks / With good strong water" (1.1.6–7), the "water" is a corrosive acid which he holds in a vessel; see *The Alchemist*, p. 12. In this excretory context, however, we might imagine the acid to be urine—since Subtle does cast waters as part of his quasi-medical practice.

61. The best short treatment of the subject of male homosociality remains the introduction in Eve Kosofsky Sedgwick's *Between Men: English Literature and Male Homosocial Desire* (New York: Columbia University Press, 1985), pp. 1–5.

services—cosmetic, quasi-medical, and even sexual—to nearly all ranks of men in the social order. The desire to appear before the world without blemish, to conceal any marks that might signify a history of syphilis or other infectious disease, becomes symptomatic of a more generalized insecurity about new possibilities of social exposure and bodily shame, about the critical gaze of others in the unrelenting co-presence of a densely crowded metropolis.[62]

Subtle and Face do not invoke the scatological in order to accuse each other of incontinence, or to bring the other closer to a state of incontinence. The threat of this incontinence, as we have seen in *Gammer Gurton's Needle* and *A Midsummer Night's Dream*, is the characteristic state of those infantilized and feminized by the loss of bodily control. The power of insult here lies in minute knowledge of the bodily condition of the other—such awareness as Margaret Pelling draws attention to—and a shaming reduction of that body to a kind of social nullity:

> I shall put you in mind, sir, at Pie Corner,
> Taking your meal of steam in, from cooks' stalls,
> Where, like the father of hunger, you did walk
> Piteously costive, with your pinch'd–horn nose,
> And your complexion, of the Roman wash,
> Stuck full of black and melancholic worms,
> Like powder corns, shot, at th'artillery yard.
>
> (1.1.25–31)

Subtle and Face each try to set before the other's memorializing imagination the image of an embarrassing earlier body, as if the past self-in-the-body were the inner, the naked, the irreducible self making the present construction shamefully transparent and inessential. They would reduce identity in the other to the regressive extreme of what the body inevitably and involuntarily produces and has always produced—its own excrement.[63] Face's phrase, "piteously costive,"

62. Margaret Pelling, "Appearance and Reality: Barber-Surgeons, the Body, and Disease," in *London, 1500–1700: The Making of the Metropolis*, ed. A. L. Beier and Roger Finlay (London: Longman, 1985), pp. 89–95, 104–5. The phrases in quotation appear on pp. 90 and 85.

63. I implicitly take issue here with Cheryl Lynn Ross, who would seek to isolate Subtle as associated with "bad smells, flatulence, and excrement." See "The Plague of *The Alchemist*," *Renaissance Quarterly* 41 (1988), 441. Certainly each seeks to associate the other with excrement, particularly in this opening dialogue.

may even imply that in cases of extreme hunger and humoral insol-
ubility the body does not even have much to excrete. In Face's narrative reconstruction, Subtle's humiliating social inconsequence seems
to have a shameful somatic signifier—a condition of humoral imbalance, an insufficiency of bodily fluid causing the cold, dry state of
melancholy.

Joubert, once again, provides a helpful gloss. He distinguishes the
human being from other animals by the quantity of its production of
excrements as the consequence of brain activity: "For experience
teaches us that there is no animal that weeps, none that blows his nose,
that spits, or that picks wax from his ears. Man among all the animals,
because he has a large brain, not only in proportion to his body, but
also with respect to his weight . . . abounds considerably in said excrements, which he releases from his eyes, nostrils, mouth, and ears."[64]
The "piteously costive" Subtle was so dried and withered as not to be
fully vital (and in this respect, if in no other, the antithesis of the
murdered Duncan: "Who would have thought the old man to have
had so much blood in him?" [*Macbeth*, 5.1.39–40]).

Thus Face and Subtle try to gain ascendancy by returning the other,
naked, to an originary dunghill, the dunghill of infantile incontinence, gluttony, and uncontrol, the dunghill of undifference: "Away,
you trencher rascal." "Out, you dog-leech, / The vomit of all prisons"
(1.1. 103–4). The dunghill here becomes almost a personal bodily
sign, an emblem of origin and return, equivalent in the emerging
bodily vocabulary of this play to the shamefully open breech in *Gammer
Gurton's Needle* or the postpurgative Bottom in *A Midsummer Night's
Dream*:

> Thou vermin, have I ta'en thee out of dung,
> So poor, so wretched, when no living thing
> Would keep thee company, but a spider, or worse?
>   (1.1.64–66)

The retrospective mirror each claims to set before the other's face is a
shameful bodily inversion, an image of the face below and behind, a
bodily site vulnerable, says Eve Kosofsky Sedgwick, because "signally
not under one's own ocular control."[65] This mirror inversion of the

---

64. Joubert, *Treatise on Laughter*, p. 98.
65. Sedgwick, "A Poem Is Being Written," p. 126.

speaking ass is like the metonymic inversion of face and ass in the hand mirrors Philip Stubbes inveighs against in *The Anatomy of Abuses*:

> The devill could never have found out a more pestilent evill then this, for hereby man beholding his face, and being naturally given to flatter hymself too muche, is easely drawen to thinke well of hymself: and yet no man seeth the true proportion of his face, but a counterfaite effigie, and false image therof in the glasse, whiche the Devill suffereth hym to see, that thereby he maie rise into Pride, and so offende the Divine Majestie. Therefore maie these lookyng glasses be called the devils bellowes, wherewith he bloweth the blast of Pride into our hartes: and those that looke in them may be said *to looke in the Devills arse.*[66]

Here, since the quarrelers' intention is so clearly to deny selfhood in the other in order to avoid incorporation by him, anal discourse functions more sadistically and aggressively than it does in *Gammer Gurton's Needle* or *A Midsummer Night's Dream*. In those plays, the threat of incorporation and the invitation to regression come from a dominant woman. But in *The Alchemist* what Face and Subtle present as the dunghill of undifference in the other is precisely at the center of what Janine Chasseguet-Smirgel has identified as the anal-sadistic universe, a perversely liberating, because antipatriarchal reconstruction of reality "where all differences are abolished" by a reduction of social, sexual, and erotogenic categories to a mass as undifferentiated as the fecal bolus.[67] What seems contradictory about Jonson's rhetorical strategy is that it proceeds by a recitation of vivid details, and yet the cumulative effect of such details is undifference, the collapse of individuation back into the chaotic urban environment.

One bodily characteristic of the undifferentiated anal universe, according to Chasseguet-Smirgel, is the fungibility of its erotogenic zones. We have seen how Subtle, in particular, seeks to defy this possibility, to reverse this threat of an externally imposed regression to anal cathexis by defining the products of his lower body as volitional, directed toward furthering rather than erasing the aims of the self: "*I fart at thee.*" Not surprisingly, then, the sign of reconciliation between the pair is a turn outward to heterosexual aggression, the restoration of ordinary phallic rather than anal competition in the erotic antic-

66. Philip Stubbes, *The Anatomie of Abuses*, ed. Frederick J. Furnivall, The New Shakspere Society (London: N. Trubner, 1877–79), p. 79n, emphasis mine.

67. Janine Chasseguet-Smirgel, *Creativity and Perversion* (New York: Norton, 1984), p. 3. I am grateful to Dr. Louis Conte for directing me to Chasseguet-Smirgel.

ipation of rivalry for Doll Common, whom "the longest cut, at night, / Shall draw" for his "Doll Particular" (1.1.178–79). To turn away from anal competition against each other is also to redirect their aggression against the urban environment, so that, instead of Face, Subtle will wish the Spanish Don had "stoop'd a little, and kiss'd our *anos*" (4.3.22).

The relationship between bodily and domestic space, the identification of the body with the house—homologies so crucial in *Gammer Gurton's Needle*—are no less so to the trajectory of action here. But the passage to social maturity in this environment—the passage Hodge found so uncertain—is far more complicated than the issue of whether or not one has a clean, whole pair of pants to go courting in. The rogues exploit the intense social competition and exposure of the urban environment by manipulating the evident insecurity of their gulls about the specialized social, bodily, and linguistic skills required in the city. Kastril, who wants to know if the Doctor "has any skill," is rebuked by Face for his naïveté and rusticity, his social immaturity in even asking: "It seems sir, y'are but young / About the town, that can make that a question!" (3.4.19–20). One source of authority for establishing standards for everyone else is the asceticism and moral purity thought to be requisite for the alchemist and those associated with him. More to my point, however, are those moments when each gull's bodily habitus is introduced as a symptom either of privilege or of disablement and vulnerability. The rogues thus construct a stringent oral and bodily discipline for the house and those like Dapper, who enter it not "costive of belief" (Surly's self-description, 2.3.26). As physiognomist or chiromancer, Subtle reads the textualized bodies of the gulls, promising Drugger for instance, on the basis of his olive-colored face and spots on the nail of his little finger, that he will be elected to office. Face promotes the aspirations of Drugger as a "neat, spruce-honest fellow" (1.3.32), who keeps a tidy, well-appointed shop, where tobacco is not "wrapp'd up in greasy leather, or piss'd clouts" (27). Not his neatness, however, but a perhaps embarrassing inability to get rid of parasitic worms was the reason for seeking out the astrological doctor's help, according to Face:

> That was the cause indeed,
> Why he came now. He dealt with me, in private,
> To get a med'cine for 'em.
>
> (2.6.82–84)

There is a greater emphasis here than in *Gammer Gurton's Needle* upon the mouth as the critical intersection of bodily and domestic protocols, thanks in part to a conception of impure language as literally polluting or contagious within the alchemical space.[68] Mammon in particular is instructed in the catastrophe that would follow upon a failure of oral discipline in his conversation with Doll, disguised as a wealthy but unstable heiress: "If you but name a word, touching the Hebrew, / She falls into her fit" (2.3.239–40). The scriptural logorrhea of her madness, moreover, is itself a contagious discourse: "You would run mad, too, to hear her, sir" (242). "The very house, sir, would run mad," says Face (4.1.13). The question, as I shall argue in more detail hereafter, is the familiar one of self-control and self-containment, not letting the wrong word out, not contaminating the atmosphere of the house and the success of its social and alchemical experiments by oral or bodily uncontrol.

Of course, this construction of disciplinary authority is the means by which Subtle and Face prepare to escape retribution for the inevitable frustration of their gulls' hopes. My point is that the image of authority they construct works like the authoritative image of society in general, to enforce conformity and, in particular, to focus psychic attention, both positive and negative, upon the sensations of bodiliness, especially bodily boundaries. Even the resistant Surly seems to conform to this aggressively disciplinary ethos even though he rejects Subtle and Face's authority in favor of his own. He hypothetically constructs his own self-shaming ritual as the consequence of failing in cognitive self-control and shrewdness:

> If my eyes do cozen me so (and I
> Giving 'em no occasion), sure, I'll have
> A whore, shall piss 'em out, next day.
> (2.1.43–45)

At one level, Surly seems merely to be introducing a vivid urinary variation upon the opening theme of anal aggression. Here, he places the burden of shame and the stain of pollution on a rejected part of himself, rather than project it upon an opponent as Face and Subtle

68. The irony of this construction is palpable, since, as Cheryl Lynn Ross has asserted about the moral and symbolic economy of the play, "the alchemical enterprise involves manufacturing the philosopher's stone, or elixir, and then transmuting base metals into gold by touching them with the magical, purified substance—in other words, it works by contagion." See "The Plague of *The Alchemist*," p. 444.

did in their opening quarrel. Since his quarrel is with himself, with his own cognitive and sensory processes, he would arrange for his own punishment, asserting self-mastery through the signifiers of sexual and economic mastery: "I'll *have* / A whore." This way, he would manage both to punish himself and to retain imaginative control over that punishment, thus ostensibly preserving the crucial sense of self-agency we later see Dapper surrender. Yet the image would seem to contain its own contradiction. Though Surly claims to limit and control his sense of shame, to invent his own punishment, he nonetheless imagines shame as socially applied. Shame for him, as for Hodge, is physical subjection to and punishment by a powerful, if debased, female.

What ought to catch our attention as well in this image of self-blinding is the odd specificity of its shameful means—the urine of the whore. To perceive the logic of the punishment it is necessary to return to the now-obscure semiotics of urine and whores at which I glanced briefly in Chapter 1 in discussing urine troped as the physician's strumpet. The harlot was a conventional sign of both verbal deceit and deceptive appearance, attributes Doll Common shares with other fictive courtesans of the period, such as Middleton's Frank Gullman in *A Mad World, My Masters* or even Shakespeare's Mistress Quickly, whose name plays complexly on just these bodily and linguistic signifiers. In the discourses of popular medicine, the whore is associated with urine because of urine's unreliability as a diagnostic tool, its propensity to change color from day to day and generally to deceive the investigator who tried to read it. Equally crucial to the metaphor is a construction of the whore's unchaste body as grotesquely open and hypereffluent. The whore was the leakiest of all female vessels in part because of her tendency to linguistic overflow, in part because her vaginal cavity, full of her customers' seminal outpourings, was moister than other women's. A more obscure connection between whores and urine is to be found in the practice among prostitutes of urinating after copulation as a contraceptive measure (discussed briefly in Chapter 1).[69] All these associations link urine and whores in a particular, if coarse, semiotics of bodily debasement and what we might call the transgressive eroticism of urinary function.

69. On the whore's linguistic overflow, see Peter Stallybrass, "Patriarchal Territories: The Body Enclosed," in *Rewriting the Renaissance*, pp. 126–27. On urination, see Henke, *Gutter Life and Language*, p. 192; and E. J. Burford, *Bawds and Lodgings: A History of the London Bankside Brothels, c. 100–1675* (London: Owen, 1976).

Here, by way of hyperbolizing his disinclination to be gulled and the protection he thinks his skepticism earns, Surly imagines his eyes to have cozened him aggressively—"(And I giving'em no occasion)"— as whores cozened their clients by flattery and false appearances. Yet, in its self-dramatization, the image exposes the anxiety and bodily insecurity it seems to intended to deny. Though Surly would separate his eyes from his self-in-the-body—with an oppositional rhetoric of *them* and *me*—to punish them is to punish the whole bodily self with shame and belittlement. Graphically and crudely imagined, for Surly to put his eyes where they can be pissed out is to be straddled by a whore urinating in the male posture. The whore has almost become a female colossus, whose size and bodily posture dwarf the body of her shamed victim as Caesar in his uncontainment dwarfed the bodies of the conspirators.[70] Hence, for Surly the essence of imagined, if not experienced, shame bears the familiar gender inflections of regression and denial, and an unconvincing assertion of male control through the conventional scatological debasement of the whore.

Later in the play this aggressive image of debasement and self-punishment is recalled in Jonson's overtly scatological parody of Titania with Bottom. I want to concentrate on the particular semiotics of the privy into which Face and Subtle thrust the unfortunate Dapper instead of fulfilling his erotic dream of regressive reunion with his aunt of Fairy. The coarse substitution in the play's overall economy of desublimation—of the privy as an alternative site of return to a degraded mother/aunt/bawd—attends Jonson's reading of the central scenes of the earlier play and undergirds my broader concern with the scatological signifiers of gender discourse.

It is the same substitution we have already seen in the passage I quoted earlier from Harington's *Metamorphosis of Ajax*. The choice there between the experience of a "good, easie close stoole" and the pleasure of sexual intercourse is also a comparison of erotic sites, a choice between the privy and the brothel, between "this house I mind to speak of" and "those which they so much frequent." As Harington's discursive caution and euphemistic self-monitoring implies, his comparison actually sets out to construct the privy as a

70. In particular, his self-directed rage reminds me of Cassius imagining his own shame and belittlement in the political magnification of the colossus Caesar: "Why, man, he doth bestride the narrow world / Like a Colossus, and we petty men / Walk under his huge legs, and peep about / To find ourselves dishonorable graves." (*Julius Caesar*, 1.2.135–38).

particularly felicitous site for the resolution of contradictory desire. The privy is both a house of office and a house of pleasure; it is a site of lawful transgression, a place of necessary pleasure taking, which is nonetheless solitary and regressive. But not surprisingly, given the close relationship I have already established between anality and misogyny, Harington's praise of the privy seems to require a bifurcated image of woman and the debasement of part of that image through associating her with excrement. Thus, after declaring that no one should "disdaine the comparison" between the privy and the brothel, he seeks rhetorically to mask his own ambivalence about moral judgment and excrement by moving to indirect discourse. He repeats a moralistic fable told by the "grave & godly Ladie" his mother-in-law:

> An Hermit being caried in an evening, by the conduct of an Angell, through a great citie, to contemplate the great wickednesse daily and hourely wrought therein; met in the street a gongfarmer with his cart full laden, no man envying his full measure. The poore Hermit, as other men did, stopt his nosthrils, & betooke him to the other side of the street hastening from the sower cariage all he could; but the Angel kept on his way, seeming no whit offended with the savour. At which while the Hermit marvelled, there came not long after by them, a woman gorgeously attyred, well perfumed, well attended with coaches, and torches, to convey her perhaps to some noble mans chamber. The good Hermit somewhat revived with the faire sight, and sweet savour, began to stand at the gaze. On the other side, the good Angell now stopped his nose, and both hastened him selfe away, and beckened his companion from the place. At which the Hermit more marvelling then before, he was told by the Angell, that this fine courtesan laden with sinne, was a more stinking savour afore God & his holy Angels, then that beastly cart, laden with excrements.[71]

Harington's oddly defensive reconstruction of desire in the privy, which I discussed earlier in connection with Bottom, seeks to gain moral authority from his fable's ostensible teller, the grave and godly "grand-mother to all my wives children," whose own female bodiliness is separated off from the courtesan's, functionally and ethically, as reproductive, not excretory. The deodorization of the social body, or the deodorization of the corporate house of office, here takes place through a specialized degradation of the female body, replacing the

71. Harington, *Metamorphosis of Ajax,* pp. 84, 85.

privy as the site of contradiction and excremental disgust. The burden of shame and social recognition in human excrement, the product of an undifferentiated and ungendered social body, is transferred from the exposure of the dung cart to the deceptively splendid body of woman. The courtesan follows upon the dungcart and assumes its social function as a receptacle of waste and negative judgment. Furthermore, the social ability to perceive that the "woman gorgeously attyred" is not a noblewoman but a courtesan is also the ability to sense the hidden corruption of the courtesan's excremental body beneath her costume—crudely, to smell her out. If she retains any vestige of her original construction as an image of male desire, that desire has been safely distanced and depersonalized as belonging to "some noble man," who is her destination as she is his.

The Metamorphosis of Ajax is a powerful and original, though self-divided text. But in the inventive discourses of early modern misogyny this troping of the whore's body as privy is itself wholly conventional and related to the whore-urine motif in Surly's self-blinding trope. Thus Thomas Coryat, for example, rationalizes the toleration of courtesans in Venice: "For they thinke that the chastity of their wives would be sooner assaulted, and so consequently they should be capricornified, . . . were it not for these places of evacuation." In *Christes Tears over Jerusalem*, Thomas Nashe plays upon the theme of whores as the "excrementall vessels of lust," climaxing one particularly fervid passage with the rhetorical question: "What are you but sincks and privies to swallow in mens filth?"[72] His moralistic trope is underwritten by what we have already seen of the assimilation of sexual and excretory function in popular medicine. From this point of view, Nashe is merely adding a negative moral overlay to an undeniable homology of social function: the body of the whore and the privy alike serve as receptacles for bodily emissions, for the products of "like evacuations." Yet, as an "excremental vessel," the whore's body functions not only in the way of the degraded body generally, as mere

---

72. Thomas Coryat, *Coryat's Crudities* (Glasgow: University of Glasgow Press, 1905), 1:402–3. I owe this and the following references to Henke, *Gutter Life and Language*. He quotes from Coryat in the entry *Places of evacuation*, p. 193. I quote Nashe here from F. P. Wilson's revised edition of the *Works*, ed. Ronald B. McKerrow (Oxford: Basil Blackwell, 1958), 2:149, 150; see Henke, sub *Whores, as sewers and privies*, p. 289. See also, sub *the Vagina, as a privy seat* (p. 274), the following passage, which resembles Harington: "An uncivill Captaine woonted to say that he lovwed a woman and his Chamber-pot alike, neither or both but for his ease." From Anthony Copley, *Wits, Fits, and Fancies* (London: Edward Allde, 1614; STC 5741), p. 91.

container of its own excrement, but more particularly as the doubly debased receptacle of *public* excrement. What Harington's praise of the privy suggests is that in the metonymic exchange between whore and privy, the privy gains in innocence as well as desirability at the expense of the corrupted female body, here made publicly more offensive than the dungcart. Indeed, while Harington declines to spend "time to allegorize this storie," he does hope his readers will endeavor to keep their souls as clean and sweet as he will teach them to keep their privies.[73]

In *The Alchemist*, the trope of the whore as privy—as site of desire and identification—establishes a potential context both for the fictional body of Doll Common and for the actual body of the transvestite actor beneath. Our recognition of the close relationship between those two bodies—themselves complexly gendered sites of desire, display, and identification—is continually reinforced by Doll's transformations of role and costume at the directorial commands of Face and Subtle. After such transformations, and often within the parameters of her roles, Doll remains "common"—that is, sexually available—a trait she may or may not share with the boy actor whose sexual availability to a male spectator is customarily foregrounded in the double cross-dressed roles of Shakespearean comedy.

But in my reading of her symbolic relation to Dapper and the privy as an anally coded interpretation of Titania and Bottom and of the bodily cathexes of maternal nurture, Doll's one constant role as sexually available woman is a key determinant. It is Doll who first spots Dapper's arrival. Her troping of him as a "fine young quodling" (1.1.189), an unripe apple, establishes him as sexually immature and tentative—conventionally the object of desire for the sexually aggressive woman.[74] If so, Dapper is also established as socially or professionally immature, and this vulnerable combination of attributes positions him in relation to the triad of two males and a female, much as Bottom is positioned in relation to Oberon, Puck, and Titania. Like Bottom, Dapper has crossed over the threshold of a liminal space, controlled by beings whose powers he does not comprehend but who seem intent on imposing a kind of bodily privilege on him.

Gradually Face and Subtle construct for Dapper a flattering self-image separated off from the conventional structure of differences in

73. Harington, *Metamorphosis of Ajax*, p. 85.

74. The trope may pun as well on "the *quods* and *quids* of legal phraseology." See Mares, *The Alchemist*, p. 24.

the Jacobean social fabric. First Face, accusing Subtle of knowing "no
difference of men," must describe who Dapper is *not* by way of assur-
ing him on the contrary that Dapper is "a special gentle, / That is the
heir to forty marks a year" (1.2.44, 50–51). Dapper's initiation proceeds, like Bottom's, by foregrounding the issue of a bodily discipline
of self-containment. (It is also worth recalling the terms of Diccon's
engagement with Hodge since Subtle, too, professes to be worried
about Dapper's ability to be contained.) Face has to assure the doubt-
ing alchemist that Dapper will keep the secret of Subtle's magical gift
to him of a familiar:

> 'Slight, I bring you
> No cheating Clim o'the Cloughs, or Claribels,
> That look as big as five-and-fifty and flush,
> And *spit out secrets*, like hot custard—
>
> (1.2.45–48, my emphasis)

Dapper himself swears by the physical self-mastery of his profession,
the technical mastery of the skillful writing hand, as the sign of his
bodily containment:

> By this hand, of flesh,
> Would it might never write good court-hand more,
> If I discover.
>
> (1.2.23–25)

Subtle and Face go on to "read" the text of Dapper's body, decoding
the marks of its history, a uniqueness constructed as an astrological
narrative of privileged birth. Thus he has "a gaming mouth," "the
only best complexion / The Queen of Fairy loves," and was "born with
a caul" (1.2.101,105–6,128). Subtle even finds contained in him the
special power of other alchemists: "The spirits of dead Holland, living
Isaac, / You'd swear were in him" (1.2.109–10). The clerk's body, duly
affirmed in its attributes of physical containment, hermetic power,
and social privilege, is accorded the competitive social power to open
up the bodies of others and take away the material substance, including the substance of even the corporate body. Thus Dapper will "blow
up gamester after gamester, / As they do crackers in a puppet-play,"
Subtle tells Face. "Not a mouth shall eat for him / At any ordinary";
"he'll draw you all the treasure of the realm" (78–79, 99–100, 102).
    The effect on Dapper of such bodily attention is ultimately as re-

gressive as it was for Bottom—promising pleasure but delivering a far
more ambiguous mixture of pleasure, humiliation, helplessness, and
punishment. The narcissism that Dapper, like the other gulls, must
have in order to believe his good fortune as recipient of the alchemist's operations is, in his case, particularly regressive, for it rests
upon a romantic fantasy of mysterious origin and privileged affinity,
the "rare star" reigning at his birth and allying him to the Queen of
Fairy. The construction of such a narrative of return to the originary
moment thus functions for the rogues as a displacement of the aggressive return they earlier wished upon each other to what I called
the dunghill of incontinence.

As with Bottom, led to Titania's bower, regression proceeds by way
of bodily, particularly anal, cathexis. Subtle, insisting that Dapper "be
bath'd and fumigated" (145) before the crucial reunion, sends Dapper "forth, by the back way" (163) with a disciplinary agenda, an
apparently ritual clarification of the sensory organs:

> Sir, against one o'clock, prepare yourself.
> Till when you must be fasting; only, take
> Three drops of vinegar in, at your nose;
> Two at your mouth; and one, at either ear;
> Then bathe your fingers' ends; and wash your eyes;
> To sharpen your five senses.
>
> (1.2.164–69)

Face's additional reminder—"And put on a clean shirt: you do not
know / What grace her Grace may do you in clean linen" (1.2.174–
75)—suggests the real function of these instructions: not so much to
"sharpen" Dapper's senses as to provoke in him a bodily anxiety rein-
forcing their power over him. The fairies' popular reputation for
·fastidiousness" rests upon a lore of punishments meted out to country girls for slovenly housekeeping:

> Wash your Pailes, and clense your Dairies;
> Sluts are loathsome to the Fairies:
> Sweep your house: Who doth not so,
> *Mab* will pinch her by the toe.[75]

75. Robert Herrick, "The Fairies," from *Hesperides*, in *The Complete Poetry of Robert
Herrick*, ed. J. Max Patrick (New York: New York University Press, 1963), p. 267. See the
commentary on Jonson's *Entertainment at Althorp* in *Ben Jonson*, ed. C. H. Herford and
Percy Simpson (Oxford: Clarendon, 1925–52), 10:395, for several passages about fairy
punishments.

For Dapper to decide to act upon an invitation of natal return—
"Captain, I'll see her Grace" (1.2.162)—is also to relearn the lessons of
early socialization, the paradoxical maternal messages of bodily privilege and bodily unworthiness. A blissful return to the mother is simultaneously the introjection of a disciplinary regimen that first requires
an astringent marking of the bodily boundaries, particularly the sensory thresholds. That the fairies' punishments fleetingly evoked by
the mention of "clean linen" are most often visited upon the bodies of
country *girls* heightens the suggestion of Dapper's retreat from adult
male heterosexuality to the more ambiguous gender identifications of
adolescence.

Like the readers of almanac verse, and signally unlike Bottom, Dapper is initially allowed to perform his own purgations—to bathe, to
wash, to fast, to "cry hum" and "then buzz" (169–70)—as the condition of return. But once he has recrossed the Blackfriars' threshold,
enacting his regressive desire, Face and Subtle proceed to enforce
Dapper's regression by requiring him to cast off the social possessions
of adulthood—his purse, his ring, his love tokens—and put on the
sumptuary signifiers of infancy. Thus he is robed in a "petticoat," the
garment of women and children, and blindfolded with a rag they
identify as a piece of his own swaddling band—torn from the Fairy
Queen's smock. The regression we traced in Bottom's experience in
Titania's bower is here a more explicit return to the genital site and
moment of birth, as Dapper's head is wrapped, his eyes darkened by
the female undergarment. "Though to Fortune near be her petticoat," Subtle reports, "Yet, nearer is her smock" (3.5.9–10).[76] But
one of the signal differences between the two contexts is the physical
and material coercion practiced upon Dapper here—a coercion re-
ified by the introduction of the talismanic maternal objects of robe
and petticoat to ensure his passivity, the coercive stimulation by tickling him, and of course the "privy" destiny of Dapper's erotic regression.

We should also note the differences between Bottom's bodily experience with the fairies and Dapper's. Titania coerces Bottom into a
dreamlike experience of apparently pleasurable passivity and a subjection encoded in, perhaps even masked by the cultic imagery and
deference accorded royalty. Though the diet she administers to Bot-

76. Mares sends the reader to Hamlet's first interrogation of Rosencrantz and
Guildenstern, who confess to being the genital intimates of the strumpet Fortune:
"Faith, her privates we" (2.2.234). See Mares's gloss to 3.5.9–10, p. 119n.

tom seems to enforce laxation, the apparent erotic effect was—as I argued—indistinguishable from coital release and fulfillment. But the only stimulation and release poor Dapper is shown to experience is produced by a pinching testifying to Dapper's objectification and complete reduction to body. Such ticklishness is one attribute of infancy the susceptible body cannot outgrow, resist, or discipline; it is a body sign of subjection and vulnerability akin to Hodge's open breech in *Gammer Gurton's Needle*. We watch as Dapper becomes that infantile body, giving up its identifying possessions and social attributes under the irresistible external pressure of its own complex but not uncomic hurt: "O, O," cries the helpless Dapper, capable of articulation only in the intervals between pinches, the pinches that result from any resistant subjectivity and "equivocation." There must be limits to the discomfort Dapper can be seen to suffer here. Even so, the sadistic structure of the pinching episode—in its excessive display of agency and subjection, in the simultaneous self-enlargement of the tricksters and the self-betrayal of their victim—resembles the agential structure of torture.[77] Dapper must finally attest to his surrender to regression, swearing "not by the light, when he is blinded" but "by this good dark" (3.5.42–43)—the dark of the blinding, enfolding smock, the dark of the prohibited, transgressive return to the mother.

That this tickling does indeed signify the successful invasion of Dapper's body space—as itself a token of regression—is suggested by the rogues' description of him as "this same puffin . . . o'the spit" (3.5.55–56).[78] It is not at all clear what further material use or value Dapper, without his portable possessions, can have for the alchemical trio, *except* as sadistic object. Stripped and infantilized, he has become one with the undifferentiated anal sadistic universe, as undifferentiated as the fecal bolus. He is destined for the privy offstage in part because of narrative exigency, for a bigger gull in the person of Sir Epicure Mammon arrives to deprive him of room and importance in the playing space and to co-opt the sexual services of Doll. More crucial for my argument, he is destined for the privy because Face and Subtle have already reduced him to a human waste product—the whole become the fecal part or, less politely, Dapper as a piece of shit.

77. See Elaine Scarry's brilliant work in *The Body in Pain: The Making and Unmaking of the World* (Oxford: Oxford University Press, 1985), pp. 18 and 36.

78. Mares's citation of Nashe's description of "the puffin, that is half fish halfe flesh (a John indifferent, and an *Ambodexter* betwixt either)" (p. 121n) aptly focuses upon the process of undifferentiation to which Dapper has been subjected.

This is the sadistic response to the dreams of erotic privilege and uniqueness with which Face and Subtle had tempted Dapper and an oblique response on Jonson's part—I would argue—to the sublimations of *A Midsummer Night's Dream*. Further, by returning Dapper to the originary dunghill of undifference and infantile incontinence, the pair succeeds in displacing onto him the anal aggression against each other they had earlier resolved to surrender.

Given the identification between the body of the whore and the privy, it is significant that Doll, rather than Face and Subtle, names the privy as the place to bestow Dapper, thus leaving Subtle to reiterate the conventional sexual and scatological pun: "Come along, sir, / I now must shew you Fortune's privy lodgings" (3.5.78–79). The exchange establishes the privy's significance as a genital symbol, hence as an erotic site, and here as the site of what we now might call anally coded discipline and bondage since Dapper is both blinded and gagged as the precondition of his thoroughly regressive return: "Gape sir, and let him fit you," advises Face (3.5.77). To gag Dapper is thus to impose a familiar discipline on the body's orifices, what Mary Douglas calls compulsory policing of the boundaries.[79] The stuffed mouth is not only the sign of enforced silence, equivalent to the tied-up tongue in *A Midsummer Night's Dream*; it is also the sign of enforced excretory control—a symbolic recollection of the earliest social disciplines on the body. Seen from this perspective, the scene expands symbolically to become a parodic reenactment of the Augustinian notion of birth between urine and feces—"Inter urinas et faeces nascimur"—which Freud memorably appropriated in his analysis of Dora.[80] Instead of acting in the role of midwife to extract Dapper from the excremental site of birth, the trio acts collectively to return him there, where "the fumigation's somewhat strong" (3.5.81). The house as body has excreted its superfluous contents.

To see the privy as a displacement for the female body is to be able to understand Dapper's trajectory as both extrusion and return, to see Dapper as both feces and baby. This is perhaps his ultimate signification as the most passive and regressively coded of the gulls, becoming assimilated as fecal object within the common infantile fantasy of defecation as giving birth. So degraded is he that only when he is on the point of being stifled by the privy's fumes does he break the

79. Douglas, *Purity and Danger*, pp. 114–15.
80. Sigmund Freud, "Fragment of an Analysis of a Case of Hysteria ['Dora']," reprinted in *The Freud Reader*, ed. Peter Gay (New York: Norton, 1989), p. 186.

injunction of silence to cry out for release—not from the fantasy but from the privy. His brief meeting with Doll as the Queen of Fairy is marked by reinscription within the regressive fantasy of erotic privilege. The Queen of Fairy "is with you everywhere!" Subtle tells the ecstatic clerk, in part to reinforce his sense of privilege, in part to internalize an atmosphere of surveillance: "Her Grace would ha' you eat no more Woolsack pies, / Nor Dagger furmety" (5.4.43, 40–41). They set him on a course of high-stakes gaming and imminent financial exhaustion, emblematized by the gift of a fly he is to wear in a purse around his neck and let out only once a week in order to feed on his blood. The final kiss Subtle orders him to bestow on the "departing part" of his "kind aunt" works as a reminder of the anal metonymies of power and powerlessness established in the opening quarrel, especially since it leads directly to Dapper's own departing promise to sign away his forty marks a year.

In the terms of my argument, this final joke at Dapper's expense is another example of how Elizabethan scatology, devoted to defending against the contradictory affects of bodily procedures, can serve as a specialized discourse of power relations as well as of bodily discipline and shame. Dapper's experience thus becomes a reduced and distanced version of the kindred bodily experiences of Hodge and Bottom—moments when scatological vocabulary and action instantiate ambivalent male fantasies of infantile regression and exposure, fantasies in which a dominant female both stimulates and threatens the bodily boundaries of a passive male subject. In this discourse, the alimentary purge occupies a culturally central place, but not because it *determined* Elizabethan psychic structures in any documentable way, or produced "a population of anal erotics." To draw that kind of conclusion is to indulge in a cultural positivism Mary Douglas has warned against: "If anal eroticism is expressed at the cultural level we are not entitled to expect a population of anal erotics. We must look around for whatever it is that has made appropriate any cultural analogy with anal eroticism."[81]

It seems to me the significance of the purge as a bodily habit of everyday life is that it offered an alluringly ambivalent bodily experience—of pleasure and shame, of erotic release within the sanctioned precincts of current therapeutic practice—which, through its power to recall memory traces of infantile sensation, becomes a signif-

81. Douglas, *Purity and Danger*, p. 122.

icant symbolic nexus in contemporary discourses of power and gender. I am not arguing that Elizabethans felt on the whole less shame than we do about eroticizing excretory function, though certainly that is an inference to be drawn from uncritical adherence to Elias's too-rigid vision of the ever-expanding domain of the superego. But because of practices such as the purge and because of the kind of changes in canons of bodily propriety documented by Elias, scatology and anality became a discursive site where contradictions in the early modern culture of the body were legible. Once we have dispelled our own resistance to the presence of such "low" material in the canonized texts of Elizabethan drama, once we have stopped accepting as "natural" earlier cultural definitions of the "low," we can begin to understand the social impulses embedded in the scatological language of the purge.

COMPLYING WITH THE DUG

Narratives of Birth and the

Reproduction of Shame

B irth, like all events of the lower bodily stratum, has a larger part to play in the history of shame than in the history of representation. That it does can be explained in part by the negative influence of what we might call the dark theological view of child-birth, summed up in the Augustinian phrase I have already quoted: "Inter urinas et faeces nascimur." Childbirth is especially invisible in dramatic representation, where the act of giving birth has been an offstage event, as unstageable as the other forms of bodily evacuation it so embarrassingly resembles. Infant feeding, however—the theme of Hamlet's expressively contemptuous remark paraphrased in the title of this chapter—*has* been frequently, even obsessively repre-sented, particularly in the visual arts of pre-Reformation Europe. Perhaps by way of compensation or displacement for the invisibility of birth, breasts with infants *at* them have been a central icon of devoted maternity, or its demonic opposite. In either case, as more and less visible emblems of our earliest object relations, they are represent-able, whereas, except in the case of medical textualizations, "the shameful parts" with infants at *them* are not.[1]

1. Margaret R. Miles has wondered about the intensity of the interest in the Virgin's breast in Renaissance Italian art: "The visual emphasis on the breast that nourished the infant Christ—and by identification with him, all Christians—is star-

Early modern culture, I have been saying, increasingly sought to regulate and regularize a subject's experience of his/her own body and relations with the bodies of others. The rigors of the civilizing process, however, did not exempt the individual subject's earliest, presocial relations with the body of another—the maternal body. The meaning of that relationship could not be civilized without also reconfiguring the maternal body.[2] It is not surprising to find that a number of early modern plays do encode a crisis in the institutional practices of reproduction, particularly a crisis of relations with and signification of womb and breast. This is signally the case in Shakespearean romances such as *The Winter's Tale*, where the structure of action follows often discontinuous episodes in the familial narrative of parents and children. But this crisis of relations with the maternal body also subtends a generically more eclectic assortment of plays—my examples in Chapter 5 are *Antony and Cleopatra* and *The Witch of Edmonton*—where the bodily signifiers of birth and suckling become the privileged sites of ambivalent cultural fantasies of rejection and return.

The differing shame quotients of womb and breast, of birthing and suckling suggest something of the ambivalence toward the maternal body this chapter seeks to interrogate. The affective and discursive transformations in the signs of womb and breast are linked to other changes in the canons of bodily propriety I have been tracing. My main concern here is to discover the effect early modern protocols of birth and infant feeding had on psychic formations—and on the subject positions of child, sibling, mother, or father which the socialized infant comes eventually to occupy. As we will see, gender is not the only shaping influence on reproductive subjectivity in early

tling." See "The Virgin's One Bare Breast: Female Nudity and Religious Meaning in Tuscan Early Renaissance Culture," in *The Female Body in Western Culture: Contemporary Perspectives*, ed. Susan Rubin Suleiman (Cambridge: Harvard University Press, 1986), p. 193. Marina Warner has a less historically specific treatment of the theme in *Alone of All Her Sex: The Myth and the Cult of the Virgin Mary* (New York: Knopf, 1976), pp. 192–205.

2. Some of this chapter's assertions have been anticipated in Valerie Traub's essay, "Prince Hal's Falstaff: Positioning Psychoanalysis and the Female Reproductive Body," *Shakespeare Quarterly* 40 (1989), 456–74. Certainly I agree with her that Shakespearean drama and Freudian and post-Freudian psychoanalytic paradigms work alike to repress the maternal figure, to place it outside of cultural determination. The reader of that essay will note, however, that Traub is much less interested than I am in the consequences for the construction of subjectivity (and thus the writing of drama) of the *specific* social protocols that govern the earliest relations of mother and baby.

modern England; class shapes destiny in birthing and nurture too. The many variables of social ascription signify—even as they are signified by—the changing states and processes of the bodies signally involved in birth.

The structure of social and bodily events surrounding reproduction and lactation, then, is important not only to the psychic economies of individual subjects. The different episodes of reproduction intersect with various other economies, symbolic and material, continually at work in culture because every stage in the reproductive process engages a different nexus of material and gender interests and of ethical responsibility. Since women in early modern Europe ordinarily gave birth under conditions monitored only by other women, childbirth in the period has been interpreted as an inversion of customary gender hierarchies—one of those instances of temporary but genuine female empowerment Natalie Davis has called "women on top."[3]

To some degree, that picture of strategic inversion is reinforced by theories of the carnivalesque which Davis draws upon. Bakhtin, for example, makes childbirth a central activity of the grotesque body, a key interaction of sexual and excremental functions.[4] In the process, however, as we shall see in more detail, Bakhtin reconstructs childbearing more as a social position or point of view than as a critical, life-and-death experience that most women could not choose *not* to undergo. More helpfully, Bakhtin and Davis, taken together, imply that to write about birth and nurture is necessarily to write within and about the available discourses of power, to participate in the sometimes ambiguous cultural assignments of empowerment or shame. What I hope eventually to make clear is that whereas pregnancy and childbirth *were* instances of female empowerment, that empowerment was constrained by a whole host of stratagems, both real and symbolic, designed to counter an understanding of the maternal body as polluted and polluting.

3. See her chapter with this title in Natalie Zemon Davis, *Society and Culture in Early Modern France: Eight Essays* (Stanford: Stanford University Press, 1975), pp. 124–51. The influence of this essay is foregrounded by Adrian Wilson in "The Ceremony of Childbirth and Its Interpretation," in *Women as Mothers in Pre-industrial England: Essays in Memory of Dorothy McLaren,* ed. Valerie Fildes (London: Routledge, 1990), pp. 68–107.

4. Mikhail Bakhtin, *Rabelais and His World,* trans. Helene Iswolsky (Bloomington: Indiana University Press, 1984), pp. 316–22.

In this chapter I want to talk not just about birth (whether we construe that to mean giving birth or being born) but about the complex sequence of events surrounding childbirth, in which different pairs of physically and socially linked bodies unite and separate. This sequence begins at conception with two biological parents and their offspring, extends through the period of infant dependency, and ends at weaning. Such is the historicity of nurture, however, that weaning, too, requires preliminary definition. Because an influential segment of parents during this period sent their babies out to wet nurses soon after birth, weaning in those cases occurred separately for mother and child. I am interested, then, in a narrative of gestation, birth, and two possible weanings—the early weaning of mother from child, the later one of child from wet nurse.

The events I want to talk about as a single, if complexly faceted, social phenomenon are prolonged in duration and radically decentered, extending out beyond the mother-child dyad to include foster parents, foster and biological siblings, and the father, whose erotic and material interests are in place at a child's beginning. These events do have a fairly constricted focus upon two key bodies, a focus on the physical transformations and movements of mother and child, including the physiological dependency of the suckling child and the memorial record of that dependency in the adult. In social terms, these two bodies are the axiological center of the sometimes conflicting, even self-contradictory interests of woman herself, her sexual partner, her child.

How to reconcile and manage such material and psychological interests was—and still is—a major cultural task in which multiple symbolic economies participate. But recovering the meanings of reproductive processes within those economies is only partly facilitated by the ensemble of critical practices currently available. Thus, how to theorize that history as an aspect of historically specific being-in-the-body and how to find that history reproduced in dramatic texts are the tasks of this chapter.

ȥ

Recent accounts of reproductive biology in early modern culture have emphasized a politics of erotic equality/parity and unity. Before the advent of the ovum theory late in the seventeenth century, both men and women were thought to produce and ejaculate the seminal fluid essential for conception. This belief, Thomas Laqueur maintains, made female pleasure as requisite as male.[5] It is easy to be attracted to Laqueur's account, for it historicizes an ideology of sexual pleasure and offers women an apparently egalitarian space within it. Too, it offers another, less-demonizing ideology to set beside the notorious myth of vaginal insatiability. But this account may also be unduly optimistic in its overall appraisal of early modern attitudes toward the female body's role in reproduction. I find in the period's materials on reproduction another narrative, founded upon sexual difference, giving institutional expression through humoral theory to a deep ambivalence toward the maternal body. This counternarrative, unlike Laqueur's, is deeply committed to and dependent upon the signifiers of class, whereby female bodies are distinguished not only from male bodies but from the bodies of other females too. By giving the authority of theoretical discourse to their correlation of bodily habitus and social distinction, medical writers reinscribe these two key variables, gender and class, and naturalize theories of social difference as theories of physiological difference. More important, they emphasize a gendered assignment of responsibility—and thus potentially a gendered distribution of credit and blame, praise and shame— throughout the extended sequence of reproductive events from conception to weaning.[6]

My counternarrative of reproduction begins with the reminder that, in its complex relation to the physical environment, the body of humoral theory was thought to change from day to day, moment to moment, as it took in, concocted, and released elemental humors. As I noted in the Introduction, sexual intercourse was understood in the humoral economy as the bodily expenditure of seminal fluid, to be regulated in both men and women for the maintenance of health. Doctors had the support of humoral theory in prescribing therapeu-

5. This position has been most powerfully stated in Thomas Laqueur, "Orgasm, Generation, and the Politics of Reproductive Biology," *Representations* 14 (Spring 1986), 1–16; and more fully in *Making Sex: Body and Gender from the Greeks to Freud* (Cambridge: Harvard University Press, 1990), pp. 98–103. But see an earlier statement by Audrey Eccles in *Obstetrics and Gynaecology in Tudor and Stuart England* (Kent, Ohio: Kent State University Press, 1982), p. 32; and Patricia Crawford, who distinguishes among several theories of conception in "The Construction and Experience of Maternity," in *Women as Mothers*, pp. 6–7.

6. The credit and blame I mean have little to do with questions of sexual potency or barrenness; as Linda Pollock has pointed out, "Barrenness was believed to be the fault of the woman." See "The Experience of Pregnancy in Early-Modern Society," in *Women as Mothers*, p. 41. I need hardly point out that the gendering of credit and blame in reproduction is not peculiar to the Renaissance.

tic sexual intercourse for sexually mature men and women since the unnatural retention or expenditure of seed could produce humoral imbalance or disease. And when it came to reproduction, humoral theory again brought an economy of expenditure to bear in order to assure the best obstetrical outcome or explain a less desirable one.

Timing and moderation seem to have been the watchwords for reproductive theorists. They explained that the sperm or seed produced by the body varied greatly in reproductive efficacy, characteristics, and strength. Its nature depended, for example, on the soundness of the blood from which it was concocted; how long it had been retained in the seminal vesicles, internal or external, common to men and women; and of course, which sex had produced it. "This foresaid seede," asserts physician-printer Thomas Raynalde with something like tautological force, "is nothing so firme, perfect, absolute and mighty in woman as in man."[7] Possible variation in the quality of the seed was so great that James I's physician, Edward Jorden, explaining the causes of hysteria, describes the "divers sortes of alteration, and likewise of corruption" of seed in the agonistic idiom of heroic tragedy:

> For as it is a substance of greatest perfection & puritie so long as it retayneth his native integritie: So being depraved or corrupted, it passeth all the humors of our bodie, in venom and malignitie. For it must needs be a vehement and an impure cause that shal corrupt so pure a substance, which would easily resist any weake assault: and a substance so pure and full of spirits as this is, must needes prove most malitious unto the bodie when it is corrupted.[8]

At the moment of a baby's conception, the bodily state of *both* parents was crucial in determining such important variables as the baby's sex, viability, normality, vigor, temperament. What brought two bodies to the reproductive act, after all, were motives and states of desire subject to moral judgment at one level and, at another, to bodily mechanisms imperfectly controlled and understood. Why were

7. As Audrey Eccles notes, Raynalde was the second English translator of Eucharius Roesslin's early textbook *Der swangern Frauern und Hebammen Roszgarten* (1513); Raynalde's version, titled *The Birth of Man-kinde: Otherwise Named the Womans Booke*, saw thirteen editions from 1545 to 1654 (Eccles, *Obstetrics and Gynaecology*, pp. 11–12). I quote from the Folger Library's copy of the 1626 edition, STC 21163, p. 38.
8. Edward Jorden, *A Briefe Discourse of a Disease Called the Suffocation of the Mother* (London, 1603; STC 14790; rpt. Amsterdam: Da Capo Press, 1971), p. 20.

monsters born? What determined the sex of the fetus? What caused miscarriage? The answers to such questions tended to rest on and, Tristram Shandy–style, to be traced back to the parents' mental and physical states at conception.

In reproductive discourse, as in humoral theory generally, no stable semantic demarcation separated ethics and physiology. The over-determined ethical signifiers in Jorden's tragic narrative of corruption of seed make clear that conceptualization of bodily states was inseparable from moral judgment. Here, the seed Jorden is ostensibly referring to is, like blood, produced by both men and women, but because his context is diseases specific to the uterus, or "mother," depravity and corruption of seed becomes thoroughly implicated by gender. Immoderate, inappropriate, or untimely desire in male or female was thought to have manifold, even disastrous obstetrical consequences. The birth of monstrously deformed babies, for example, could result from problems in the amount of male seed (too much, too little) or from an undesirable state of the uterus.[9] Monstrous birth was also thought to result from coition during menstruation, a flagrant violation not only of Levitical taboo but of the right ordering of bodily mechanisms of implantation and fetal nurture. As the Flemish physician Lemnius explained: "For when a man lyeth with his wife that hath her courses, he stops her flux, and the blood is forced back again. . . . Yet it is not necessary nor fit to stop the blood running forth, when as the mans seed mingled with such filthy moisture, cannot make a perfect man. For the matter is naught and unfit to receive a decent and proper figure." Failure to observe the proper time for coition because of immoderate desire is punished, whether by God or by nature Lemnius doesn't say: "It can hardly be expressed what contagion and mischief comes thereupon, when men do not refrain from women that are impure."[10]

This explanation for monstrous births was not universally admitted, though coition during "the time of separation" was usually

9. Ottavia Niccoli, "'Menstruum Quasi Monstruum': Monstrous Births and Menstrual Taboo in the Sixteenth Century," trans. Mary M. Gallucci, in *Sex and Gender in Historical Perspective*, ed. Edward Muir and Guido Ruggiero (Baltimore: Johns Hopkins University Press, 1990), p. 5. Robert Muchembled discusses the popular beliefs governing conception and birth in rural France in *Popular Culture and Elite Culture in France, 1400–1750*, trans. Lydia Cochrane (Baton Rouge: Louisiana State University Press, 1985), pp. 76–78.

10. Levinus Lemnius, *The Secret Miracles of Nature* (London, 1658; Wing L1044), p. 23; also quoted in Niccoli, "'Menstruum Quasi Monstruum,'" pp. 1, 2.

The figure of a monster that came forth of a maides belly.

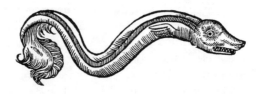

The shape of a monster that came forth of a womans wombe.

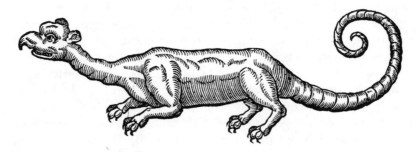

Two monsters from women's wombs. Detail, from Ambroise Paré, *Works*, trans. Thomas Johnson (London, 1634), p. 764. By permission of the Folger Shakespeare Library.

thought to leave bodily markers on children. The midwife Jane Sharp writes that such children "will be Leprous, and troubled with an incurable Itch and Scabs as long as they live."[11] Jacques Guillemeau, citing Galen, thought that such acts of coition resulted in the formation of false conceptions, "fleshy Mole[s] . . . bred when the mans seede is weake, barren, imperfect . . . and for the most part choked through the abundance of the menstruous bloud, which is grosse and thicke,

11. Jane Sharp, *The Midwives Book* (London, 1671; Wing S2969B), p. 51. She is repeating an old belief, articulated for example in Jacob Rüff's *De conceptu et generatione hominis*, translated into English as *The Expert Midwife* (London, 1637; STC 21442); for this belief, see p. 191.

unfit for the framing of a child."[12] Laurent Joubert, however, thought that "a woman cannot conceive during her flowers" because the "blood would carry the sperm away with it like a torrent flooding from every direction." But in matters of successful reproduction he too was convinced of the importance of timing and moderation of desire: "The longer sperm remains in its vesicles and is not spilled or spread about prodigally, the more it is fecund and prolific."[13] Nicholas Culpeper has a word of warning about the consequences for female fertility of immoderate desire, arguing that too frequent copulation "makes the womb more willing to open then shut. Satiety gluts the womb, and makes it unfit to do its Office."[14]

Joubert is not unaware of the irony that timely retention of seed had the rare effect of promoting healthier conceptions among the lower classes than among their betters. For the upper classes, devoted only to their pleasures, "any time is a good one." Their idleness promoted the too frequent expenditure of sperm, by which "they foreshorten their lives considerably," weaken their seed, and impair their offspring.[15] Moderation and timeliness were naturally enforced among workers, however, who were usually interested in intercourse only after nourishing themselves and resting from their work and whose moderate expenditure of sperm was repaid by large numbers of children "stronger and lustier of body, and usually longer lived than such as live idly, and fare deliciously." Indeed, laments Nicholas Culpeper, "tell me else, What becomes of all our Citizens Children, there being scarce so many of them to be found now, as may be proved have been born in half a years time? I am confident not so many of them are now to be found of seven years of age." In particular, "such

12. Jacques Guillemeau, *Child-birth, or The Happy Deliverie of Women* (London, 1612; STC 12496; rpt. Amsterdam: Da Capo Press, 1972), p. 14.

13. Laurent Joubert, *Popular Errors*, trans. and ed. Gregory David de Rocher (Tuscaloosa: University of Alabama Press, 1989), pp. 108–9, 105, 112. This taboo, though widely reiterated in sermons and medical literature, may have been ignored in practice, particularly if sexual partners believed conception could not occur. Linda Pollock quotes Arthur Stanhope's remarkably detailed letter of sexual advice to his nephew, including the suggestion that "you finger my lady espetially att this time now she has her flowers for I assure you those parts are most apt to delate and widen when she is in thatt condition." See "The Experience Of Pregnancy," pp. 41–42.

14. Nicholas Culpeper, *A Directory for Midwives* (London, 1671; Wing C 7492), p. 97. Culpeper was also convinced that unusual coital positions, perhaps especially entry a tergo affected conception: "Apish wayes and manners of Copulation, hinder Conception," p. 97.

15. Joubert, *Popular Errors*, p. 112.

women that live idely (as most of our City Dames do)" are singled out as having few children, or children who do not live.[16]

Moderation and timeliness of desire also had the effect of promoting the conception of a boy, a result many theorists of generation assumed that both parents and nature desired. Joubert recommends allowing sperm to remain overnight in the spermatic vessels, becoming less "raw" over time. He comments that "those who go at it less often make more males, and that by knowing their wives as soon as they are in bed they are making daughters instead of sons. For such sperm is not at that moment as well provided with everything required for its perfection. . . . the morning is more appropriate for producing sons." Conception of a girl, therefore, evidenced either some imperfection in the sperm or some accident in the timing or manner of conception. Girls, he says, are most often begotten either by drunks or on feast days. Even an hour's difference in the timing of coition mattered: "When one sees some lusty girl, more manly in manners and strength than her consorts or companions, one can well say that if she had been engendered an hour later, she would have been a boy; as, on the contrary, of a soft and effeminate boy, that one hour sooner, he would have been but a girl."[17]

But opinion differed on this subject. Nicholas Culpeper, assuming that the seed of male and female naturally desired to reproduce itself, understood the conception of boy or girl to be dependent on whose seed predominated at that moment: "Nature strives to beget its like, men to beget men, women to beget women; but for men to desire Girls, and Women boys, is Appetite not Nature." The age of the parents, too, affected the sex of their offspring. Young women, "because they be hoter then the elder women," said Guillemeau, more "commonly are with child rather of a boy then of a wench." In one chapter titled "Whether It Is True That an Old Man Cannot Beget Sons," Joubert enumerates the conditions under which the cold constitution of an old man can still produce male children.[18]

As these strongly class-based descriptions of the timing and fre-

16. Culpeper, *Directory for Midwives*, pp. 39, 91.

17. Joubert, *Popular Errors*, pp. 114, 115. This is, in effect, another instance of what Stephen Greenblatt has called "an internal power struggle between male and female principles" in generation and conception; see "Fiction and Friction," in *Shakespearean Negotiations: The Circulation of Social Energy in Renaissance England* (Berkeley: University of California Press, 1988), p. 78.

18. Culpeper, *Directory for Midwives*, p. 49; Guillemeau, *Child-birth*, p. 9; Joubert, *Popular Errors*, p. 115.

quency of intercourse suggest, early modern reproductive theory reproduced the structures of difference in class and gender, those explanatory paradigms of the culturally natural. Though one could never be sure of the particular state of one's body at any given moment, reproductive theory offered guidelines and prescriptions for ensuring the particular outcome most often desired. More to the point, in an area of experience where lived practices may have diverged significantly from theory, theory offered an explanation when things went wrong. "Excess in either meat or drink," said Nicholas Culpeper, "causeth crudities; crudities cause ill blood; of ill blood cannot be made good Seed; and by this means Parents often come to the death of their infants, even in their infancy, and know not of it."[19]

My interest in citing such material, even briefly, is not to compare the state of empirical knowledge in reproductive theory then and now. Nor is it to suggest, naively, that scientific theories become less ideological as they become more strictly empirical. The point, rather, is to note how thoroughly early modern reproductive theory was permeated by the ideologies of class and gender and thus how we can expect to find marked out in it the ideological fault lines of early modern culture. One of those fault lines, feminist historians have been suggesting, is the deep-seated misogyny on which patriarchal culture depends. In the almost exclusively male-written reproductive discourses—even those genuinely devoted to promoting the social and medical interests of the woman in travail—that misogyny is legible as discomfort with the fluids and processes of female physiology and, as I shall argue later, with the technical events of birth. In reproduction, the female body was not only different *as usual* from the male body but different from itself in a way that, at its most dangerous, threatened contamination of self and baby. Humoral theory in this way coincided with what Julia Kristeva has labeled "the semiotics of biblical abomination."[20] Thus, Culpeper instructs women who would conceive how *"to preserve the Womb in a due Decorum"*: "If you would have Children, see that the Menstruis come down in due order, the colour of them will shew you what humour offends; purge it out." The *"Instruments* of *Generation,"* he insisted, must be kept "pure and clean."[21]

19. Culpeper, *Directory for Midwives*, p. 33.
20. This phrase is the title of chapter 4 in Julia Kristeva, *Powers of Horror: An Essay on Abjection*, trans. Leon S. Roudiez (New York: Columbia University Press, 1982), but on the question of maternal defilement, see pp. 99–101.
21. Culpeper, *Directory for Midwives*, pp. 96, 32.

As Culpeper's vehemence suggests, a chief difficulty to the theory of reproduction certainly and perhaps also to the interpellating experiences of pregnancy, was that the womb was so suspect and unstable, even so paradoxical an obstetrical environment—in Joubert's phrase, "unclean, filthy, and foul."[22] On the whole, early modern physiology accepted Galen's denial of Plato's assertion that the womb was an independent, animate entity capable of smell and violent movement.[23] Treatment, however, continued to assume the womb's attraction to sweet smells, its antipathy to foul smells. Simon Forman, for example, repeats the conventional wisdom that "all noisum thinges doth troble the matrix and makes her vomite up those humors or excrementes that ar in her. And againe the matrix dothe encline and drawe to all swete and savorie thinges.[24] Such characterizations focus upon the womb a kind of fetishistic attention only partly attributable to the actual gynecological sufferings of the female patient population or even, I would argue, to the high rate of maternal mortality. Culpeper, for example, quotes Jean Fernel in a phrase that seems to have the force and memorability of adage: "As *Fernelius* saith, The place from whence comes life, is also the breeder of the most deadly poison."[25] Edward Jorden's account of the *general* disease-proneness of women, "especially in regarde of that part," was virtually medical commonplace:

> For as it hath more varietie of offices belonging unto it then other partes of the bodie have, and accordingly is supplied from other partes with whatsoever it hath need of for those uses: so it must needes thereby be subject unto mo infirmities then other parts are: both by reason of such as are bred in the part it selfe, and also by reason of such as are communicated unto it from other parts.[26]

22. Joubert, *Popular Errors*, p. 178.
23. See Ian Maclean, *The Renaissance Notion of Woman: A Study in the Fortunes of Scholasticism and Medical Science in European Intellectual Life* (Cambridge: Cambridge University Press, 1980), pp. 40–41; also Ilza Veith, *Hysteria: The History of a Disease* (Chicago: University of Chicago Press, 1965), pp. 31–37.
24. Simon Forman, "Matrix and the Paine Therof," ed. Barbara H. Traister, *Medical History* 35 (1991), 443.
25. Nicholas Culpeper, *Directory for Midwives: The Second Part* (London, 1671; Wing C7498), p. 114.
26. Jorden, *Suffocation of the Mother*, p. 1ʳ. Lucinda Beier has suggested, too, that the special relation to illness which their physiology gave women seems to have been a well-developed social attitude. See *Sufferers and Healers: The Experience of Illness in Seventeenth-Century England* (London: Routledge and Kegan Paul, 1987), pp. 211–41.

Many diseases of the womb were in fact intractable given contemporary therapeutic practices. Thus Jorden's emphasis on the pathology of the womb does have empirical support in the suffering women who fill the casebooks of practitioners such as Richard Napier or Simon Forman.[27] At stake both socially and psychologically, however, is the collectively internalized figuration of a body organ of such demonstrable material importance to society at large—in what was called its public action—being capable of the autonomous malevolence, the will to do harm, implied and authorized by a characterization of the womb as "breeder of poison."[28]

One can see the womb functioning metonymically in such locutions for the culturally feared maternal power of women in general. More interesting, it seems to me, is the suggestion that the womb seems to function as a kind of quasi-independent force in the female body, like an agent within. Such a characterization, while it elevates the womb to a potentially threatening importance, offers the counteradvantage of representing the womb as a political entity, a potentially disorderly force needing pacification and colonization but capable of negotiating terms of external control and regulation. Such empowerment does not necessarily extend, however, to the female bearers of wombs, subjected by the power within. Treatises on diseases of the womb by male practitioners, even as they recommend treatments often to be administered by women to themselves or to other women, have the effect of making the womb knowable not only to the women who have wombs but also to a variety of men. These include the men who write about and treat wombs, the men who establish technical discourses, the men who reproduce the wombs in medical illustrations and thus allow the female gazer a textualized image of her internal bodily self.[29] That that image may be construed as shameful is often power-

27. For Napier, see Michael MacDonald, *Mystical Bedlam: Madness, Anxiety, and Healing in Seventeenth-Century England* (Cambridge: Cambridge University Press, 1981).

28. Margaret R. Miles has discussed the connection between representations of childbirth and the cultural terror of female reproductive organs in *Carnal Knowing: Female Nakedness and Religious Meaning in the Christian West* (New York: Vintage, 1991), pp. 145–62. For literary treatment of the theme, see Janet Adelman, "'Born of Woman': Fantasies of Maternal Power in *Macbeth*," in *Cannibals, Witches, and Divorce: Estranging the Renaissance*, ed. Marjorie Garber (Baltimore: Johns Hopkins University Press, 1987), pp. 108–9.

29. As Laqueur has pointed out, anatomical illustrations of both male and female reproductive organs were widely distributed "well beyond the bounds of the learned community to midwives, barber surgeons, and laypeople" (*Making Sex*, p. 110). Thus it is clearly too simple to suggest that such texts merely operate to effect the erotic

An Explication of the Figures, shewing the difference of the Parts of a Child in the Womb, from those in a Person of Years.

The Second of the Figures in this Brass Plate, shews the Form the Child lies in, in the Womb, according to the Opinion of Hippocrates, *and* Bartholinus.

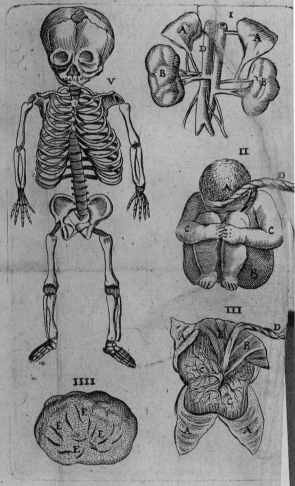

FIG. I.

A A *The Deputy-Kidneyes or Vice-Kidneyes, called in Latin* Renes Succenturiati.

BB *The True Kidneys, as yet distinguished by divers kernels; but ill expressed in point of Scituation, by the Gravers mistake.*

C *The great Arteria from which the Branches go to the Kidneyes, and* Capsulæ, *or Cases.*

D *The Vena cava, from whence spring the Emulgents, and the small Twigs of the* Capsulæ, *or Cases.*

FIG. II.

Shews the Scituation of a Child in the Womb, howbeit in some it differs.

A *The Head bending forward, so as the Nose may be hid between the Knees.*

BB *The Buttocks, to which the Heels are close set.*

CC *The Arms.*

D *The Band or Rope carried along by the Neck, and bended back upon the Forehead, and continued with the* Placenta, *expressed in the following Figure, at the Letter* D.

FIG. III.

AAA *The Membrane* Chorion, *divided.*

BB *The Amnios Membrane, as yet covering the Band.*

CC *The inner Concave part of the* Placenta, *or Womb-cake, which lyes next the Infant with twigs of the Vessels.*

) *A portion of the Band or twisted Rope.*

Situation of the child in the womb. From Nicholas Culpeper, *A Directory for Midwives* (London, 1671), foldout frontispiece. By permission of the Folger Shakespeare Library.

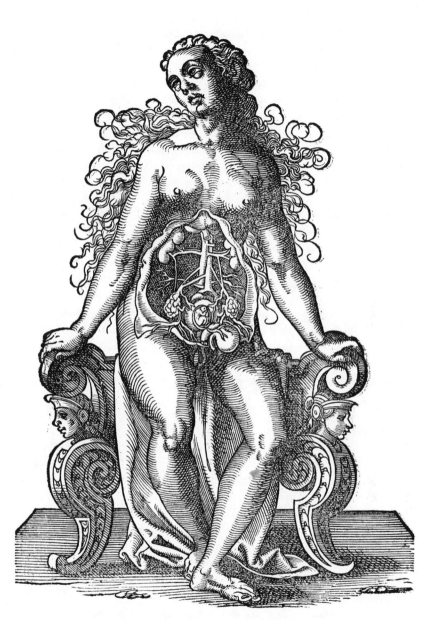

Pregnant woman, viscera exposed. From Jacob Rüff, *De conceptu et generatione hominis* (Frankfurt, 1580), p. 10ᵛ. By permission of the Folger Shakespeare Library.

fully suggested by the abashed posture of the infant in the gravid womb, who bends his head and holds his hands before his face as if to hide himself from the gazer.

In Jorden's representation, the womb becomes the protagonist in an ethical drama, burdened with both responsibility and disease. It has "more varietie of offices" than other parts, peremptorily drawing what it needs for those offices from elsewhere in the body, yet subject by that very power to "mo infirmities." Simon Forman has a yet more wonderful locution in the treatise he devoted to pains of the womb. He speaks of the womb as "*a world of yt selfe* lying betwen the bowells and the bladder spredinge yt selfe to bothe sides of the belly," and he insists that it cannot be treated like the rest of the body with medicines taken in by mouth. Effective treatment must be done through the vulva because "ther is noe waie into the matrix but one." Nor will the womb long retain what it receives, for "the matrix doth exempte himself of any thing that yt receyveth of man more then once in a month or noe." And like the watery world of which it was a kind of emblem, the womb was subject to tidal forces, waxing and waning in a majestic harmony with the lunar cycle: "For as the tyde doth flowe soe doth the matrix begin to flowe and open and *spred her selfe* & the humors doe gather in the matrix."[30]

Forman's evident awe of menstrual majesty to the contrary notwithstanding, part of the problem for uterine reputation and a major rationale for medical colonization came not from just its proximity to other excretory organs but from the fact that excretion was one of its variety of offices. I have already noted how in one degraded sexual rhetoric the wombs of whores were seen as sewers and privies. Even in the more decorous discourses of reproductive theory, just as the bowel and bladder stored waste products, so the womb, created by nature "to be the said receptacle & house of office," stored and released waste menstrual blood before pregnancy and lochial flow in the period after delivery.[31] Even apart from events directly connected to reproduction, the womb was notoriously subject to other forms of more or less pathological flow—the leucorrheal discharge popularly

---

exposure of a female torso to an implied male gazer. My point is rather that such illustrations, like other forms of emergent technological reproduction, construct a discourse of knowledge alienating women from their own bodies and bodily self-experience, making them subject to those bodies and to those who can represent it.

30. Forman, "Matrix and the Pain Therof," pp. 442–43, emphasis added.

31. I quote here from Raynalde, *Birth of Man-kind*, p. 48.

known as "the whites," for instance, which the midwife Louise Bourgeois described as "an inordinate eruption of an excrementitious
humor collected together through some vitiousness of the blood."[32]
The deep cultural ambivalence surrounding menstrual blood has
been well documented; as I suggested in Chapter 3, its production is a
central attribute of the grotesque body and a potentially ominous
symptom of gender ambiguity.[33] A similar ambivalence by women
toward their own bodily flowings, particularly to kinds of discharge
other than menstrual, is far harder to document historically but is
contextually persuasive.

The cultural ambivalence generated by menstrual blood carried
over into reproduction, since it was thought to be the source of fetal
nurture. In order to recuperate blood in this form as food, reproductive discourse has to work hard to decontaminate it from its unstable
social meanings. Raynalde insists that "this bloud is even as pure and
wholesome as all the rest of the bloud in any part of the body else."[34]
Culpeper contradicts such authorities as "*Columella, Pliny, Columbus,*
and *Fernelius*," who contend that the fetus cannot be nourished by so
evil a substance: "This Blood which a Woman voideth once a month, is
not so bad *as they make it to be*, nay, simply in it self considered, not bad
at all, but very good, for if the womans body be in good temper, her
blood must needs be good."[35] Jane Sharp admits that menstrual blood
"hath strong qualities indeed, when it is mixed with ill humours. But
were the blood venomous it self, it could not remain a full month in
the womans body, and not hurt her; nor yet the Infant, after conception."[36] Joubert acknowledges that the blood the body "rejects each
month is the least fine and smooth of all her blood," but still sees
"nature's great and marvelous providence" at work. Indeed, "the
crudest [blood] suffices, especially since the conceived sperm has a
great digestive virtue. . . . Once the child is formed, his liver is the
first to receive it, consuming and making from it very refined blood

---

32. See R. C., *The Complete Midwife's Practice Enlarged* (London, 1680; Wing C99.2),
p. 213. This is the English translation of the second part of the famous French midwife
Louise Bourgeois's *Observations diverses*.

33. See Patricia Crawford, "Attitudes to Menstruation in Seventeenth-Century En-
gland," *Past and Present* 91 (1982), 47–73; but see also Angus McLaren, *Reproductive
Rituals: The Perception of Fertility in England from the Sixteenth to the Nineteenth Century*
(London: Methuen, 1984).

34. Raynalde, *Birth of Man-kind*, p. 56.

35. Culpeper, *Directory for Midwives*, p. 56, emphasis added.

36. Sharp, *Midwives Book*, p. 289.

for the nourishment of the body."[37] The child's body, in other words, compensates for the systematic failings of its mother's. Though even here the results could be imperfect: Guillemeau explains childhood skin rashes as the surfacing of "reliques of the impurer part of the bloud, wherewith the child was nourished in his Mothers wombe." And even after the cessation of menses in pregnancy, the womb continued to be a container for excrement since amniotic fluid was usually regarded as fetal excrement, the baby's sweat and urine.[38]

Apart from its unattractive excretory function, its tendency to bleed and flow, and its proneness to disease, the womb was also suspect as an obstetrical environment because of its odd capacity to house other things besides babies (such as the "false conceptions" called moles), its susceptibility to effects of the psyche, and its threatening association with bizarre longings. Obstetrical texts and diary records alike abound with anecdotes of mothers whose frights or longings during pregnancy were thought to have marked their babies with harelips, blood- or wine-stained markings, hairy moles, or other deformities.[39] In such accounts, responsibility for avoiding a poor outcome comes to rest heavily upon the mother, who must submit herself quietly and submissively to her state. *"Content of Mind,"* says Culpeper, "dilates the Heart and Arteries, whereby the vital blood or Spirit is sufficiently distributed throughout the Body, and thence arise such affections as please, recreate, and refresh the Nature of man."

But this contentment, imposed as a condition for success in conception and pregnancy, comes suspiciously to resemble the subordination and submission enjoined upon all women, pregnant or not:

> the imagination of the Mother operates most forcibly in the Conception of the child. How much the better then were it for women to lead *contented* lives, that so their imaginations may be pure and clear, that so their conception may be well formed, than to vex, and fret and fume, and fling and throw, and murmure and repine, and fill their minds all full of distracting cares and fears, as an Egg is full of meat, making a tumult in

37. Joubert, *Popular Errors*, p. 100.
38. Jacques Guillemeau, *The Nursing of Children* (London, 1612; STC 12496; rpt. Amsterdam: Da Capo, 1972), p. 99. Guillemeau suggests that the newborn may have roughness or "nitrosity" about the eyes "through his long swimming and lying in his owne sweat and Urine, while he was in his mothers wombe" (p. 12).
39. To cite one example of many, Alice Thornton records seeing a penknife, "which was nigh to have hurt me," causing the baby to be born with "a mark of a deep bloody colour upon [its] heart." Quoted in Beier, *Sufferers and Healers*, p. 233.

their spirits, and bringing all their thoughts into such a confusion, that they look more like beasts then women, so that if they could but see themselves, they could not *but be ashamed* to see how like Anticks they are.

Culpeper's point here—much more conventional than his vehement, energetic prose might suggest—is that the anxious, complaining woman has no one to blame but herself for the difficulties in her pregnancy or the hazards in its outcome. He recommends "content of mind" not only for its obvious psychological benefit but, more authoritatively, for its physiological one ("content of mind dilates the Heart and Arteries"). Discontent alters the blood, thus altering "the very nourishment wherewith the child is nourished in the Womb."[40] Guillemeau, similarly, uses pregnancy to warn women of the hazards of psychological and bodily openness or receptivity: "Discreet women, and such as desire to have children, will not give eare unto lamentable and fearefull tales or storyes, nor cast their eyes upon pictures or persons which are uglie or deformed, least the imagination imprint on the child the similitude of the said person or picture. . ."[41]

Reproductive writing uses physiology, in other words, to reinforce a conventional construction of the female body as dangerously open and the female imagination as dangerously impressionable and to contest the social privilege that pregnancy gave to the mother-to-be "to have her longing." Some of those longings, it was understood, could be deeply irrational, bizarre, or even pathological, and Culpeper was sure they also reflected the structure of class difference: "Those which live idlely (as the Gentry and Citizens Wives, that seldom use their bodies to any exercise, unless it be playing with their Dogs) and keep not good diet, are most pestered with such Longings." In the recognized danger that denying those longings posed for the fetus lay the empowerment of and incentive to desire. In the case of pregnant women's cravings to eat "absurd things," Culpeper recommends a dialogue beginning "with fair words, to abstain from them," but finally counsels surrender: "If the appetite will not be allayed, rather grant them, than suffer an abortion or mark upon the Child."[42] Thus for many, if not most, women, a desired pregnancy could open up a space within the confines of patriarchal

40. Culpeper, *Directory for Midwives*, pp. 93, 94. The first set of italics in the long quotation is Culpeper's, the second mine.

41. Guillemeau, *Child-birth*, p. 26.

42. Culpeper, *Directory for Midwives*, p. 120; *The Second Part*, p. 105.

marriage for the expansion or even momentary hegemony of female desire. William Gouge, advising "*an husbands provident care for his wife about her child-bearing*," tells the readers of his treatise "of husbands particular duties" to procure "for their wives to the uttermost of their power and abilitie, such things as may save their longing, in case they doe long."[43]

As such cautions suggest, the interaction between the mother's rapidly altering body and the growing fetus sheltered in her swelling womb was both dynamic and portentous. Even more, perhaps, than other physical conditions peculiar to women, pregnancy partook of what Mary Ann Doane has described as the logic of the symptom: "The symptom makes visible and material invisible forces to which we would otherwise have no access; it is a delegate of the unconscious."[44] Perceivable as a complex of constantly changing symptoms, pregnancy was a rare type of bodily event knowable as to cause and desired effect but radically unknowable even in its visibility for the long months in between. In the attention pregnancy necessarily focused on the apparent concavity and expandability of the womb, it typified the body's aspect as container, so crucial to humoral corporality's self-experience. The difficulty in pregnancy, however, was that the pregnant womb, instead of containing merely its own humors and waste products, housed and was accountable for the production of a baby in whom patriarchy claimed the presiding interest.

Even more frightening perhaps for patriarchal interests was that on the whole even normal, survivable pregnancy was conceptualized as a disease state. "The greatest disease that women can have," wrote Guillemeau, "is that of the nine Moneths, the *Crisis* and cure whereof consists in their safe deliverie." Perhaps pregnancy was perceived this way because it entailed so many physical changes within a bodily paradigm where change was cause for fear, perhaps it was because the baby itself could be regarded, like an unwonted growth, as an alien presence altering the humoral balance of its mother and destined for evacuation and release. Birth was called a "great evacuation," a great emptying-out, which not only configured the baby as excretory product but, more to my purposes here, construed birth as a violent purgation not unlike the purges central to humoral therapy. The "extraordinarie delight" the womb was said to experience at conception, "a

43. William Gouge, *Of Domesticall Duties* (London, 1622; STC 12119; rpt. Amsterdam: Theatris Orbis Terrarum; and Norwood, N.J.: Walter J. Johnson, 1976), p. 399.

44. Mary Ann Doane, "The Clinical Eye: Medical Discourses in the 'Woman's Film' of the 1940s," in *The Female Body in Western Culture*, p. 154.

shaking or quivering (such as we commonly find presently upon making of water)," was soon followed by early signs of pregnancy, any one
of which in other bodily contexts would signify the imbalance of humoral disease. Guillemeau enumerates vomiting, spitting, loss of appetite, bizarre cravings, and a "fallen" belly, "which makes them often-
times to complaine and say they be quite fallen away."[45]

If, as I have suggested, class behaviors were thought to affect conception in ironic and to us perhaps surprising ways, gender organized
a differential perception and experience of the nine months' illness
that was pregnancy. The sex of the fetus altered and oriented the
mother's body, *made it different* from what it had been before pregnancy or would be again in a differently gendered gestation. According to
Hippocrates, gestation proceeded differently for males and females,
the male fetus, with its greater heat, taking thirty days to be completely formed, the female forty-two. Perhaps it is not surprising that
the sex of fetuses, according to some experts, could be read on mothers' bodies by a whole host of opposed bodily signs, hierarchically
ordered by hot/cold, right/ left, up/down, hard/soft. Guillemeau
listed some of these:

> *Hippocrates* saith, that a woman which goeth with a boy hath a good
> colour, *for a woman in her case*, but if it be of a wench, she will have a worse
> complexion. Likewise if the right breast be harder and firmer, the nipple
> hard, red, and more eminent, the milke white and thicke . . . and if you
> make a cake with the said milke and flower, and in the baking it con-
> tinues firme, and close, it is a signe the woman is with child of a boy. . . .
> The Male child lyeth high above the Navell by reason of his heate, and
> the Female at the bottome of the belly, because of her coldnes and
> weight.[46]

The naturally greater heat of the male fetus had the distinct advantage of counteracting the cold, moist temperature of its mother's
womb, whereas the colder female fetus, unfortunately, could only
intensify it. Reproductive theory seems to have coincided with popular belief.[47] From both, women could have drawn an expectation of

45. Guillemeau, *Child-birth*, pp. 81, 4, 5.
46. Ibid., p. 9.
47. Joubert begins his chapter "If There Is Certain Knowledge That the Child Is
Male or Female" (3.4) by citing Hippocrates but moves on to the "signs given by
laymen" (*Popular Errors*, pp. 152–53). He regards none of these signs as predictive since
pregnancy could coexist with other bodily states that would serve to complicate a
woman's health.

differential health and well-being in pregnancy, profoundly gender-based. "They which be with child of a boy are more quicke and nimble in all their actions, and be in better health of body, without being subject to many infirmities, which commonly happen to women with child of a wench," Guillemeau explained. Even her mental state was affected, he said, the woman carrying a girl being "wayward, fretfull, and sad," no doubt from cold moisture breeding melancholy.[48]

The clarity of such differential accounts of pregnancy in reproductive texts, I hasten to add, is not borne out by diary records. Ralph Houlbrooke includes some diary predictions about the sex of a baby in his anthology of family life but maintains that "their basis is unknown, and they were not always accurate." He does include Nehemiah Wallingford's expostulation of relief after his wife's safe delivery of "a man child, contrary to our expectation," which may suggest some such differential understanding. The sympathetic and attentive Ralph Josselin records his wife Jane's predictions, which change frequently enough during pregnancy to suggest some correlation on her part between her health and the baby's gender. Jane found one of her labors "very strange to her" and concluded, perhaps on that basis, "It would be a daughter, contrary to all her former experience and thought."[49] But the diary makes clear that the Josselins, like their contemporaries, understood their bodies in humoral terms and would presumably have so understood Jane's pregnancies.

Pregnancy was an unusual "disease" in being so often anticipated and delighted in, particularly by upper-class women, whose absence from economic production led—so Patricia Crawford has argued—to an increased emphasis on their reproductive labor.[50] If pregnancy was experienced as disease—and even for the many women who survived multiple childbirths, it was often a time of discomfort and anxiety—that disease was uniquely tied to duty, whether that duty is constructed socially or theologically.[51] My point, however, is not to reconcile reproductive theory with a complex and as yet incomplete social record but to show how pregnancy was *inscribed* as disease even as it was required for most women.

ﺰ▰

48. Guillemeau, *Child-birth*, p. 10.
49. Ralph A. Houlbrooke, ed., *English Family Life, 1567–1716: An Anthology from Diaries* (Oxford: Basil Blackwell, 1988), pp. 101, 117.
50. Crawford, "Construction and Experience of Maternity," p. 14.
51. See the diary accounts excerpted in *English Family Life*, pp. 101–32.

It may well be the case, as social historians of childbirth in early modern England have argued, that in pregnancy and childbirth married women enjoyed their greatest power and autonomy. Adrian Wilson, in particular, has found evidence for this argument in the ritual exclusivity of childbirth. "Before childbirth belonged to medicine," he says, "it belonged to women"; they constructed "a coherent system for the management of childbirth, a system based on their own collective culture and satisfying their own material needs." The picture of childbirth emerging from Wilson's upbeat account is of a ceremony, carnivalesque to the degree that it is structured by gender inversion and focused upon the material satisfaction of bodily need, in which women invited to participate in a childbirth would rapidly reorder domestic space and restructure household activities. The marital bedchamber, ordinarily under the more or less firm control of patriarchal prerogative, became a different space both socially and physically, a darkened and shuttered birthing chamber closed to men, full of women, and presided over by a midwife paid for her services. This neighborliness, the companionship of other women and the familiarity of their ritualized activities of preparing caudles and linens presumably helped to allay the fears, and thus the pain, of the woman in travail.[52] The period of female hegemony extended throughout the lying-in from the onset of labor to a time about four weeks later, when the newly delivered mother would publicly reemerge from her house for a "churching ceremony" celebrating her safe delivery, perhaps a successful birth, and her full return to social existence.

What Wilson wishes to make clear is how powerfully and effectively these rituals of the collective female culture of childbirth functioned within the overall confines of seventeenth-century patriarchy. I have no wish to dispute the general outlines of his account, or even the relevance of carnivalesque theory to birth practices in the period. I would like to consider childbirth less synchronically than Wilson does, however, not as a relatively static social practice but as an emergent field of discourse and technical knowledge. In this emergent field, the regulatory mechanisms of shame threaten the female enclosure of the birthing chamber and the privileges of the laboring woman. The interpellation of shame turns the ritual practices of childbirth into not-always-successful female defenses against the cultural ambiguation of female bodily changes and physical properties of birth.

52. Wilson, "Ceremony of Childbirth," pp. 70, 71–75. In more modest domestic circumstances a separate room might not be available, but some ritual demarcation of space would socially separate birth from the household structure.

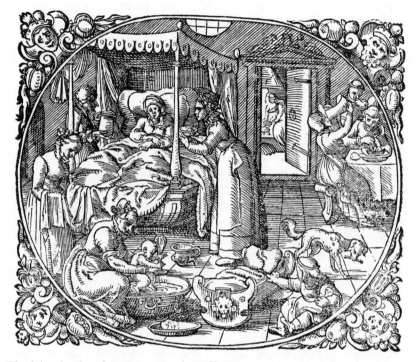

The lying-in chamber. From Jacob Rüff, *De conceptu et generatione hominis*
(Frankfurt, 1580), title page. By permission of the Folger Shakespeare
Library.

What I earlier described as the womb's general unsavoriness of
reputation, functions, and mysterious effluences—so apparent in the
rhetorical coloration of medical literature—has the effect of attaching
shame and obscurity to the birth process, even as ceremonially ordered by women's culture. It is in order to theorize the relation between the invisible forces at work in reproduction and their visible
and material effects that medical representations of conception and
birth occur. But in early modern England, cultural unease about representing these events registers powerfully in the vernacular medical
texts devoted to the subject. Even physicians who wrote or translated
works on birth, such as John Banister (*The Historie of Man*, 1578) or
Richard Jonas and Thomas Raynalde (first and second translators of
The Birthe of Mankynde, 1552), worried that detailed description in

English of the reproductive organs, male and female, would commit
"indecencie agaynst the office of *Decorum*."[53] Raynalde, who as
physician-printer translated one of the first two works in English on
midwifery, was also worried that knowledge of birth processes would
contribute specifically to female shame and male disgust about female
reproductivity:

> Some alleaging that it is shame, and other some, that it is not meete ne
> fitting such matters to be intreated of so plainely in our mother and
> vulgar language, to the dishonor (as they say) of womanhood and the
> derision of their owne secrets, by the detection and discovering whereof,
> men it reading or hearing, shalbe moved thereby *the more* to abhorre and
> loath the companie of women, and further in their communications to
> jest and bourd of womens privities, not wont to be knowne of them.

The culturally available pun on "privity" here signifies women's
secrets as the shame—the pudenda—of female reproductivity.
Raynalde uses the pun to assert that men without benefit of Latin—
that is, literate but nonprofessional men—are "not wont" to know the
secrets of women's reproductive organs, their names and their functions in gestation and birth. Raynalde takes great pains to assure his
readers, however, presumably on his authority as physician, "that *I
know* nothing in woman so privie ne so secret" to make an honest man
"conceive a certaine loathsomnesse and abhorring towards a woman."[54] But his rhetorical emphasis is suspect, overdetermining the
"loathsomnesse and abhorring" of the female body he imagines as
already present in patriarchal culture. He may well be contributing
"the more" to the derision of women in defending so strenuously
against it and offering the facile hope that dispelling secrecy may be
one way of dispelling shame: he knows nothing "so" secret that it will
conduce to male loathing. Seventeenth-century writers—Nicholas
Culpeper and the midwife Jane Sharp, for example—were less timid,
but as Charlotte Otten points out, nearly all vernacular writers on
human reproduction betray their uncertainty about writing in a new
and culturally unprotected discourse that will expose women's re-

---

53. John Banister, *The Historie of Man* (London, 1578; STC 1359), sig. Bbiiiiᵛ. I owe
this reference to Charlotte Otten.
54. Raynalde, *Birth of Man-kinde*, pp. 8–9, 12. Current information about
Raynalde's occupations was made available to me by Peter Blayney.

productive organs and the events of birth to the uncontrolled internal gaze of male imaginations.[55]

Writing about birth in English, however, opens up a textual space from which men—and their erotic interest in women's bodies—cannot be excluded. What Raynalde is particularly worried about, paradoxically, is that reading will serve both to eroticize and deeroticize interest in the female body by the greater arousal of disgust: the "secrets" of women can only be shameful. Fearing unwarranted, unauthorized results of textualization, Raynalde weakly tries to limit and control the discursive and social circulation of knowledge of birth processes by redefining textuality as an elect community of the silently knowledgeable. To the men into whose hands his book should come, he writes: "I counsell and exhort, that they take not upon them to *talke* of any things herein contained, but onely where it may edifie, and be assuredly well accepted."[56] At the very least, however, textualizing birth during a time when literate men far outnumbered literate women discursively reconstitutes the practices of childbirth as a field of theoretical knowledge, neutralizes its strong gendrement as female, and participates in what was to become in the later seventeenth and eighteenth centuries the medical professionalization of birth.

Joubert notes, condescendingly, that it is "very good and reasonable" for midwives to "share among themselves their usual little remedies." But he insists that "women have never invented a single remedy; they all come from our domain or from that of our predecessors."[57] Culpeper, recognizing no professional boundaries in the dissemination of knowledge, begins his *Directory for Midwives* by inveighing against "the notable injuries offered to Men and Women . . . by absconding the Rules of Physick from them." He seeks to assure midwives of their continued control over birth as a practice: "To whom doth the *Practical Part* of it belong, but to your selves?" Even so, he too is committed to conceptualizing childbirth as, first, a field of theoretical knowledge, hence a male preserve to be transmitted by means of a patriarchal process of formal, intellectual endowment from on high. Custom—the social transmission and regulation

55. Charlotte Otten, "English Medical Texts: The Vocabulary of Medical Writing on Sexuality in the 16th and 17th Centuries," unpublished manuscript, pp. 3–4. Otten's point, unlike mine here, is not gender specific.

56. Raynalde, *Birth of Man-kinde*, p. 13, emphasis added.

57. Joubert, *Popular Errors*, pp. 172–73.

of behaviors instantiated in the behaviors themselves—is replaced by textuality, the inscription in a "directory" of what the birthing practitioner always already should have known before entering a female enclosure no longer secret or simply female: "Many of you are ancient, but if you be too old to learn, you are as much too proud. God speaks not now by voice to men and women as formerly he did, but he speaks in, and by men; and 'tis no part of wisedom for men and women to stop their ears against it."[58]

By and large, as Wilson and others make clear, the practice of birth in the seventeenth century remained one of "womens privities." The ritual enclosure of the birth chamber offered the laboring woman quiet, freedom from distractions, and the support of other women who had survived or would themselves face the substantial risks of childbearing. Thanks to the textual reiterations of the immodesties of birth, however, this aura of protection becomes hard to distinguish from one of concealment and shame, from the isolation ordinarily granted to acts of bodily evacuation. If metaphors of visibility/invisibility lend ethical and physiological ambiguity to that symptom which is pregnancy, so ideologically charged metaphors of opening and closing dominate birth. After conception, the womb, which opened sexually to receive male seed, closed decisively in order to reject the entrance of further male seed in any subsequent acts of coition. (The closure of pregnancy was usually but not always final: hence the superfetation represented by the birth of twins. Too, the egregious bodily openness associated with the prostitute meant that her womb rarely closed tightly enough to retain seed and made her deliveries suspiciously easy. Joubert says that whores and other lascivious women have an easier time in childbearing because the "shameful parts are so much in use that it is easy for the child to come through the well-worn passageway".)[59] At birth, the female body opens again even more dramatically and decisively to expel the baby.

We have seen how threatening such bodily openness is to a dominant ideological configuration that always valorizes enclosure of the female body. By ritually sealing off the birthing chamber, even stopping up the keyholes, women at a birth offer an ideologically weighted countersign to the bodily opening and emptying enacted in birth. The birthing chamber thus becomes a symbolic outer body

58. Culpeper, *Directory for Midwives*, sig. A2^r, A3^r, A3^v.
59. Joubert, *Popular Errors*, p. 168.

envelope or, to paraphrase Forman's wonderful figure, "a world of yt selfe" where women alone controlled physical exit and entrance. Birth rituals sought also to limit access to and exposure of the inner thresholds of birth, the bodily thresholds of cervix, vagina, and labia through which the baby must emerge. According to Wilson, only the midwife herself "was entrusted with the *right to touch*" these thresholds.[60] The sense of taboo operating here is corroborated by Joubert despite his insistence that physicians know better everything that midwives know. He adds, "We leave to them this branch of surgery involving childbirth because it is more decent that this treatment be administered woman to woman in their shameful parts." Guillemeau, who as a surgeon would usually have been called only to deliver prominent women or in cases of difficult presentations or obstructed births, orders the hips and knees of a woman he will deliver manually to be covered so that no one present will "see what the Chirurgion toucheth, or doth: and likewise, that the woman bee not afraid of him, when he shall be about his businesse."[61] Even most illustrations of the birth scene obscure the bodily thresholds of birth; the midwives are shown thrusting their hands up beneath the heavy draperies of the laboring woman's skirts to check the progress of labor. Once birth and the birth chamber are given over to depiction, the dark spaces beneath the laboring woman's skirt must do the necessary cultural work of enclosure and concealment.

Humoral theory offered rational, empirical support for birthing rituals designed to offer concealment and enclosure, for the explanations of danger in childbirth focused precisely on the exposure of bodily thresholds ordinarily concealed from view and the traumatic opening of bodily thresholds ordinarily closed. In pregnancy, according to Guillemeau, "there be divers winds and vapours, that are shut up, and inclosed in the neather belly of a woman with child." The great evacuation of birth released those winds and vapors, but of course it also opened the mother's body to the entrance of yet other humors or cold air, causing afterpains. Guillemeau offers instructions for swathing the belly with "linnen cloth foure times doubled" not only to keep the "Matrice in his place" but to prevent air from getting in to the womb, "which being emptied of such a burthen, will easily receive it, and this might bee a meanes to make it swell, and puffe up."

60. Wilson, "Ceremony of Childbirth," p. 73.
61. Joubert, *Popular Errors*, p. 172; Guillemeau, *Child-birth*, p. 126.

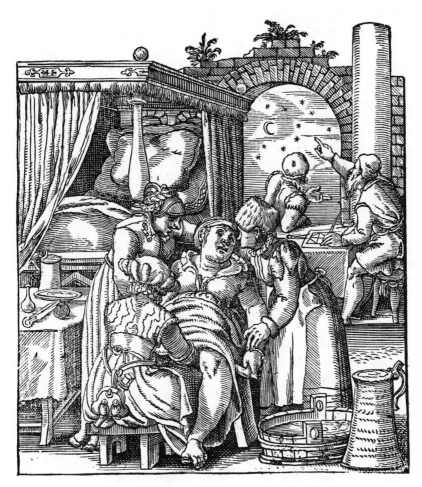

Woman in labor. From Jacob Rüff, *De conceptu et generatione hominis*
(Frankfurt, 1580), p. 3. By permission of the Folger Shakespeare Library.

The need to keep this newly emptied body from unknowingly absorbing dangerous humors may also lie behind Guillemeau's insistence
that the new mother "must be kept from sleeping, though shee bee
very desirous thereof." Culpeper thought labor weakened even the
eyes, "by a Harmony between the Womb and them," and urged the
parturient woman to avoid the light. But the dangerousness of bodily
opening is epitomized in Joubert's characterization of the mother's
body as wounded: "One could not more aptly compare a woman who

has just delivered than to a person who has just been severely wounded." The chief similarity here is not the risk of death but the fact of flow.[62]

Even more than the suspiciously effluent female body in other states, the parturient body flowed—with the fluids released at birth, after birth, and in lactation. Thus Joubert's notation of the *difference* between bodily opening at birth and in injury suggests how the changes in bodily flow which began for the parturient woman after delivery seemed—at least in medical discourses, as in the scriptural discourses they seemed to rationalize—to signify uncleanness and thus to require ritual purification. After injury, "bleeding is stopped immediately because the blood is good," says Joubert, "whereas in the case of the woman this cannot be done because this blood [of the afterbirth] is not worth anything."[63] This body must be allowed to flow; this blood ought not to be retained. Although the filth of birth washes quickly off the baby, it seems to remain a signal attribute of the newly delivered woman. Thus, the placenta in this model was by definition the waste of the waste, the least of the least, because it represented menstrual blood that not even the baby could turn to use: "This blood is not *worth anything.*"

Even in an age without a modern conception of sepsis, retention of the placenta was recognized as dangerous, and the placenta itself became another excretory object of shame and disgust, "a thing contrarie to nature." Texts emphasize a thorough and complete purging after birth or, says Guillemeau, "the dead, (which is the after-birth:)" will kill "the quicke (which is the wombe)." You may easily perceive "if the Womb be foul," Culpeper instructs, "by the impurity of the blood, it either coming away in gobs, or stinking." Raynalde advises the midwife to "take diligent heede that she be *exactly and utterly purged.* To this be agreeable all such simples the which provoke urine, and open the vaines, making free way for the blood to passe, and send the humours & matter downeward."[64] Besides bleeding in the ankle vein, he also recommends sneezing and holding the breath to ensure complete and utter purgation! "Suffocation after Child-bearing," notes

---

62. Guillemeau, *Child-birth*, pp. 52, 102–3; Culpeper, *Directory for Midwives*, p. 145; Joubert, *Popular Errors*, p. 186. Joubert's analogy may have been commonplace, since Guillemeau also makes use of it in terms of postpartum diet. See *Child-birth*, p. 190.

63. Joubert, *Popular Errors*, pp. 186–87.

64. Guillemeau, *Child-birth*, pp. 176–77; Culpeper, *Directory for Midwives*, p. 146; Raynalde, *Birth of Man-kind*, pp. 120–21, emphasis added.

Culpeper, "is from the stinking after blood, which sends up stinking vapors which kill many." The point was to eliminate all the fluids and tissues that had collected in the bodily enclosure of pregnancy without allowing humors to flow into the newly opened body of the woman after birth. Any way the body could be stimulated to flow and purge—in order that all such flows should cease—was encouraged. Guillemeau thought retention of the lochia caused ague, and he prescribed clysters to keep the belly loose and emetics, "if she can vomit easily." The new mother was also fed lightly, in order not to promote the production of *more* impure blood, until eight days passed, "about which time commonly the wombe is well purged, and cleansed."[65]

Not all bodily fluids were quite as subject as retained placenta to charges of stinking putrefaction and thus to powerful affect-formations of disgust. But as with birth itself, they may have been regarded as publicly undiscussable. In his wedding sermon, *The Bride-Bush*, William Whately alludes to this period—the "larger and longer emptying" after birth—as one of the times scripturally forbidden for sexual relations, and as one women wrongly find shameful: "Neither let women thinke themselves disgraced, because I have laid this matter open in plaine, but modest speeches."[66]

But all the first flowings after birth from womb or breast represented waste products that had to be removed, "sent forth," in order for the parturient body to return to something approximating its less effluent, nonpregnant state. Lochial flow, too, attracted a negative attention that—like so much else in these constructions of pregnancy—is strongly affected by gender. Here, the sex of the baby often determined the extent of its mother's uncleanness, the amount of her flow: "*Hippocrates*, doth proportion the time, in which a woman in child-bed should be purged, according to the time wherein the child is shaped or formed: which is 30. daies for a man-child, and 42. at most for a woman child." Guillemeau, looking for less gendered symmetry in the protocols of bodily return, suggests "the time may bee also measured according to that ordinary time of purging, that is omitted in the nine moneths she goes with child."[67] In Leviticus, of

65. Culpeper, *Directory for Midwives: Second Part*, p. 194; Guillemeau, *Child-birth*, pp. 232, 193.

66. William Whately, *A Bride-Bush, or A Wedding Sermon* (London, 1617; STC 25296; rpt. Amsterdam: Theatrum Orbis Terrarum, and Norwood, N.J.: Walter Johnson, 1975), p. 44.

67. Guillemeau, *Child-birth*, pp. 220–21.

course, the disparity is even greater—thirty-three days in the "Blood of her Purification" after delivering a boy, sixty-six for a girl.[68]

Like other first flowings after birth, the milk of a woman who had just begun this process of purification partook of her unclean state; thus, there was a widely reiterated prohibition on colostrum, the first milk, or "beestings," which, until the end of the seventeenth century, was regarded as so impure and harmful to the baby that most writers recommended it be drawn off—even by putting newborn puppies to the breasts! Valerie Fildes suggests that colostrum may have been suspected because it differed from breast milk in color and consistency.[69] Her view is supported by the attention the birth manuals give to evaluating the differential worth of breast milks by color, temperature, consistency, and "age." The uncleanness of the womb could not but contribute to the impurity of the milk. For one thing, a great sympathy or consent was thought to exist between the breast and womb; for another, breast milk was concocted from uterine blood. First milk is "naught," says Culpeper. "If the blood be impure, how can it breed good Milk? Dirty water will make but dirty Pottage."[70]

The prohibition on colostrum may be one instance where practice may have conformed to theory; certainly women who had grown up with the "familiar age-old taboo," Valerie Fildes argues, would not have defied it and would have offered their babies other possible first foods, including another woman's "older" breast milk, along with a laxative purge. Women farther removed from professional medicine may well have had no choice but to feed the newborn "beestings," but even they may have come under the influence of the taboo.[71] In either case, this rhetoric of unclean flowings from breast and womb immediately after birth can be understood as at least partially relevant to the ritual practice of "churching," the end point of the parturient woman's gradual reemergence from the hermetic enclosure of the birthing chamber. The lying-in, known as "her month," was effectively ended when the new mother went "abroad" to church, wearing a white veil and accompanied by her midwife and gossips.

---

68. Culpeper quotes Leviticus even though the rule does not conform to his own understanding of postpartum flow, which is determined rather by whether a mother nurses her baby or not: "Women that gave their children suck themselves, have them not so long as those that do not" (*Directory for Midwives*, p. 150).

69. Valerie Fildes, *Breasts, Bottles, and Babies: A History of Infant Feeding* (Edinburgh: Edinburgh University Press, 1986), pp. 84–85.

70. Culpeper, *Directory for Midwives*, p. 150.

71. Fildes, *Breasts, Bottles, and Babies*, pp. 83–85.

What churching may have meant to its participants and observers has come into dispute among social historians of the period. Keith Thomas has contended that the ceremony must presuppose the defilement of birth and the uncleanness of women because opposition to it was "one of the surest signs of Puritan feeling."[72] Adrian Wilson has insisted instead on the gendering of attitudes toward churching, noting the rite's great popularity among women across the religious spectrum despite the disapproval of Puritan husbands. He thus interprets it as a rite not of purification but rather of highly visible self-congratulation by the new mother and her birthing cohort, a female rite of thanksgiving and celebration after the physical and psychological challenges of childbearing. And it is true that the liturgical text for "the Churching of Women" emphasizes the "great pain and peril of childbirth," the great mercy of safe deliverance, without mentioning the need to purify the mother's body ritually.[73]

Powerful cultural motives do not always find textual expression, of course, particularly of matters as condemned to silence as the changing bodily states of childbearing women. What the medical literature does articulate, and powerfully, is a widespread cultural definition of the fluids emanating from the childbearing woman as highly unstable in quality and effect—capable of harm and good. In this context, the ceremony's popularity among women may argue just as forcefully for their internalization of shame and embarrassment as for their pride, relief, and self-congratulation; indeed, the two affects may be inextricable in explaining the survival of the practice despite Puritan effectiveness in removing or altering other ceremonies. Though theologians such as Thomas Comber insisted that churching could take place as soon as the new mother felt able to come to church, the ceremony's timing at the end of the lying-in month remained constant and thus continued symbolically to mark—if not explicitly to signify—a moment of bodily restoration, the cessation of flow, a social return (however temporary) to a nonpregnant state of wholeness given high cultural value.

In a culture that saw the lowering of the shame threshold in matters

---

72. Keith Thomas, *Religion and the Decline of Magic: Studies in Popular Beliefs in Sixteenth- and Seventeenth-Century England* (1971; rpt. Harmondsworth, England: Penguin, 1978), p. 69.

73. Wilson, "Ceremony of Childbirth," pp. 88–93. I quote here from John E. Booty's modern-spelling edition of the *Book of Common Prayer, 1559: The Elizabethan Prayer Book* (Charlottesville: University Press of Virginia, 1976), p. 315.

of bodily bearing and management and a widespread textualization of gynecology and obstetrics by male writers, the question of religious beliefs may have seemed irrelevant to shamed women defending against—even as they continued to internalize—the textualized constructions of bodily shame. What is clear is that a ceremony originating as a ritual of purification retained its popularity in seventeenth-century England despite the massive cultural changes wrought by the Reformation, perhaps because those changes did not include a recategorization and reconceptualization of female bodies or a reformed aesthetic of bodily beauty tolerant of changes wrought by frequent childbearing. Nor was liturgy completely silent about the reproductive capacity of an individual woman, since that section of the wedding ceremony inscribing oaths based on reproductive fertility was omitted for a woman "past the age of childbearing."[74]

Thus Guillemeau, even as he details postpartum regimens for "belly, breasts, and nether parts," thinks wistfully of a category of childbearing women completely unlike any he knows, antipodean women with a magical bodily elasticity that unwrites obstetric event, undoes the changes of birth:

> If our French Ladyes, were (in this point) like unto those, which *Vesputius Florentinus* doth write of: it would then be needles to prescribe so many medicines, for the restoring them to the same state they were in before their beeing with child. There are women (saith he) that dwell beyond the Antartique Pole, whose bodies are entire and Virgin-like, even after often child-bearing, and in whom there is perceived no difference from them that are Virgins, as they that have opened them, having made diligent search, doe testifie: But since there bee no such women found in our quarters, (though I dare boldly say, there be some, *not much different*) therfore will it be very necessary to have a care what is to be done, to their belly, breasts, and nether parts.[75]

Perceived as "not different" by whom, and "opened" (or *re*-opened) for whose purposes? In this fantasy of a female body that is not, female desirability is notable for surviving even the "often childbearing" incumbent upon "Ladyes." Absent these "Virgin-like" mothers of perpetual restoration, whose bodies in defying even the final intrusions of diligent anatomists retain this element of desirability after death, Guillemeau can only recommend old standbys for treat-

74. *Book of Common Prayer*, p. 296.
75. Guillemeau, *Child-birth*, p. 195, second emphasis added.

ing the strained and "changed" postpartum body and acknowledge the difficulty of repair: "But it is not enough onely, (especially in great Ladies) to make the foresaid parts firme and hard, and keepe them from hanging and flagging down: But it is also very fitting, and likewise much required by them, to have their skin made faire, smooth, and delicate."[76]

If for seventeenth-century men and women churching signified a ritual of purification, the purification it marked was that of the postpartum womb—the end of its postpartum flow, the complete and successful expulsion of the bodily materials stored and gradually released after birth. In the postpartum body, of course, flow from the womb is replaced by flow from the breast; but despite cultural prohibitions on the first flowings of colostrum, the lactating breast would seem in comparison to the womb the object of a far more positive, far less ambivalent affect. It appears to be part of the decorous upper bodily stratum, not the demonized lower; and (even apart from psychoanalytic theory in which it plays so large a part as first object of desire) it has always signified the infant's first source of gratification.

This is precisely what Caroline Walker Bynum has argued for medieval culture: that whereas the breast is for us primarily an erotic object, to medieval people the breast, flowing or not, signified food.[77] Because safe alternatives to mother's milk did not exist, it may have also signified health. Because of its great digestibility, breast milk was used in feeding the sick and elderly; because of its reputation for purity, it was used as an ingredient in medicines taken internally or, like eyewashes and burn ointments, applied topically. Thus, even if we allow for eroticism in the sight of a woman giving suck, Anne Hollander maintains, "its basic eroticism is always reassuringly transcended by the everyday sanctity of mother's milk. Breasts bring pleasure to everyone, and sight of them brings its own visual joy besides; and so images of breasts are always sure conveyers of a complex delight."[78] And the cultural visibility of the breast, which I noted at

76. Ibid., p. 204.
77. Caroline Walker Bynum, "The Body of Christ in the Later Middle Ages: A Reply to Leo Steinberg," *Renaissance Quarterly*, 39 (1986), 405–8. See also her *Holy Feast and Holy Fast: The Religious Significance of Food to Medieval Women* (Berkeley: University of California Press, 1987), pp. 269–70.
78. Anne Hollander, *Seeing Through Clothes* (1978; rpt. Harmondsworth, England: Penguin, 1988), p. 186.

the beginning of this chapter, would also seem to imply its safe distance from the cultural mechanisms of bodily shame.

But as recent work in the history of infant-feeding practices has made clear, the lactating breast is not simply the source of a "complex delight," and mother's milk, sanctified or not, is not only the first of foods. In lactation, even more than in the events surrounding conception, gestation, and birth, early modern culture constructed a complex hierarchy of differences between women based on social evaluations of their bodies, body products, and the aesthetic, commercial, erotic, and reproductive uses to be made of them. Both breast and milk were highly semiotized signs that, when they became part of the relations of production, were at the axiological center of several cultural economies. As such, they were no less infiltrated by the discourses of class—and thus, potentially, the cultural mechanisms of shame—than the maternal figure and its overdetermined womb.

Besides its ideological and psychological complexity, the rhetorical energy aroused by the question of maternal breast-feeding also suggests that in social classes that had a degree of personal choice, agency, and wherewithal in the matter, any infant-feeding practice was capable of contestation and challenge on a number of grounds. In religious discourse, a woman's ability to suckle her baby was promoted as separable from, but an important extension of, her ability to bear children, "the blessing of the breast" devolving from the "blessing of the womb."[79] In religious discourses, particularly after the Reformation, the mother's obligation to nurse her own child was clear; to send a child away to a nurse, in Erasmus's colloquy "The New Mother," was equivalent to "exposure": "Or isn't it a kind of exposure to hand over the tender infant, still red from its mother, drawing breath from its mother, crying for its mother's care . . . to a woman who perhaps has neither good health nor good morals and who, finally, may be much more concerned about a bit of money than about a whole baby?"[80] In seventeenth-century England, women of "stricter protestant sects" were, Fildes suggests, likelier to breast-feed.[81]

The opinion of humanist-physicians, too, was virtually unanimous

79. In *Of Domesticall Duties*, William Gouge quotes from Genesis on the two blessings: "*God shall blesse thee with the blessing of the breasts, and of the wombe.* By the blessing of the wombe, what can be meant, but children? By the blessing of the breasts, what, but milke, whereby those children are nourished?" (p. 508).

80. *The Colloquies of Erasmus*, trans. Craig Thompson (Chicago: University of Chicago Press, 1965), p. 273.

81. Fildes, *Breasts, Bottles, and Babies*, p. 99.

in recommending maternal suckling, not only because a mother's milk was thought to be naturally the correct temperature and complexion for the baby but also on the grounds that maternal suckling promoted infant-mother bonding. The *quantity* of a mother's milk might be problematic (and was a matter often addressed in popular medical texts), but its *quality*, its suitability, usually went unquestioned. Despite such injunctions, however, only aristocratic women who were "enlightened and defiant" routinely suckled their own children; most families of means sent their newborns away for a period of up to three years and visited them only occasionally during that time.[82]

Breast-feeding was an action differing semiotically from itself, depending on the class and relationship of the persons involved, on whether or not it had entered the means of production. The majority of mothers nursed their own babies out of custom and economic necessity; in so doing, they were serving food, satisfying nature, rather than exercising choice. Their action is not the topic of discourse and does not signify ethically or morally. But maternal breast-feeding becomes an ethical act as soon as it implies choice, as soon as it implies financial means to do otherwise. The upper-class mother who *chose* to nurse her own baby was performing a virtuous act of love and sacrifice, giving the "sweete milke of your owne breasts, to your owne childe."[83] The woman nursing another woman's child was engaged in remunerative labor, performed more or less faithfully, more or less responsibly. In hiring her services, parents leased exclusive rights to her lactating breasts and their milk. During the period of hire, the wet nurse was expected not to suckle another child and to maintain an adequate supply of milk. She was expected not to menstruate, not to become pregnant, and if she did, to notify her nurse-child's parents.[84]

As such details suggest, even though the breast was closely related to the womb by the physiological theory of sympathy and consent of parts, its characteristic function to give milk could be assimilated into a competitive marketplace economy, as the womb's in giving birth could not. The womb could never function as surrogate, could never be leased out; it was never, in a word, a fungible resource. As

82. I quote here from Dorothy McLaren, "Marital Fertility and Lactation, 1570–1720," in *Women in English Society, 1500–1800,* ed. Mary Prior (London: Methuen, 1985), pp. 27–28.

83. I quote here from Elizabeth Clinton, *The Countesse of Lincolnes Nurserie* (Oxford, 1628; STC 5432; rpt. Amsterdam: Theatrum Orbis Terrarum; and Norwood, N.J.: Walter Johnson, 1975), sig. A2r.

84. Fildes, *Breasts, Bottles, and Babies,* pp. 175–78.

purchasable commodities, lactating breasts and their milk possess what I would call limited fungibility. The lactating breast never completely loses the class and other attributes of the body of which it is part, thus never becomes *completely* fungible with any other woman's breast. As soon as it was offered to a baby other than the mother's own, breast milk became a commercial product that, like any other commodity, varied in quantity, quality, and availability. Medical texts, recognizing that the families they address used wet nurses despite injunctions to the contrary, specified the temperature, consistency, color, and taste of the ideal milk, even its ideal "age" calculated by the distance from the nurse's last delivery. Some of those characteristics could be determined from a nurse's complexion and coloring, others by the normality of her pregnancy and the sex of the baby she had borne, others by a series of tests on the milk itself. Nurses' breasts and nipples, too, came in more or less ideal sizes and, of course, nurses' moral and ethical qualities mattered since these were believed to be transmitted through the milk.[85] ("Thy valiantness was mine," says Volumnia to Coriolanus, "thou suck'st it from me" [3.2.129].)

In these cases, breast-feeding signified as a uniquely gendered form of labor, which, like other forms, was more or less alienable from the laborer herself and had a fluctuating, highly contingent commercial value.[86] Records of charity nursing do survive, and wet nurses would accept lower fees to nurse a child "on the parish" than they took from a paying family, especially if by doing so they would maintain their milk supply. But that a motherless newborn from a poor family was at greater risk than a wealthier orphan may be inferred from a story Joubert tells, on the reliable authority of a "learned and expert physician" friend, about the five-month-old orphan of a poor woman saved from inevitable starvation by being nursed miraculously for a year by its young cousin. Joubert wants to show "that a virgin is able to produce milk," not—as his narrative

85. Ibid., p. 168–78.
86. It is much easier to demonstrate this contention for Renaissance Florence, where wet-nursing was a highly regulated institution and, thanks to the obsessive record keeping of Florentine heads of households, thoroughly documentable from the quattrocento on. See Christiane Klapisch-Zuber, "Blood Parents and Milk Parents: Wet Nursing in Florence, 1300–1530," in *Women, Family, and Ritual in Renaissance Italy*, trans. Lydia Cochrane (Chicago: University of Chicago Press, 1985), pp. 138–39, for a statistical correlation of nurse's wages and length of service with sex and birth order of her nurselings.

suggests to me—the thorough commodification of breast milk.[87] Thus, the important question of who fed whose baby what in this period—a question, crudely put, of who controls the use and management of any woman's breast and its milk as social, aesthetic, or erotic resources—is one that cannot be easily answered without recourse to complex variables of a family's class and location, the baby's sex and birth order, and the sometimes ambiguous erotic or even narcissistic investments of its parents. The management of infant feeding becomes no less a question of patriarchal disposition and power than the question of female fertility to which it is intimately, and causally, related.

Indeed, it is a telling irony in the history of childbearing and infant feeding in the period that the childbirth practices of married women in the lower and middling classes may have been healthier, that is, more conducive to an early return of health, strength, and muscle tone, than those of women hierarchically above them, and may have promoted physically healthier intergenesic intervals. This is true primarily for two reasons, one being the invalidism enforced on, if not also sought by, upper-class women but clearly not available in the same degree to women returning perforce to household tasks. The other is the class-based practices of infant feeding that by and large discouraged upper-class women and those who would imitate them from nursing their own babies. In fact, the institution of wet-nursing enforced a major, paradoxical difference of empowerment between women of different stations, since women from wet-nursing classes had the opportunity to use lactation to control their own family size and limit the number of babies they would bear.[88] Prolonging the period of lactation by accepting a nurse-child and suckling it not on schedule but on demand, the lactating woman effectively minimizes her chances of conceiving again soon, while adding to her household income. The aristocratic woman, belonging to a class that valued and praised high fertility, would experience many more pregnancies than her lower-class counterpart during the same reproductive span—

87. Joubert, *Popular Errors*, pp. 207, 204.
88. The historical basis for these claims—if not the sense of irony to be drawn from the evidence—is the groundbreaking work of Dorothy McLaren in a series of stunning articles: "Fertility, Infant Mortality, and Breast Feeding in the Seventeenth Century," *Medical History* 22 (1978), 378–96; "Nature's Contraceptive: Wet-Nursing and Prolonged Lactation: The Case of Chesham, Buckinghamshire, 1578–1601," *Medical History* 23 (1979), 426–41; and "Marital Fertility and Lactation," pp. 22–46.

perhaps as the desired effect of a choice, more or less passive, more or less her own, not to breast-feed, a decision not to be barren even temporarily; but she would risk a higher rate of mortality for herself and her babies.[89]

Breast-feeding was widely assumed to be more difficult as well as more burdensome for the aristocratic woman. To make herself totally available to nurse an infant on demand—the most common form of breast-feeding in the period—was to remove herself from social circulation, and to risk the premature aging and wrinkling that was commonly associated with suckling.[90] Writers recognized that lower-class women by and large ignored—or could not obey—the prohibition on suckling their babies soon after birth with first milk, apparently without harmful consequences. We now realize the valuable properties of colostrum in promoting the excretion of meconium and in protecting newborns against gastrointestinal distress. Medical writers, however, Joubert especially, tended to perceive this social difference as natural, as the physiology of class objectively at work:

> These children are of a robust constitution, born of mothers and fathers who were nourished coarsely. Such nursing cannot harm these people. But for city people, who are nourished more delicately, and for all who have the wherewithal to give their children better nourishment, this observation is most important and must be followed: for two days at the very least the child must not be nursed by its mother.[91]

Such recommendations may sound strange to late twentieth-century Americans, who are not only thoroughly acculturated to the primary erotic signification of the breast but may also be ideologically attuned to the breast-feeding movement of the past few decades. It is therefore useful to be instructed in the physical and psychological complexities of breast-feeding in the centuries before antibiotics and modern lingerie, when another woman could be paid to do it. As

89. McLaren, "Marital Fertility and Lactation," pp. 27–28.

90. Fildes, *Breasts, Bottles, and Babies*, p. 100. Note the complaint voiced in 1603 by Fulke Greville the elder to Lady Anne Newdigate that "you wyll styll contynew a nurse & by [that] meanes hold backe from such as much love & desyre your company: Ytt wyll besydes make age grow upon you & I wyshe you alweys greene & floryshinge as you wer when you were in your pryme"; see *Gossip from a Muniment Room: Being Passages in the Lives of Anne and Mary Fytton, 1574 to 1618*, ed. Lady Newdigate-Newdegate (London: David Nutt, 1897), p. 52.

91. Joubert, *Popular Errors*, p. 202.

Valerie Fildes has suggested, the number of pages in seventeenth-century receipt books and medical and midwifery treatises devoted to care of the breasts and nipples implies a high incidence of breast infections and indicates the number of painful and potentially disfiguring diseases breasts and nipples were prone to. Breasts became marked by infections and abscesses, nipples scarred over because of infected cuts or might even be completely lost either because of ulceration or because "older children chewed them off." When milk supply is insufficent, a hungry baby will "mump," or bite, the nipple. Popular medical texts included instructions for the rebuilding of nipples, a process which may or may not have been successful, and suggestions on how to continue nursing even without them. Though complete loss of the nipple may have been unusual, the painful experience of nursing with cracked or bleeding nipples cannot have been. Furthermore, if a new mother waited the recommended eight days or so before nursing her baby, she would have experienced a great deal of pain from engorged and distended breasts, as would postpartum women trying to suppress lactation altogether. Having such a breast or seeing such a breast, perhaps even feeding from such a breast, would not simply "bring pleasure."[92]

The point I wish to make is that Anne Hollander's idea of the lactating breast in representation as the visual signifier of even a *complex* delight works to occlude an important material and medical history, not to mention a series of competing psychoanalytic paradigms, all of which work to call that delight into question or at least to implicate it in the discourses and practices of class difference. Cultural forces may influence even the ostensibly anatomical: the unusually high number of English women reportedly unable to nurse because of inverted nipples may be the result of fashion in the fashionable classes, the practice of corseting the bosoms of even little girls and flattening the bodices after puberty. The preacher Henry Smith, though, is skeptical that genuine physical difficulty was ever a function of class. "But whose breasts," he asks sarcastically, "have this perpetual drought? Forsoothe it is like the goute, no beggars may have it, but citizens or Gentlewomen."[93]

There is no way to ascertain if breast disease or disfigurement in the period can be significantly correlated to class (beyond the possible

92. Fildes, *Breasts, Bottles, and Babies*, pp. 100–102.
93. Henry Smith, *Four Sermons* (London, 1598; STC 22747.5), quoted in Fildes, *Breasts, Bottles, and Babies*, p. 101.

effects of costume just noted), certainly by comparison to the clear correlation between social rank and infant-feeding practices. Furthermore, as Guillemeau's emphasis upon the cosmetic measures required by great ladies in a passage quoted earlier suggests, the bodily changes, including lactation, wrought by childbearing may have been experienced differently—or weighted differently—by women in different classes. The return to bodily beauty which is the desired result of the French doctor's "many medicines" may have been of much greater consequence to the woman of rank. Even the return to health—though presumably important to any woman—would matter in different ways to women of leisure or labor. And it seems reasonable to infer that aesthetic and erotic investment in unblemished breasts might also signify as a matter of social difference. Joubert acknowledges the conflict between the breast's erotic and nurturing functions in his "exhortation" to mothers on behalf of maternal breast-feeding: "There are also some husbands who do not wish to allow their wives to nurse so that their breasts will not sag but stay prettier, the way they want them to be for caressing. There are others who hate the smell of milk on their wives' bosoms." But this disgust does not extend, he argues, to the body of the nurse, whose erotic appeal seems to be a function of her maternal bodiliness: "Most of those who say such things make love to the nurse more often than to their wives. The sagging breasts of the *nurse*, or the smell of milk on *her*, do not disgust them."[94] Such a husband has the means to exercise erotic choice, even if he does so (according to Joubert) hypocritically. He has made the breasts on his wife's body an exclusively erotic object of desire, without foreclosing the erotic potential or sexual availability of the maternal body of the nurse in his employ. In both cases, the breast is a resource under his patriarchal management and definition in a way that suggests a potential class inflection in female desirability.

Joubert's fiction reflects what Anne Hollander, in her history of the representation of the breast, describes as a newly eroticized interest and signification, a new deemphasis of the maternal agencies of the breast. In representation, the ideal breast became larger, rounder, altogether more emphatic in the seventeenth century. Extreme decolletage, which before had flattened the bosom, now sometimes bared it altogether. One might think of the emphatically displayed breasts and semiexposed nipples of the masquing ladies depicted by

94. Joubert, *Popular Errors*, pp. 200–201, emphasis added.

Inigo Jones, or even of the unusual, controversial fashion for complete breast exposure in the years just before and after 1610. In sixteenth-century visual conventions, furthermore, nipples became "another paired element of feminine decor, like earrings or false eyelashes," cosmetically reddened to contrast more sharply with the artificially whitened face and breast.[95]

Even with such changes in erotic signification, however, the beautiful breast throughout the Renaissance and the baroque period was always "delicate and minimal." Heavy, sagging breasts, Hollander remarks, "are shown to be characteristic of ugly old women and witches."[96] Images such as the one wrinkled breast with its long nipple which is bared by Albrecht Dürer's witchlike allegorization of Avarice, an obvious inversion of the visual trope of the single bared breast of the idealized female figure, imply that having heavy, sagging breasts is shameful. Their display is also potentially comic, as in the parade of half-dressed women flocking to Eleanor Rumming's "wyth theyr nake pappes, / That flyppes and flappes, / It wygges and it wagges, / Like tawny saffron bagges."[97] In his dictionary, Cotgrave gives the large, heavy breast semiotic distinction and particularity by identifying a cluster of separate signifiers in French related to *tete* or *tetin*. The powerful negative affect of this breast as an emblem of deeroticization and bodily debasement underlies the rhetorical energy of his definitions. Thus, he lists *tetasse*, "a long, swagging, flaggie, withered, and filthie dug; whence, *Avallé en tetasse de vielle*. Hanging down like the wrinckled, and ouglie breast of an old hag." Or his definitions for *tetassier* or *tetineux*, meaning "duggie, having great or long dugs."[98] The large breast is the female metonymy not only of age but of shame and thus of a specifically gendered form of social and bodily inferiority.

95. Hollander, *Seeing Through Clothes*, pp. 194–99; the quotation appears on p. 198. On the fashion for complete breast exposure, see Donald W. Foster, "'Shall I Die': Post Mortem: Defining Shakespeare," *Shakespeare Quarterly* 38 (1987), 71–73. I am indebted to Barbara Mowat for this reference. James T. Henke, too, refers to this fashion; see his entry for *Naked paps*, in *Gutter Life and Language in the Early "Street" Literature of England: A Glossary of Terms and Topics Chiefly of the Sixteenth and Seventeenth Centuries* (West Cornwall, Conn.: Locust Hill Press, 1988), pp. 170–71.

96. Hollander, *Seeing Through Clothes*, p. 98.

97. From the anonymous "Pimlyco, or Runne Red-Cap" (1609), included by James Henke, sub *Naked paps*, in *Gutter Life and Language*, pp. 170–71. The author attributes the lines to Skelton.

98. Randle Cotgrave, *A Dictionarie of the French and English Tongues* (London, 1611; STC 5830; rpt. Menston, England: Scolar Press, 1968). When citing Cotgrave, I have retained his usage and spelling.

Focus upon the attributes of the ugly breast is a feature, as well, of the counterblazons of courtly verse, which work dialogically against the counterposed praise of the idealized mistress's beautiful breast.[99] But while this emphasis on the ugliness of the heavy, sagging breast seems disproportionate, it suggests an expansion of the disciplinary regime from the lower parts upward to include the breasts, perhaps in order to protect so visible an erotic site from metonymic contamination by association with reproduction. This is precisely what is suggested by the contrasted images of the "good" and "bad" breasts of Charissa and Duessa in *The Faerie Queene*. So overdetermined are sagging breasts that Spenser gives them to the disrobed Duessa, whose "dried dugs, like bladders lacking wind, / Hong downe, and filthy matter from them weld" (1.8.47).[100] Metonymy transforms these breasts into the lower parts, an oozing, excretory bladder-womb, an image of disease and projected oral frustration and deprivation. And Duessa's body represents a second biological stage of mother Error, suckling her "thousand yong ones" with "poisonous dugs" (1.1.15). Duessa's breasts replace the reproductive organs that Spenser refuses to describe: "My chaster Muse for shame doth blush to write" (1.8.48). Charissa, by contrast, is an image of conspicuous maternal display and boundless availability: "Her necke and breasts were ever open bare, / That ay thereof her babes might sucke their fill" (1.10.30). It is hard to imagine that such impossibly bountiful breasts would *not* sag or otherwise betray the signs of aging so feared by socially conscious opponents of maternal breast-feeding; but by denying them the particularity of description he devotes to Duessa's "bad" breasts, Spenser effaces the issue altogether and allows Charissa's breasts to be beautiful, and maternal, and perhaps even erotic. Medical history suggests, however, that unblemished, beautiful breasts like Charissa's might not have been easily obtained by *any* childbearing woman in the seventeenth century, whether or not she suckled her own children. And possessing them, in order to approach an ideal of female beauty so powerfully and widely inscribed, positively and negatively, might well have been a matter of far greater

99. Laqueur makes this point about the contrasted breasts as well in a somewhat different context, in *Making Sex*, p. 130. We are both indebted here to the work of Nancy Vickers, especially to "Diana Described: Scattered Woman and Scattered Rhyme," in *Writing and Sexual Difference*, ed. Elizabeth Abel (Chicago: University of Chicago Press, 1982), pp. 95–109.

100. I quote here from *The Faerie Queene*, ed. A. C. Hamilton (London: Longman, 1977).

importance to the frequently pregnant woman in high or aspirant ranks.[101] One seventeenth-century gentlewoman's household compendium, in addition to its conventional prescriptions for sore breasts, includes a recipe for how to keep breasts small.[102] For such women, the constantly available naked breast of Charissa may have been as fearsome a prospect as the dried and oozing bladder-dugs of Duessa.

Thus, though it was much more visible than the reproductive organs, perhaps *because* it was more visible, the breast is not protected, semiotically or discursively, from the negative affects attaching to the bodily changes of reproduction. The breast, by virtue of its great "sympathy" with the womb, becomes implicated in the mysterious changes and events that made the womb so threatening and unstable an environment. Like the womb, the breast was thought capable of housing bizarre objects: Culpeper cites the authority of Lemnius for breasts containing "hair, stones, and worms."[103] Gynecological texts narrate stories of women pissing milk and lactating menstrual blood; they elaborate the conditions, such as immoderate desire, which trouble milk. And Joubert even compares milk to semen, "the benign excrement, as the substance of semen is that of members." Even nipples are subject to distinctly problematic semiosis. According to Joubert, they were popularly thought to be telltale signifiers of socially critical changes in a woman's sexual status or age.[104] He denies that they are, but Culpeper confidently reports that nipples are "blew in them that give suck; black in old women; and in them that have known Venery, it is natural, and red as a Strawberry." Discoloration of the nipples, moreover, is a reliable sign of disorder in the womb.[105]

At this point, it is possible to ask whether such ambivalent attention to the breast implies a new anxiety: if breast and nipples can be made more beautiful through cosmetics, then breast and nipple au naturel become plain and less erotic. More crucial, the literature of medicine and "popular error" links the breast with threatening forms of bodily

101. See Ellen Chirelstein's discussion of the "pearl-like" white skin and exposed left breast of Lady Elizabeth Pope in her wedding portrait: "Lady Elizabeth Pope: The Heraldic Body," in *Renaissance Bodies: The Human Figure in English Culture, c. 1540–1660*, ed. Lucy Gent and Nigel Llewellyn (London: Reaktion, 1990), p. 47.

102. Katherine Packer, *A Book of Very Good Medicines for Several Diseases Wounds and Sores both New and Old* (1639; Folger Ms. V.a. 387), f. 10. I owe this reference to Patricia Crawford.

103. Culpeper, *Directory for Midwives*, p. 216.

104. Joubert, *Popular Errors*, pp. 206, 209.

105. Culpeper, *Directory for Midwives: Second Part*, p. 223.

mutability. To protect the breast from such mutability is the characteristic impulse of Petrarchan discourse, invoking metonymies—lilies, ivory, snow—that eroticize the beloved's breasts by keeping them from the unstable contaminations of milk, of flow, of change. The larger point is that the question with which I began—who fed whose infant what—was never a personal, medical, economic question only. It was always a function of competing interests that were aesthetic, social, class-based, medical. The aristocratic woman had a whole set of material choices her social inferior did not, but a set of ideological constraints as well. For her, breast-feeding signified as an act of choice, as it did not for most women, but the nature of that choice is extremely difficult to reconstruct historically. She also had the expectation—her own, her husband's, her status group's—of being frequently pregnant. She may have chosen *not* to suckle her infants because to do so would delay a next conception, or would involve her in what had come increasingly to signify remunerative labor, or to avoid the risk of having less beautiful, much larger breasts, of becoming a prematurely old woman with shamefully great dugs. In making such a choice, such a woman undertook the reproductive labor only she could do and allowed the work of the womb to supplant the work of the breast.

ᕲ

An unstable oscillation between shame and celebration, I suggest, constitutes the affective polarities of pregnancy, birth, and infant-feeding practices in early modern culture. One way to test out this thesis (and introduce the thematics of birth in English dramatic literature) is to look at a Renaissance narrative that plays boldly with representational conventions of birth—the "strange nativity of Gargantua"—and at two modern readings that, by making Rabelais's narrative symbolic of large-scale ideological struggle, fail to account for the local, material contests to which even the most textualized of births refer. The two readers are Mikhail Bakhtin and Stephen Greenblatt, whose accounts of Rabelais's obstetrical carnival I want to complicate and ironize. I offer instead a deliberately literal and unamused feminist rereading of this episode, which I hereby rename "the strange lying-in of Gargamelle."[106]

106. I quote here from François Rabelais, *Gargantua and Pantagruel*, trans. J. M. Cohen (Harmondsworth, England: Penguin, 1955), pp. 48, 51–52. Subsequent quotations will be cited parenthetically. Bakhtin's reading occurs in *Rabelais and His World*, pp. 225–27; and Greenblatt's in "Filthy Rites," *Daedalus*, 111 (1982), pp. 1–16.

The scene early in Rabelais's novel begins with the Shrovetide feast of a slaughtered calf and a labor brought on by Gargamelle's enthusiastic consumption of tripe. It ends—at least for our vision of Gargamelle herself—when the baby Gargantua, finding his passage down the birth canal blocked by his mother's prolapsed lower bowel, makes his own way out of the maternal body through the left ear. In Rabelais's celebration of "the merry, abundant, and victorious bodily element" here engaged in a parodic reenactment of heroic birth, Bakhtin sees emergent humanism's triumph over "the serious medieval world of fear and oppression." The labor of Gargamelle's womb, like other events in the novel, becomes the token of an ideological struggle between popular-festive cultural forms and the variously repressive forces of officialdom, here thwarted by the indisputable carnality of birth itself and by the celebratory frankness of Rabelais's insistent identifications of shitting with the birth of heroes, animal tripe with human tripe, feces with baby hero.[107]

But within Bakhtin's account of that triumph, the laboring woman herself seems to play little part. Bakhtin displays no interest in Gargamelle as a possible subject-in-the-body—however limited and exteriorized a subject she may be—in part because he fails to see the relevance of gender to his account of the lower bodily stratum:

All the images develop the theme of the feast: slaughter of cattle, disemboweling, dismemberment. The images continue to unfold along the lines of a banquet: devouring of the dismembered body. They are later transferred to the anatomic description of the generating womb. These images create with great artistry an extremely dense atmosphere of the body as a whole in which all the dividing lines between man [sic] and beast, between the consumed and consuming bowels are intentionally erased. On the other hand, these consuming and consumed organs are fused with the generating womb. We thus obtain a truly grotesque image of one single, superindividual bodily life, of the great bowels that devour and are devoured, generate and are generated.[108]

That Rabelais was both humanist and physician cannot be coincidental to his informed account of birth processes, or to the scatological punishment he invokes for anyone who finds it implausible. Bakhtin's reading of the lying-in of Gargamelle, however, almost explicitly ignores the meaningful features of anatomical difference be-

107. Bakhtin, *Rabelais and His World*, p. 226.
108. Ibid.

tween the "representative" male body and the specific reproductive organs of the female. His erasure of gender as an ascriptive category within carnivalesque theory simplifies the possible complex of meanings for, contested interests in, this childbirth carnival.[109] Certainly for Bakhtin, the comic force of Rabelais's image of the all-generating womb triumphantly subsumes any meaning framed by or grounded in individual consciousness. Furthermore, he finds the loss of distinction here between belly and womb, digestion and reproduction affirmative for popular partisans of the festive body, as part of the general imagery of the feast. But this loss also serves to erase the gender-specificity of the womb's function, the exclusively female aspect of carnival. Men and women gorge on tripe at Shrovetide feasts like this one, but only women give birth. Eating too much tainted tripe could give almost anyone indigestion or even a prolapsed bowel, but the bellyache can stimulate the greater pain of labor only in pregnant women. Thus, the contest for evacuation from Gargamelle's body—a contest between the baby and the tainted tripe for different bodily thresholds, here collapsed into one—registers for Bakhtin not as a seriocomic image of the birth pain that only women feel but as an image of cosmic process: "Looming beyond Gargamelle's womb [is] the devoured and devouring womb of the earth and the ever-regenerated body of the people."[110]

I think we should resist a reading that so easily elides one woman's laboring womb with the symbolically abstract "womb" of mother earth and tacitly privileges what does remain visually distinct in the Rabelaisian image of birth—the phallic upthrusting of the individualistic baby boy who chooses *not* to be born through his mother's vagina. If Gargamelle's womb is a signifier for the abstract, life-affirming signifieds of earth's womb, it also functions as a textual signifier for *actual* wombs and their hard, painful work in giving birth. It is thus not clear on what basis Stephen Greenblatt excuses either Rabelais or Bakhtin from the charge of celebrating "transcendence of the human condition—*inter urinas et faeces nascimur.*" He says, "The birth of Gargantua celebrates a primal, animal energy, difficult to moralize

109. This is not a novel complaint against Bakhtin. See Peter Stallybrass's acknowledgment of Bakhtin's assumption of an "'ungendered,' i.e., implicitly male body," in "Patriarchal Territories: The Body Enclosed," in *Rewriting the Renaissance: The Discourses of Sexual Difference in Early Modern Europe*, ed. Margaret W. Ferguson, Maureen Quilligan, and Nancy J. Vickers (Chicago: University of Chicago Press, 1986), p. 125.
110. Bakhtin, *Rabelais and His World*, p. 226.

conventionally, and impossible to contain."[111] Something else seems equally clear to this feminist reader: the site so elegantly identified and erased through Latin allusion is the only bodily threshold peculiar to woman. Although woman is not responsible for the location of the birthing site, she may still find shame in it. As Nicholas Culpeper notes tendentiously: "The neck of the womb is seated between the passage of Urin and the right Gut, to shew fond man what little reason he hath to be proud and domineer, being conceived between the places ordained to cast out excrements, the very sinks of the Body, and in such a manner that *his Mother* was ashamed to tell him how."[112]

Whereas Rabelais's representation of birth comedy may celebrate the products of the lower bodily stratum, it does so by setting carnival within, not against the hierarchical structures of gender difference. The episode of Gargamelle's labor and Gargantua's birth thematizes the opposition of male culture against female nature, male control and individuation against female uncontrol and the undifference of bowel and womb. Furthermore, Bakhtin's symbolic reading converts the local, material contests surrounding childbirth and lactation into large-scale structural oppositions. Thus the lavish hospitality incumbent upon Grandgousier as host and master of the feast requires him to encourage the appetites of his guests, but his patriarchal interest in his wife's pregnancy seeks to limit her consumption, to discipline her appetite: "Anyone who eats the bag . . . might just as well be chewing dung" (48). Gargamelle's refusal to curb festive appetite for the sake of her pregnancy becomes an effect of the notorious gluttony and irrationality of pregnancy itself, rendered clearly symptomatic by the swelling of tripes within her. Two modes of bodily license—the license of carnival and the license of pregnancy—converge here. Even in so primitive a society, the privileges of the pregnant woman destabilize the hierarchy that pits patriarchal restraint against female desire. What was once a union of the sexes—the union in coitus—leads to separation at childbearing, as when the conversation between the giant king and queen at the onset of labor contrasts the mutuality of their pleasure to the gendered separation of pleasure from pain nine months later: "I shall have trouble enough to-day, unless God helps me," Gargamelle tells her husband, "all on account of your member and just because I wanted to please you" (51–52).

111. Greenblatt, "Filthy Rites," p. 7.
112. Culpeper, *Directory for Midwives*, pp. 25–26, emphasis added.

Rabelais insists on two comic inversions in this birth—both of them focusing attention on changes in Gargamelle's womb. The midwives first mistake the prolapse of Gargamelle's lower bowel—presenting as "some rather ill-smelling excrescences" (52)—for the crowning of the baby. Then, in responding to the birth obstruction the chief midwife applies too powerful an astringent to Gargamelle's sphincter muscles. The womb next door overreacts, closing its lower passage and opening at the upper end, so that Gargantua's escape up through his mother's body is, at least inferentially, an escape from the messy scatological drama going on below. To the degree that such scatological mess is an obvious comic substitution for the normal "mess" of childbirth, Gargantua may be said to have escaped the Augustinian shame of ordinary birth between urine and feces, a shame his mother's delight in tripe particularized. Such a clean birth is the result not of the womb's expulsive powers—here much compromised by Gargamelle's gluttony and her midwives' mishandling of the prolapsed bowel—but of the rebellious, upward thrust of the phallic hero.

Bakhtin's lack of interest in the experience of Gargamelle merely follows the narrative's shift of focus away from laboring mother to upwardly mobile child. Its effect is to occlude the obstetrical drama of an impeded delivery, an obstetrical drama that—as the humanist-physician knew well—was the unhappy, often unavoidable fate of ordinary women in travail. One way to counter Bakhtin's reading is thus to complicate his simple picture of Rabelais's celebration of bodily function. However implausible Gargantua's route to daylight may be at one level, Rabelais does not set aside physiological "facts" or the gendered rivalries of Renaissance medical practice between university-trained male physicians and the *saiges femmes* who attended at births. I noted the narrative use he makes of the monstrous appetites of pregnancy. Though the sudden and unexpected onset of Gargamelle's labor results in an unusual delivery *sur l'herbe*, many ordinary birthing procedures, such as the exclusion of male witnesses, seem to obtain. The host of midwives who suddenly appear, summoned as if by instinct on hearing Gargamelle's cries, displace the father at the scene; take instruction from their senior member, "a dirty old hag of the company" with a reputation "of being a good she-doctor" (52); experience difficulty in recognizing birth processes or managing complicated presentations; and intervene too aggressively in response to obstetrical obstruction. The violent reaction of

Gargamelle's womb follows Galenic understanding of uterine behavior in response to unpleasant local applications: "The Matrice flyeth from any thing that is of a bad savour."[113]

And Gargantua's upward passage through his mother's body gains some anatomical plausibility from the understanding that the passages of the womb were thought to communicate more or less directly with the cranial passages, the nose and mouth above. In one test for conception, "if she receive below any strong or stinking oder or smell, . . . and the sent pierce not up into her nose, she hath conceived."[114] A garlic placed in the vagina could not be smelled the next morning on the breath of a pregnant woman.

It is not accidental, then, that the baby born so energetically and willfully at the tripe feast is a boy or that his phallicly modeled purposiveness is so clearly contrasted to the "extremely dense atmosphere" (in Bakhtin's phrase) of his mother's blurry lower parts. I cannot imagine that Gargamelle's *daughter* would have had the option of so privileged an escape. Here is yet another difference, one the obstetrical texts could not account for, of the manifold differences the baby's sex makes in the entire birth process from conception to weaning. Here the fact of Gargantua's maleness powerfully genders the contrast between his Herculean routing of his own birth and his mother's loss of bowel control. The increasingly depersonalized Gargamelle is not the subject of her own obstetrical drama, and she is only barely responsible for the production of her own shit. And if she is rendered invisible as an agent in her own body (the process key to her son's subsequent education), that body is itself subject to an unusual, perhaps not entirely comic exposure at a moment of acute physical challenge ordinarily barred from public view or textual encoding. We might even suggest that such comic exposure of women's "privities" is precisely what printer-physician Thomas Raynalde worried so anxiously about in the preface to his gynecological tract. Thus to say with Bakhtin that this is exactly the point of Rabelais's creation of "an extremely dense atmosphere of the body as a whole" simply ignores the difference gender makes even in the midst of carnival and reproduces the occlusion of mother in the triumphant emergence of son.

Just as Gargantua's strange nativity must also be Gargamelle's strange lying-in, so the experience and meanings of bodily processes

113. Guillemeau, *Child-Birth*, p. 244.
114. Ibid., p. 6.

at birth cannot be understood solely within the critical framework of carnival. The collisions of patriarchal restraint and female privilege, the determinacy of gender, the nature of personal agency, even the sometimes radical uncertainty of any obstetrical outcome—themes that work powerfully in Rabelais's comedy to complicate the meaning of carnival—also provide the central problematics for understanding early modern birth and infant-feeding narratives. It is to their representation in drama that I now, finally, turn.

CHAPTER FIVE

QUARRELING WITH THE DUG,

or I Am Glad You Did Not Nurse Him

E arly modern culture in England and elsewhere, I have been arguing, constructed pregnancy as disease, birth as evacuation, and lactation as a possibly demeaning form of labor. Within this general paradigm, women were offered a deeply ambivalent image of their own reproductive functions and their control of birth and infant-feeding practices. Recent comparisons of reproductive rituals to the structure of carnival, seeking to devalue the depth and significance of this ambivalence, serve to explain it instead. As Adrian Wilson and others have argued, carnival does offer a theoretical model of female empowerment at the scene of birth. But as my critique of Bakhtin's celebratory reading of Gargantua's "strange nativity" in the previous chapter sought to make clear, carnival necessarily implies the contingency of that empowerment. Even within the hermetic enclosures of the womb, the birthing chamber, and the nursing dyad, patriarchy continued to deploy the disciplinary mechanisms of shame and thus to manage the female bodiliness so visible in the symptomatology of pregnancy and lactation.

In this chapter, I want to consider what dramatic encodings of maternal functions may signify in a historical context provided by the practices of wet-nursing, the institutionalization of parental surrogacy, and the complex, ambivalent semiosis of breast and womb I

have constructed. Many Elizabethan-Jacobean plays could be—
indeed, have been—deployed in such an interrogation, *Macbeth* perhaps being the most familiar, thanks to Lady Macbeth's unforgettable
image of murderous weaning:

> I have given suck, and know
> How tender 'tis to love the babe that milks me;
> I would, while it was smiling in my face,
> Have pluck'd my nipple from his boneless gums,
> And dash'd the brains out, had I so sworn as you
> Have done to this.
>
> (1.7.54–59)

But instead of the imagery of nursing, weaning, and loss of the breast,
I want to concentrate on the sometimes obscure emplotment of birth
and other key reproductive sequences within the overall structure
and paradigmatic social inversions of the carnivalesque. The social
space for desire and bodily need which pregnancy and birth open up
for reproductive women within patriarchal culture endures to include the baby born into it. The medical texts devoted to obstetrics
and gynecology regularly end with a section, or add a concluding
book, devoted to the "nursing" of children, the discursive field having
been constituted to define both categories of subject bodies as alike.
And midwives were assumed to have responsibility for the initial care
of mother and infant both. But what is true of the desires of pregnant
women is true for the material and psychological needs of the baby as
well: they are not privileged without contestation, nor do they take
place completely away from patriarchal regulation and definition. In
the many-sided contest among and between parents, parent surrogates, and children for the gratifications of desire—the first form of
which comes at the breast—the carnivalesque opportunity for dramatic signification occurs.

Ambivalent social constructions of reproduction and infant feeding, taken together, give discursive particularity and material form to
the fear of maternal agency and competition for the maternal body so
pervasive in Elizabethan-Jacobean drama.[1] By bringing psychoanalyt-

---

1. This point has been most powerfully argued by Janet Adelman in "'Born of
Woman': Fantasies of Maternal Power in *Macbeth*," in *Cannibals, Witches, and Divorce:
Estranging the Renaissance*, ed. Marjorie Garber (Baltimore: Johns Hopkins University
Press, 1987), pp. 90–121.

ic interest in the formation of the individual subject into relation with the material and discursive history of reproductive practices, I want to suggest drama's role in shaping cultural and psychological narratives of birth and infant feeding. The plays I want to focus on here to sketch out possibilities for this role—*Romeo and Juliet, The Witch of Edmonton, Antony and Cleopatra,* and *The Winter's Tale*—either overcode aberrant forms and functions of the maternal body or defend against the regressive desire for oral dependence and symbiotic union with the maternal body. As Joel Fineman has argued, plays "constitute strategies of psychological defense, defending, that is, against the very fantasies they represent."[2] The fantasies I am most interested in concern not only the infant's earliest relationship to its care givers, a relationship centered upon the breast, but also more conscious, if no less controllable, fantasies on the part of the care givers themselves about their own and the infant's experiences. Once we allow for the psychological implications of medical and material history, these fantasies come to seem no less embedded in historical difference than the reproductive practices themselves.

If, for example, the attention medical texts paid to the care of breasts and problems of supply and demand in lactation is indicative, and given what we know of maternal mortality rates and the widespread practice of wet-nursing in the period, babies must have experienced a significantly high incidence of inconsistent, difficult, or ruptured nurture. The "benign circle" of early mother-child interactions, around which salutary being-in-the-body forms, would have been importantly affected, too, by prohibitions on maternal suckling in the first days after birth or by a baby's extrusion from the birthing chamber in the first weeks after birth to a second, and also temporary, site of nurture—the home of its nurse and her family. Furthermore, routinely to deny babies colostrum and feed them instead the "older" milk of a woman months or even years from her last delivery is to deny them important immunological protection and put them at increased risk of chronic gastrointestinal distress even before the critical weaning period. From the medical point of view alone, Valerie Fildes suggests, sending a baby out to the different ecosytem and germs of its host family would expose it to significant physical stress. No wonder the first stage of life in Jaques's Seven Ages of Man speech has the

2. Joel Fineman, "Fratricide and Cuckoldry: Shakespeare's Doubles," in *Representing Shakespeare: New Psychoanalytic Essays,* ed. Murray Schwartz and Coppélia Kahn (Baltimore: Johns Hopkins University Press, 1980), p. 73.

representative male infant "mewling and puking in the nurse's arms" (*As You Like It*, 3.1.144). Since the baby is held not by its mother but by its nurse, the image not only characterizes the satirist as disgusted by physical existence but also implies the extended gastrointestinal trauma experienced by that significant minority of wellborn infants, male and female, being sent out to nurse.[3]

Even without a theory of the unconscious and despite the empirical shortcomings of humoral medicine, some recognition of the physical and psychological significance of these effects is documentable in the controversy over maternal breast-feeding and in the lore surrounding breast milk. Nurses' milk was regularly praised or blamed for adult health of all kinds; children were known to form deep, even lifelong ties to their nurses; and at least one Jacobean will leaves a larger bequest to the daughter who was maternally breast-fed. Alice Thornton attributed her own good health as a child to the "fresh" milk of her wet nurse, who had "had a child betwixt the nursing of my brother and myself." In her own (ultimately futile) desperation to limit her losses in childbearing, she nursed her last four babies.[4] Such evidence cannot be said to document characteristic forms of early modern subjectivity or recurrent cultural narratives in any recoverable way. But the likelihood of problematic early nurturing experiences, on the part of children and their care givers, must be regarded as a significant factor in cultural hermeneutics, particularly for narrative encodings that give fetishistic attention to female reproductivity and nurturance, representing those key processes as magically enhanced, deficient, or threateningly self-enclosed.

But the desire to conceal such preoccupations is also clear: in a culture increasingly using the disciplinary mechanisms of shame to regulate physical gratification and the expression of physical need,

3. For an account of the recursive stages of what he calls the "benign circle," see D. W. Winnicott, "The Depressive Position in Normal Emotional Development," in *Collected Papers* (London: Tavistock, 1978), p. 270. Valerie Fildes gives an authoritative account of the immunological risks to the baby in *Breasts, Bottles, and Babies: A History of Infant Feeding* (Edinburgh: Edinburgh University Press, 1986), pp. 194, 200–202. That *all* babies "mewl and puke" and *have always done so* is of course true. But this baby, and other wet-nursed babies like him, have an additional, historically specific reason to do so. Most English babies of the period would have been held by their mothers; hence Jaques's speech, even at its beginning, silently excludes many English babies, male and female, from its picture of representative "humanity."

4. For the larger bequest, see E. M. Symonds, ed., "The Diary of John Greene (1635–57), Part 3," *English Historical Review* 44 (1929), 116; I owe this reference to A. R. Braunmuller. See also Fildes, *Breasts, Bottles, and Babies*, p. 100. Alice Thornton is quoted in Lucinda McCray Beier, *Sufferers and Healers: The Experience of Illness in Seventeenth-Century England* (London: Routledge and Kegan Paul, 1987), pp. 226, 232.

even unconscious fears about the loss of nurture could produce embarrassment and denial. These are precisely the motives Janet Adelman finds at work in *Coriolanus* in the protagonist's rejection of food and nurture and in associations of eating with dependency.[5] These preoccupations make historically specific psychological sense in early modern England not only because of high maternal mortality but also because, from wet-nursing right through apprenticeship, the culture so widely employed surrogacy as the institutional model for parenthood. Thus, the loss and magical return of children structuring the Jacobean romance plots may really mask a suppressed anxiety originating not from the subject position of grieving parent but from that of grieving child. That is, the romance plot may memorialize a pervasive, though clearly somewhat shameful anxiety about the loss and magical return of mother and breast, a loss for which the infant may feel in part responsible. And of course, to the wet-nursed infant, restored to his/her parental home after weaning, return may really mean a disappointing, even shaming replacement since, as I argued in the last chapter, breasts had only a *limited* fungibility even within a structure of commodified exchange and for the infant none at all.

The suspicion of withheld nurture legible in Elizabethan constructions of the Amazon, the embarrassment in needing nurture inscribed in *Coriolanus*, may well inform almost any extended emphasis on female reproductivity, references to suckling or weaning, or the deviant female bodiliness inscribed in the figure of the witch. I want above all to insist that what may seem a disproportionate emphasis on the properties of the maternal breast is grounded in, if not determined by, physical and material conditions of a kind twentieth-century Anglo-Americans may find hard to conceptualize— particularly the irreplaceability of breast milk, hence of lactating breasts, in a preindustrial age. Joubert comments on the great indulgence shown by employers to a wet nurse: "They become proud and haughty because of the great need one has for them, and this forces one's indulgence more than in the case of other servants, out of love for the child."[6] Clearly, a constraining triangulation of desire and dependency is already in place, a resentment by the employer of dependence on the essential bodily equipment of the employed.

Without being drawn into narrow overliteralism, one may infer that

5. In her now-classic essay, "'Anger's My Meat': Feeding, Dependency, and Aggression in *Coriolanus*," in *Representing Shakespeare*, pp. 129–49.

6. Laurent Joubert, *Popular Errors*, trans. and ed. Gregory David de Rocher (Tuscaloosa: University of Alabama Press, 1990), p. 230.

Miranda is said to be three years old when she and Prospero are cast adrift because that age would signify to a wet-nursing culture her graduation from physical dependency on a nurse's breast milk, an age when she could be given to and fed by her father. Indeed, the odd specificity of this detail in Prospero's narrative, along with the vagueness of Miranda's memory of female nurture and perhaps even the early abandonment of the orphaned Caliban when Sycorax dies, could be said to precondition Prospero's implicit claim to be the complete biological and social parent—sole civilizer, sole nurturer, jealous patriarch on the motherless island.[7]

Thus, the powerful male fantasy of escape from the condition of being born of woman, which surfaces so powerfully in *Macbeth*, is twinned by the equally necessary fantasy of escape from infant suckling, from dependency on the breast. The shamefulness of such dependency is widely current, as in the proverbial metonymies of dephallicized uncontrol and delayed maturation: "His mother's milk is not out of his nose."[8] The overt engenderment of this proverb, like many another, may be worth comment, for in my reading of Elizabethan culture there is nothing comparably shaming about the same proverb differently gendered—"mother's milk not out of *her* nose." (When it comes to engenderment, nose is not a nose is not a nose.) Thus, just as it is unimaginable that Gargantua's sister would be given the privilege of her brother's magical phallic escape from ordinary childbirth—or that such an escape would signify—so the gender system suggests why a naturalistic, nostalgic, ostensibly comic, but nonshaming account of a Shakespearean protagonist's weaning would be that of a girl, the three-year-old Juliet:

> 'Tis since the earthquake now aleven years,
> And she was wean'd—I never shall forget it—
> Of all the days of the year, upon that day;

7. Some of these details are mentioned by Stephen Orgel in "Prospero's Wife," though not the possible significance of Miranda's age in relation to Prospero's success as sole parent. See *Rewriting the Renaissance: The Discourses of Sexual Difference in Early Modern Europe*, ed. Margaret W. Ferguson, Maureen Quilligan, and Nancy J. Vickers (Chicago: University of Chicago Press, 1986), pp. 50–51, 54–55.

8. On the fantasy of escape from dependency on the breast, see Adelman, "'Born of Woman,'" p. 98. For the proverb, see Morris Palmer Tilley, *A Dictionary of the Proverbs in England in the Sixteenth and Seventeenth Centuries* (Ann Arbor: University of Michigan Press, 1950), M1204, p. 478. Tilley cites the following line in *Twelfth Night* as analogue: "One would think his mother's milk were scarce out of him" (1.5.161–62). Note the projection of embarrassing maternal influence over one's speech in Malvolio's contemptuous dismissal of the shrewishly speaking Cesario.

> For I had then laid wormwood to my dug,
> Sitting in the sun under the dove-house wall.
> My lord and you were then at Mantua—
> Nay, I do bear a brain—but as I said,
> When it did taste the wormwood on the nipple
> Of my dug and felt it bitter, pretty fool,
> To see it teachy and fall out wi'th'dug!
>
> (1.3.23–32)

The several reasons I have to dwell on this narrative have little to do with its ostensible comic function—to stereotype the Nurse as a tediously garrulous old woman who uses the proverbial nurse's "privilege to talk."[9] One is to note that the material history implied by this narrative replicates the early domestic environment of many wellborn Elizabethan infants and conforms in key respects to the theory of infant feeding I documented in the last chapter. This nursing relationship, like most in the period, calls a quintet of actors into being: the two "blood" parents, the two surrogate "milk" parents of nurse and husband, and the infant girl in their care.[10] Juliet, of course, is herself a surrogate for the baby Susan whose (presumably very early) death brought her mother, grieving and lactating, into the Capulets' employ, along with her now-dead husband. It is likely that the Capulets sought a nurse the "gender" of whose pregnancy matched their own and whose "new" milk would be highly desirable. Though married and presumably sexually active during the three years she nursed Juliet, the Nurse seems to have borne no other children during that time (or presumably ever again). She was, she reminds Juliet, "thine only nurse," and Juliet was "the prettiest babe that e'er I nurs'd" (67, 60). Like many an English mother of her class, she held off conception—and the end of her tenure as nurse—by suckling Juliet on demand. Though Juliet, unlike most Elizabethan babies among the elite classes, was not sent away to nurse and thus did not face the postnatal trauma of physical separation from home and biological parents, the presence of the Nurse's husband creates a second parental unit, socially subordinated but potentially subversive, within the

9. "A Nurse's tongue is privileged to talk." Tilley, *Dictionary of the Proverbs*, N 355, p. 509. The most extended discussion of the Nurse's narrative to date has been Barbara Everett's in *"Romeo and Juliet*: The Nurse's Story," *Essays on Shakespeare's Tragedies* (1972; rpt. Oxford: Clarendon Press, 1989), pp. 109–23.

10. These terms come from Christiane Klapisch-Zuber, *Women, Family, and Ritual in Renaissance Italy*, trans. Lydia Cochrane (Chicago: University of Chicago Press, 1985), p. 132.

Capulet household. It is this second, highly differentiated set of parents which in effect replicates the social circumstances of many Elizabethan nurse-children. I want to question what their inclusion here, shadowing the social outlines of the Capulets themselves, might signify. I especially want to query the distinctly gratuitous textual existence granted the Nurse's husband and his role within the two very separate, even incommensurate experiences of nurse and baby inscribed in the narrative.

That is, rather than construe the narrative typically, as symptom and proof of an old nurse's garrulity, I take it as socially expressive of a complex structure of relations in and between the members of the nursing quintet. And the social role of each member would have a valence probably far more recognizable to a wet-nursing culture than to us, for whom the most likely surrogates for mother's breast and mother's milk are a bottle and any number of substitute milks. The Nurse, hired because of her body's reproductivity, speaks a denial—conscious or not—of the fungibility of her breast or her milk, a denial that nurture can be commodified without consequence for the child or adults invested in significantly different ways in its welfare. Paradoxically, however, this denial is embedded within a narrative and a familial event representing and depending on that very fungibility—that the surrogate mother was and is a member of the household.

The narrative is paradoxical in at least one other way. A narrative of weaning, particularly a weaning by means of aversion techniques such as applying wormwood to the nipple, is almost by definition a narrative of disjunction and rupture, prima facie evidence of what has been called "woman's treachery in the feeding situation."[11] But the Nurse's reminiscence takes on perlocutionary force by embodying her silent claim to be present when mother and daughter must talk "in secret" (1.3.08). It is particularly significant for the Nurse's narrative that Juliet's parents were absent at, also perhaps oblivious to, her weaning—a biological event widely and correctly regarded as physically critical and marked here by its timing on her third birthday.[12]

11. The phrase, referring to Lady Macbeth, belongs to David B. Barron, "The Babe That Milks: An Organic Study of *Macbeth*," in *The Design Within: Psychoanalytic Approaches to Shakespeare*, ed. M. D. Faber (New York: Science House, 1970), p. 255.

12. Fildes, *Breasts, Bottles, and Babies*, pp. 200–202, 365–66. On demographic evidence for a mortality crisis at weaning, see Roger Schofield and E. A. Wrigley, "Infant and Child Mortality in England in the Late Tudor and Early Stuart period," in *Health, Medicine, and Mortality in the Sixteenth Century*, ed. Charles Webster (Cambridge: Cambridge University Press, 1979), pp. 69, 90–91. Klapisch-Zuber also devotes a section to the late weaning of wet-nursed Florentine babies, pp. 153–59.

Juliet's weaning forms a nostalgic narrative that is her nurse's alone to tell, because the weaning, which marked a far more crucial change in Juliet's relationship to her nurse than in her relationship to her parents, seems to have been her nurse's decision in timing and design. In this respect, it is hard to know whether the weaning was unusual (in ways other than its lateness, to which I shall return). The pattern of evidence suggests a baby's return to the birth parents well before the third birthday, after a decision by the parents themselves.[13] Perhaps we should understand Shakespeare's noting of this parental absence as another buried narrative of lost parents, an additional symptom of loss in a distancing narrative that seems to remember the infant's loss and trauma only as comic.

That by contemporary standards Juliet was weaned late is also susceptible to a contextual reading, for the age at weaning seems to have been emerging as a significant point of dispute. Seventeenth-century writers were increasingly less tolerant of prolonged suckling, perhaps because of an emergent sense of its incompatibility with new demands for self-mastery and self-discipline.[14] Culpeper in particular regards suckling after the first year, except for the weak child, as an unnatural dependence on the breast caused by maternal possessiveness:

> If a child be strong and lusty . . . a year is enough in all conscience for it to suck. Experience teacheth the inconvenience of childrens long sucking; Suck being ordained for children no longer, then until they can digest other food. The fondness of Mothers to children doth them more mischief then the Devil himself can do them: one part . . . of which appears in letting of them suck too long. *Unnatural food* in their infancy, and cockering in their youth will . . . make a Devil of a Saint.[15]

Woman's treachery in the feeding situation can come not only from weaning but, as Culpeper's vehemence here suggests, from the failure or even refusal to wean, transforming children from saints into devils.

13. I infer from Valerie Fildes's evidence that weaning tended to occur by prearrangement between nurses and their employers. See *Breasts, Bottles, and Babies*, pp. 379–80. Evidence for weaning of children sent out to nurse is inconclusive in the diaries anthologized by Ralph A. Houlbrooke, *English Family Life, 1576–1716: An Anthology from Diaries* (Oxford: Basil Blackwell, 1988), pp. 103–4. Sometimes the nurse herself was removed or hidden from the baby; the Josselins took in their grandchildren at this time. See Fildes, *Breasts, Bottles, and Babies*, p. 380.

14. Fildes, *Breasts, Bottles, and Babies*, p. 368. For an early application of weaning materials to Juliet, see Maynard Mack, *Rescuing Shakespeare*, International Shakespeare Association Occasional Paper, no. 1 (Oxford: 1979), pp. 10–11.

15. Nicholas Culpeper, *A Directory for Midwives* (London, 1671; Wing C 7492), p. 159, emphasis added.

The lateness of Juliet's weaning may explain why the Nurse used the aversion technique, not much recommended by authorities except for older babies who were understood to be harder to take from the breast. Thus, as a last resort to wean a child still "very eager after it," Guillemeau advises, "You must make him loath it, annointing the Nurses breast with Mustard, or else rubbing the top of the nipple with a little Aloes, and likewise make him *ashamed* of it."[16] If we are invited to critique the Nurse's comic distance from the child's weaning—and such an invitation is possible given the length and elaborateness of her memorial narrative—we should also remember the duration of the Nurse's bodily commitment to the baby. Suckling on demand seems to have been the norm both in theory and, insofar as it can be documented, in practice. Because this practice subordinated the nurse to the baby's needs and schedule, it probably offered the greatest single motivation to both upper-class parents to send a baby out to nurse. The irony here, of course, is that the cultural requirement—so accommodating for the baby's needs—to suckle on demand rather than to institute a more or less fixed feeding schedule may have been what most worked to separate babies from their mothers and tie them to their nurses, at least until weaning and extrusion/return. The lateness of Juliet's weaning may suggest fragile health or underscore her importance as the sole surviving Capulet heir, but it certainly signifies the physical interdependence of nurse and baby or—for the Nurse herself—a physical and emotional subordination to the baby directly resulting from her social subordination to the parents. A change in the nature of that bodily subordination is what the weaning may mean for the Nurse qua nurse, a transition to the less demanding forms of nurture she has been occupied with ever since.

Perhaps more to the point, though, is that the narrative offers itself in interesting ways to two kinds of psychoanalytic readings: one, a quasi-Lacanian reading about the subject's loss of relation to the imaginary dyad, here varied (in perhaps un-Lacanian ways) to include Juliet's relation to both the Nurse and the "merry man" (1.3.40) who was the Nurse's husband; the other, a reading within an object-relations paradigm that underlines the Nurse's maternal presence, "holding the situation," as the baby experiences the successive bodily and psychic traumas of injury, weaning, and earthquake.[17] In both

16. Jacques Guillemeau, *The Nursing of Children* (London, 1612; STC 12496; rpt. Amsterdam: Da Capo Press, 1972), p. 27, emphasis added.

17. For Lacan's narrative of enculturation, see, for example, "The Signification of the Phallus," in *Ecrits: A Selection*, ed. and trans. Alan Sheridan (New York: Norton,

interpretations, however, Lady Capulet has a distinctly diminished and occluded role between the symbolic poles represented by the Nurse and old Capulet.

Thus the narrative is structured dramatically as a text occurring within the social space between the two hierarchically differentiated mothers, between the two forms of motherhood institutionalized in Elizabethan culture: the social legitimation founded in Lady Capulet as undisputed biological mother, as nonfungible, originating womb, and the surrogate nurture offered by the Nurse's body and breast between birth and weaning. Lady Capulet's absence from the scene of weaning should be taken as emblematic of her physical, hence emotional withdrawal from Juliet after birth and her replacement by the Nurse. Since a second separation from the surrogate maternal body ordinarily returned a baby to *both* her biological parents, the two sets of parents and the difference between *them* enact the Lacanian narrative of enculturation. Here, the Capulets together occupy the place of the phallocentric Law of the Father into which Juliet must fall, the Nurse and her husband the preoedipal fantasy of Imaginary symbiotic union out of which Juliet must be propelled into subjectivity or "lack-in-being." Class hierarchy, in other words, structuring the baby's movement "up" from its nursing parents to its social parents in the sequence of events from birth to weaning, takes over for or seriously complicates the phallogocentric operations of gender binarism. Because the Nurse and her husband, as a unit within the household, are subordinate, they occupy the place of woman in the binary operations of patriarchal culture. To put it the other way round, the lower class occupies the place of the body, the space of the presocial, for the wet-nursed baby in Elizabethan narratives of enculturation. The Nurse's husband becomes an extension of the economically productive body of his wife, Lady Capulet a more or less secondary effect of patriarchal rule once her womb is vacated and responsibility for her baby's survival given over to a servant.

Of course, it is also necessary to account for the difference in gender *between* the Nurse and her husband, as the baby's stand-in heterosexual parents, rather than simply the difference between the two couples. Since Juliet is the surrogate child replacing the lost Susan for the Nurse and her husband, both take up parental roles as surrogate

---

1977), pp. 281–91. "Holding the situation" is a term associated with the work of D. W. Winnicott. See, for example, "The Depressive Position," pp. 263–66, which discusses weaning.

mother and father. Yet the Nurse's dead husband, folded into the Nurse's narrative through reminiscence and quotation, exists for us primarily as a signifier of her discourse, a part of what she has lost. The Nurse may even link that loss here to her own loss in Juliet's weaning. Thematically, the Nurse's husband enters the play's textual field to voice a "natural," that is, low, view of female sexuality over against the Capulets' "high" appropriation of female desire for advantageous arranged marriages. His affectionate, familiar imagining of an inevitable sexual future for the little girl functions in carnivalesque terms to legitimate her future sexual desire as natural, indeed, as inevitable as first steps and stumbling. He stipulates that future only as the time when she will have "more wit," leaving aside patriarchy's more anxious concern about whether or not such female wit will be obedient and whether desire will be contained in marriage:

> For even the day before, she broke her brow,
> And then my husband—God be with his soul!
> 'A was a merry man—took up the child.
> "Yea," quoth he, "dost thou fall upon thy face?
> Thou wilt fall backward when thou hast more wit,
> Wilt thou not, Jule?" and by my holidam,
> The pretty wretch left crying and said, "Ay."
>   (1.3.38–44)

This joke about a future fall beneath the inclining thrust of the dominant male is, of course, gender-specific, suggesting the husband's role in instructing his surrogate daughter in the submissive posture of her engenderment even within what this play construes as the broad license of plebeian sexuality. The husband's witticism consists in constructing the two falls antithetically—forward replaced by backward, accident replaced by purpose and design, fear replaced by desire, broken forehead replaced by broken maidenhead. It is his implied equivalence of the two latter terms that reveals his "lowness," that makes him a dubious guardian of the aristocratic investment in female chastity. What we learn of his functioning as parent is carnivalesque too in aligning him with the comforting presence of the Nurse's body, since we hear of him picking Juliet up from one fall, imagining a better kind of fall, and ending her tears—helping to hold the situation, acting in loco parentis. Of course the joke could easily be altered for a baby boy's pratfalls, as in the jokes about future phallic prowess which routinely accompanied the future Louis XIII's nursery behavior when he was about the same age as Juliet here.[18] But the joke, transmuted for the boy, loses its carnivalesque function to sanction an otherwise illicit freedom of desire.

My point in teasing out the implications of the husband's presence in this narrative is to extend to *both* surrogate parents the familiar characterization of the Nurse as amoral and sexually permissive and to suggest the play's internal division about it. The contrast between these two sets of parents produces a differential narrative of nurture organized hierarchically as low/high, natural/social, physical/spiritual, appetitive/disciplined. Lady Capulet functions, then, as her husband's agent, the conduit of his dicta in the arrangement of a marriage she orders Juliet to desire as an act of obedience to custom and precedent and for the sake of great social advantage: "So shall you share all that he doth possess, / By having him, making yourself no less" (93–94). These social forces replace the biological structures of maternity, become the impersonal criteria of sexual maturity:

> Well, think of marriage now; younger than you,
> Here in Verona, ladies of esteem,
> Are made already mothers. By my count,
> I was your mother much upon these years
> That you are now a maid.
>
> (1.3.69–73)

From Juliet's place at the Nurse's suddenly distasteful breast, however, weaning is in fact surrounded and metonymized by environmental trauma—the "perilous knock" on her forehead the day before, the earthquake striking just at the moment of her loss of the good breast and her rage with the bad. It is possible to argue on thematic grounds that this pattern of sudden loss and disruption, enclosed within the Nurse's narrative of weaning, encapsulates the patterns of violent reversal, of sudden possession and apparently arbitrary or accidental loss, played out in the larger action. But because this weaning narrative is linked in so many details to the actual experience of many wellborn infants, I wish to see it as a self-enclosed textualization of the radically incommensurate experiences of surro-

18. See Elizabeth Wirth Marvick, *Louis XIII: The Making of a King* (New Haven: Yale University Press, 1986), pp. 24–25, 33–34.

gate mother and baby. In some sense the narrative presages Lady Macbeth's fantasy of maternal malevolence, though in a different key. Here the blow to the head comes before, not after and as a result of, the weaning, and the earthquake rather than the witches effects the projection of malevolence into the cosmos. Since the child experiences aversion as rejection, there may be little or no subjective difference between having the nipple plucked out and turning away from it in distaste. Lady Macbeth, in her overtly psychologized fantasy, in effect breaks the mirroring moment by turning her gaze away but she also asks the "murth'ring ministers" to "take my milk for gall"—an exchange that would reproduce the disagreeable experience Juliet had at her nurse's breast the morning of the earthquake.[19]

Infantile rage at the breast is not shocking or surprising, as unrepentant maternal rage always is. But recollection of that rage may be deeply humiliating for the adult subject, especially when it comes from without. Here, the moment of humiliation comes precisely from the distant comic gaze of the maternal spectator fixed on a drama in which she seems suddenly to have so little stake and from which she seems to have withdrawn the rest of her body—"To see it teachy and fall out wi'th'dug!" Because the Nurse remembers what the subject would repress, narrative works to identify the origin of subjectivity with an embarrassment constituted in and through maternal memory, undoing the work of repression. The child "falling out" of its fantasized symbiosis with the maternal body, falling out of the benign circle that sustains its sense of being-in-the-body, is watched, objectified, and memorialized in that moment of loss as "pretty fool." Juliet's fall into separate selfhood is mediated and made possible by the shame that comes from being watched in such a crucial rejection, the double–bound shame of finding out one's dependency at the terrible moment of its unexpected disruption.

The particular relevance of this memory for the characteristic formations of early modern subjectivity may come from the articulation of the weaning narrative within the triangulated relations of maternal

19. Adelman makes the point that "what the witches suggest about the vulnerability of men to female power on the cosmic plane, Lady Macbeth doubles on the psychological plane." In addition to, or instead of, the exchange of milk and gall—the most common reading of the line since Johnson, Adelman wonders if Lady Macbeth wants the spirits to "take her milk *as* gall . . . the milk itself is the gall; no transformation is necessary." See "'Born of Woman,'" pp. 97–98. But though the affect of the two transformations, one imagined and one remembered, is nearly antithetical for us, the experience for the baby at the breast is arguably the same.

surrogacy, told by the breast mother to the social mother, Lady Capulet, whose function here and throughout is aligned, in Lacanian terms, with the phallus, the third term of culture, which breaks into the imaginary dyad of nurse and baby: "My lord *and you* were then at Mantua." The material point to make is that weaning, particularly sudden weaning like Juliet's, has a historically specific valence of earthquakelike magnitude. Since weaning ordinarily returned a nurse-child to its biological parents, the experience of loss was magnified for the child of early modern England by the loss of an entire environment, the family among whom it had grown up and whose function, I have suggested, is metonymized here by the Nurse's (lost) husband. The Nurse, remembering what the child could not, offers a partial record of weaning as an experience the meaning of which cannot be constructed apart from subject positionality. Weaning signals the end of the Nurse's reproductive bodiliness and distances her from her own body (the "nipple of *my* dug" is followed in the narrative by "the dug"). But it is a far more critical developmental passage for the little girl, extruded—here somewhat belatedly, quite traumatically—and made "other" under the suddenly distanced gaze of her surrogate mother—into the seriocomic postures of isolate selfhood. The Nurse's emotional withdrawal from the little girl is itself a presage, of course, of her withdrawal from Juliet's grief at Romeo's banishment, the cause of Juliet's second quarrel "wi'th'dug." Thus the Nurse's narrative of weaning, which seems narratively so redundant except as a means to characterize the garrulity of an indulged family servant, suggests as well the meaningfulness of weaning as a powerful, deeply ambivalent signifier of the foundation of desire in shame and loss.

And, finally, the phrase "falling out wi'th'dug" and weaning itself may have a kind of proverbial weight for Elizabethan audiences in ways that are almost impossible to reconstruct, depending on the existence of a rich, somatic discourse about nursing, nurses, and weaning almost entirely lost to us. This loss has occurred not through the innocent processes of historical wastage but as one result of emergent disciplines that increasingly identify bodily humor as "low."[20] We should, I think, take "falling out wi'th'dug" as exactly antithetical in meaning but equivalent in force and recognizability to

20. On this theme, see Francis Barker, *The Tremulous Private Body: Essays on Subjection* (London: Methuen, 1984), pp. 17–21.

Hamlet's contemptuous dismissal of Osric as one who "did [comply], sir, with his dug before 'a suck'd it" (5.2.187–88).

Discussion of the affected courtier begins with Horatio's clearly proverbial, "This lapwing runs away with the shell on his head" (185– 86), likening Osric to the forward and bold baby bird. Hamlet's rejoinder is something like the witty play with proverbial phrases characterizing his encounters with Rosencrantz and Guildenstern, and Mercutio's with Romeo, in rejecting the demeaning characterization of ridiculous boldness but picking up on the reference to infancy.[21] The gentlest interpretation of this trope is to see it as evidence for a "commonsense" reiteration of the natural. Osric grotesquely introduces artifice and false courtesy where none is required just as Juliet misrecognizes the cause of her unhappiness—quarreling with the dug rather than its possessor. The Nurse's lack of self-consciousness in talking about her breast and the baby's behavior toward it would support such a reading.

But unlike *breast*, *dug* is a signifier Shakespeare uses rarely and usually to refer to the bodies of female animals or old women. Dugs, I infer, are breasts of the large, sagging kind, which, as I argued in the last chapter, Cotgrave and others found so unappealing. Dugs are not aesthetic; dugs are breasts whose erotic appeal has been removed by maternity and lactation. Distinctly "lower" in social register than *breast* or even *pap*, the word is now "contemptuous," says the *Oxford English Dictionary*, if used in relation to a woman's breasts and may well have been undergoing semiotic debasement in the seventeenth-century, thanks in part to the cultural repetition of such images as Hamlet's about Osric here. Contempt for the suckling cannot be separated from contempt for the maternal body to which he was in thrall. It is crucial to recognize in Hamlet's contempt a kind of projection, for what generates Hamlet's mockery is Osric's relation to and misrecognition of power, here metonymized by the dug. The play itself has dwelled insistently on the ambiguities of Hamlet's relation to and recognition of power and authority, in part represented in his mother's body, which is both demonstrably maternal and highly eroticized, mother and not-mother. The affective difference between the two memorial images—Osric as infant, complying with the dug before

21. The Arden editor glosses Hamlet's rejoinder with reference to Ulpian Fulwell's *Art of Flattery* (1576): "The very sucking babes hath a kind of adulation towards their nurses for the dug." See *Hamlet*, ed. Harold Jenkins (London: Methuen, 1982), p. 405n. For the lapwing reference, see Tilley, *Dictionary of the Proverbs*, L69, pp. 368–69.

sucking it, and Juliet, quarreling with the dug after finding it so horribly distasteful—is less important than the deep cultural ambivalence toward maternal suckling and dependency to which they testify.

The Nurse's narrative of weaning, then, assumes its full historical valency by opening up—and filling with detail—a particular semiotic space in the culture's ambivalent typology of female bodies. Thanks to the insistent deployment of Petrarchan rhetorics in *Romeo and Juliet*, that typology is structured antithetically in terms of bodily presence and absence, openness and opacity, change and changelessness. The Nurse and Lady Capulet are antithetical kinds of maternal bodies between which the upper-class infant moved in the process of enculturation, one warm, present, and responsive, the other cold, distant, and demanding. Available and unavailable, they replicate in the social sphere of maternity the contrasting female types contained within Petrarchanism and anti-Petrarchanism, those antithetical images of conflicted male desire given utterance in this play by Romeo's portrayal of the forever unavailable Rosaline, who "hath sworn that she will still live chaste" (1.1.217), and Mercutio's anti-Petrarchan hope for female grotesqueness: "That she were, O that she were / An open[-arse]" (2.1.37–38). That typology is of course both confounded and contained in the body of Juliet, in whom all the potentiality of the female body for sexuality and maternity exists and is brought to a state of active, and transgressive, desiring: "Thou wilt fall backward when thou hast more wit, / Wilt thou not, Jule?"

&.

Even in the bodily self-references of the Nurse's weaning narrative, it is clear that material differences in infant-feeding practices between early modern culture and our own are evidence of fundamental changes in understanding of the female body and its products. It is not, I would argue, the culture's widespread institutionalization of maternal surrogacy which most violates our understanding of early mother-child relations (not in this age of surrogate wombs, nannies, and day care). Rather it is wet-nursing itself and what wet-nursing presupposes—the fungibility of breasts and milk and their deployment as commodities. For us, suckling a baby is an intimate bodily act between two persons related by blood. Nursing may take place in public, though the social boundaries and rules governing the act are still somewhat blurry and highly context-specific, but nursing occurs only between a mother and her *own* child. Other people may feed the baby, of course, and may feed the baby a bottle of its own mother's milk. But I do not think we feel free to feed a baby a bottle of any *other* mother's milk, because mother's milk has been removed from the sphere of commodity exchange, excluded from its former "natural" place within the system of other commodifiable foods. In this respect, human milk and cows' milk occupy unhomologous spheres, since cows' milk is entirely commodified and completely fungible. (Even though animal milks are not themselves fungible for us, since we do not feed a child the milk of *any* animal but only that of some cloven-footed ungulates.)

A belief that, because of the caloric differences between bodies, a mother's milk best suited her own baby was an important consequence of humoral theory. But the social construction of that milk as a body product thoroughly enclosed within the (overlapping, if not identical) spheres of personal, bodily, and familial privacy did not yet exist. If it had, only very great poverty among a sufficient number of lactating women would have allowed the institution to survive. Indeed, the inscription of breast milk as personal, the redrawing of personal boundaries to exclude a contractual nursing relationship with a succession of strange families, could have emerged only as the domain of domestic privacy itself was drawn and the social and psychic distances prescribed between bodies in any given social situation increased. Whereas Elizabethans in public lodgings shared beds with strangers, a middle-class American considers clean sheets for houseguests an essential courtesy to spare the guest the "intimate" contact with another's body gained from sleeping in his/her sheets. By the same token, I would argue, the modern female subject cannot, except by overcoming some degree of resistance, imagine offering her breast to a strange baby, a stranger's baby. And it is with still greater difficulty that she imagines offering her lactating breast to a *non*-baby. The violation of this modern bodily taboo of personal boundaries and literal self-possession underlies the shock and vividness of that final moment in *The Grapes of Wrath* when Rose of Sharon, the Joad daughter whose baby has just died, offers her breast to a starving man. Her extraordinary act of charity—decided upon after a silent, intersubjective glance between mother and daughter—not only resembles that of the Virgin, to whom Steinbeck conspicuously alludes here, but also repeats what lactating women *in the wet-nursing classes* once were paid to do for the sick and elderly in the way of customary therapeutic practice.

The point in articulating this taboo is to mark a difference—just legible in the Nurse's self-distancing attitude toward her "dug"— which seems to me essential for interpreting Elizabethan semiologies of the breast. Such difference is also clear in the advice in midwifery and gynecological treatises for women with engorged breasts or new mothers lactating colostrum to put puppies, "little prettie whelpes," to the breast.[22] Either the colostrum thought to be so harmful to the child would not hurt the puppy, or no one cared if it did. In either case, the action did not constitute feeding, since the woman meant not to *feed* the puppy nourishment but to relieve her own discomfort. Nevertheless, I believe that the puppy could have signifed as child surrogate in such a case, as it did if the woman's breasts were engorged because her child had died, if only because of the physical action itself, putting the puppy where the child would be. The ingredients in Katherine Packer's recipe, mentioned in Chapter 4, "to cause the breasts to continew smalle," were also thought to work for small animals: "Herein may be washed young whelpes w*ch* you desire should wax no bigger."[23] This belief too suggests some sense of connection between women's breasts and puppies. In his *History of Serpents*, Edward Topsell describes tame Macedonian dragons "so meeke, that women feede them, and suffer them to sucke their breasts like little children."[24] Topsell doesn't bother to explain *why* the Macedonian women did this, perhaps because his reader did not need to be told; his point in citing the practice is to demonstrate the remarkable meekness of the *dragons*.

I trust I am not alone in finding these examples of what could be called cross-species suckling—whether fictional or actual—grotesque, shocking, and not a little bit kinky. But the image of women, prompted by some kind of bodily necessity, putting other than human babies to their breasts the Elizabethans seem not to have construed as monstrous. What they did think monstrous were those instances of suckling—human babies or animal babies—which seemed, however paradoxically, to threaten women's withdrawal from the maternal function that suckling makes visible. That is to say, the culture's heightened erotic investment in and signification of the female breast

22. Guillemeau, *Nursing of Children*, p.18.
23. Katherine Packer, *A Book of Very Good Medicines for Several Diseases Wounds and Sores both New and Old* (1639; Folger Ms. V.a.387), f. 10.
24. Edward Topsell, *The Historie of Serpents* (London, 1608; STC 24124; rpt. Amsterdam: Theatrum Orbis Terrarum, 1973), p. 157. I owe this reference to Miranda Johnson Haddad.

contained within it the specter of autonomous female desire. Worse, it suggested the possibility of female control of erotic practices, even an autoeroticism using suckling as its modality. Thus Joubert, explaining the erotogenic power of the breasts, inscribes an erotic motive and possibility within the suckling dyad. He compares the sensory capacity of the breasts to the erotic energy of the womb, a more familiar locus of female desire:

> Of the sympathy between the breasts and the womb we have plenty of evidence and many solid arguments. First, when the nipples are tickled, the womb takes delight in it and feels a pleasant titillation. Also, this small button on the breast is highly sensitive because of an abundance of nerve endings; and this is so that, even here, the nipples will have an affinity with the reproductive organs. For just as in these latter organs nature has set some lasciviousness so that animals, driven by voluptuousness, might be inclined to copulate in order to continue their species, so, too, has she done with the breasts, especially in their little buttons, so the female will offer and give suck to the child, who tickles them and pulls on them gently with its tongue and tender mouth. In this the woman can only feel great pleasure, especially when they are abundantly filled with milk.[25]

Joubert's is an inscription of women's erotic experience in which phallic power plays no part. I relate this exclusion of patriarchy to the widely diffused fear of withheld or grudging nurture, which, I have been suggesting, is a likely cultural trace of traumatic weanings and institutionalized surrogacy. Both are elements of the great contemporary fascination with Amazons and witches—female figures made to occupy the cultural space of the other in part because of bodily oddity, specifically the oddity of their breasts in number, size, location, and function, including cross-species suckling.

The Amazons' significance as ambivalently powerful figures of aggressive, self-determining desire is epitomized by their self-mutilation. As Louis Montrose has argued, the fascination and horror Elizabethans directed toward the Amazon was "an ironic acknowledgment by an androcentric culture of the degree to which men are in fact dependent upon women."[26] More specifically, however, the Amazon, like the self-mutilating, self-starving medieval woman saints, de-

25. Joubert, *Popular Errors*, p. 224.
26. See his extended discussion of the meaning of the Amazon: Louis Montrose, "'Shaping Fantasies': Figurations of Gender and Power in Elizabethan Culture," in *Rewriting the Renaissance*, p. 71. Montrose cites Celeste Turner Wright's survey of refer-

rived significance as a symbolic female figure whose body and body-image express her relationship to the world. *Amazon* was thought by some to mean "without a breast."[27] When Amazon girls reached the age of seven, Thomas Heywood tells us, their right breasts were seared off "that with the more facilitie they may drawe a Bowe, thrill a Dart, or charge a Launce."[28] Heywood may specify age here in order to suggest the ceremony's equivalence to the breeching ceremony, which marked the bodily engenderment of an Elizabethan boy by taking him out of the skirts of infancy and into the company of men; it presumably suggested the age when the fictional Amazon girl, like the real boy she antithesizes, could begin to learn arms and to take on the bodily markings of her particular androgynous engenderment as woman warrior.

The Amazon's morphological asymmetry, her single-breastedness, resembles the trope of the slipped chiton associated with the heroic virgin or the single breast bared by the nursing woman, both in actual practice and in visual representations of suckling.[29] But the Amazon's

---

ences to Amazons in "The Amazons in Elizabethan Literature," *Studies in Philology* 37 (1940), 433–56. Wright sees the Amazons' custom of searing off one breast—which is an accretion of the Greek legend—as symbolizing "unwomanliness" and unnatural maternity and quotes a character in John Webster's *Devil's Law Case*: "Like an Amazon lady, / Ide cut off this right pap, that gave him sucke, / To shoot him dead" (p. 452). I see these details, rather, as a particular troping on maternity and female bodiliness. For another discussion of the Amazon figure, see Simon Shepherd, *Amazons and Warrior Women: Varieties of Feminism in Seventeenth-Century Drama* (Brighton: Harvester, 1981), pp. 5–17.

27. See Noelle Caskey's discussion of the anorexic in "Interpreting Anorexia Nervosa," in *The Female Body in Western Culture: Contemporary Perspectives*, ed. Susan Rubin Suleiman (Cambridge: Harvard University Press, 1986), p. 184. On the etymologies of *Amazon*, see Wright, "Amazons in Elizabethan Literature," p. 452. Wright notes that Diodorus Siculus says both breasts were seared, p. 452 n. 236. It is interesting that André Thevet, whose *New Founde World* is cited by Wright, does not believe that the Amazons could have seared off a breast and refers to the judgment of "medicines," i.e., doctors, "whether they can burne those partes without death, knowing that they are tender, and also neere to [the] heart. . . . I wold thinke that for one that escapeth death, there dieth a hundreth." Thevet also cites, as the etymology of *Amazon*, "as those that have bene norished w[ith]out womans milke, the which is most likeliest to be true" (London, 1568; STC 23950. Rpt. Amsterdam: Da Capo Press, 1971), p. 101ᵛ.

28. Thomas Heywood, *Gynaikeion, or Nine Bookes* (London, 1624; STC 13326), p. 223.

29. For the trope of the slipped chiton, see Marina Warner, *Monuments and Maidens: The Allegory of the Female Form* (New York: Atheneum, 1985), pp. 267–93. In her several references to Amazons, however, Warner tends to see them as the generic classical female warriors and displays no interest in the self-mutilation sometimes part of their legend. Also, see Margaret R. Miles, "The Virgin's One Bare Breast: Female Nudity and Religious Meaning in Tuscan Early Renaissance Culture," in *The Female Body in Western Culture*, p. 197.

one breast, the breast she *doesn't* sear off, the breast she reserves to suckle her exclusively female young, is precisely the one she would keep from the gaze. What she *would* be thought to bare is the scar, the mark of absence, as if in this case morphological asymmetry signified her complete willingness to sacrifice beauty to function. But in this adherence to functionality, the Amazons would bear no resemblance to those maternally minded seventeenth-century women who nursed their children in willful defiance or class-based ignorance of the powerful aesthetic, erotic, and reproductive motives to suppress lactation I discussed in the last chapter. On the contrary, because the Amazons organized their bodies, individualistically, to be half maternal and half martial—hence entirely functional for a gynocratic way of life—their asymmetry suggests two kinds of difference from contemporary ideals of womanhood: on one hand, complete uninterest in an erotic appeal governed by male desire and, on the other, a certain emotional distance from or refusal to become absorbed into the personal and maternal gratifications, the social rewards, of nurture. Unlike Spenser's always available, naked-breasted Charissa, the Amazon is always only half available, only half maternal to half of her possible offspring. It is precisely this conspicuous stinginess of nurture, the withholding of food so as to coerce subjection, which Spenser emphasizes in the Amazonian society in book 5 of the *Faerie Queene*. There (we are repeatedly told) captive knights not only are forced by the Amazon queen Radigund to perform the female labor of spinning and carding but are fed only what they can earn: "For nought was given them to sup or dyne, / But what their hands could earne by twisting linnen twyne" (5.5.22).[30] The particular force of this climactic humiliation to work for what you eat may be somewhat obscured for most modern wage earners. It depends on a valorization of the warrior class as those born to deserve and dispense, not earn hospitality. But if we understand these warriors as allegorizing the subject position and powerlessness of infants, we may come closer to the text's affect inscription here and to the early experience of oral frustration and deprivation it encodes. The knights are humiliated by being dependent for inadequate food on a niggardly ruling woman.

That the cultural fantasies surrounding the Amazon were importantly focused on their bodily self-inscription is suggested by the con-

---

30. I quote here from *The Faerie Queene*, ed. A. C. Hamilton (London: Longman, 1977).

troversy over *which* breast was actually seared off and by the class-inflected resolution: noblewomen, who used shields, were said to sear off the left breast; Amazonian commoners, who used the bow, seared off the right.[31] Even Amazon women, that is to say, differed from themselves, manifested as if by nature the structure of class; but unlike European society, Amazon society did not designate a class of nurses, and all the Amazons presumably continued to offer babies milk from one breast. A single breast can, of course, produce an adequate milk supply and satisfactorily nourish a baby. But that it may have signified a poverty of milk is suggested by the fact that even healthy mothers of twins were routinely advised to give one baby to a nurse, on the assumption that they would have enough milk for only one.[32] (The potential psychic consequences of such an arrangement for *both* twins, needless to say, could have been devastating. How, one wonders, did Anne Hathaway Shakespeare feed her twins, and in a matter of parental choice, did she herself suckle the boy or the girl twin?)

Furthermore, Amazonian mastectomy, like a distortion of the Petrarchan body, with its ivory paps, its hills of snow, becomes a metamorphic trope that paradoxically half separates the Amazonian body from the contaminations of female mutability—"safe and untouched," as Heywood says, from change, flow, and sagging breasts.[33] (Though like other tropes that miraculously remove characteristic traits from the female body, this one works by replacing one form of bodily grotesqueness—the swelling protuberance of the flowing breast—with another, the flat but scarred surface of the seared upper torso.) Mastectomy also implies the Amazons' crucial bodily heresy at least by comparison with the many claims, material and symbolic, on womb and breast in early modern culture—the heresy visibly to control their own bodies, to regulate their own reproductivity, and to offer a model of female self-government in which reproduction and nurture are only two of several forms of service and productive activity.

The figure of the Amazon would, as Montrose makes clear, most threaten patriarchal culture by its inversion of that culture's system of gender and nurture.[34] But that threat also implies an anxiety, not

31. Wright, "Amazons in Elizabethan Literature," p. 452.
32. Fildes, *Breasts, Bottles, and Babies*, p. 178.
33. Heywood, *Gynaikeion*, p. 223.
34. Montrose, "'Shaping Fantasies,'" pp. 71–72.

unrelated to the practice of wet-nursing, about the foundations of subjectivity in early object relations. On the asymmetrical, half-breasted, fantastic figure of the Amazon living on the edges of the known world, a cultural projection of the infant's ambivalent experience of maternal nurture is legible. Her body visibly gives and withholds itself, promises and frustrates both oral *and* aesthetic satisfaction, defines nurture and aggression as equal aspects of its nature; it is vulnerable in the possession of one breast while toughened by the absence of the other. In this it only too clearly instantiates the good breast/bad breast dichotomy so crucial to the developing infant's focal object relation, with this proviso: that even the Amazon's one "good" breast is, by virtue of its anomalous, threatening, *grudging* singularity, perhaps none too good. More to my purposes in this chapter, interest in the Amazon's regulation of her body's nurturant function by the removal of the one breast is part of what I see as cultural preoccupation with experience of loss of the breast or its equally terrifying opposite, protracted dependence on the breast.

Both of the images I have described thus far—cross-species suckling and the bodily self-determining of the Amazon—come together in *Antony and Cleopatra* in the powerfully autoerotic sign of Cleopatra putting the asp to her breast. Interpretation of this final action has focused on the meanings to attach to the asp, particularly the erotic suggestiveness of this and other serpent references in the play which make Cleopatra a bisexual maternal figure, hence the object of unattainable, self-destructive desire. Constance Brown Kuriyama has made the Freudian case that "the association of Cleopatra with biting and devouring creatures strongly suggests the fantasy of the *vagina dentata*," with the serpent representing the fear of castration and its symbolic denial.[35] Such Freudian interpretations, of course, silently assume a male reader or viewer who identifies ambivalently here with Antony's emasculating, hence incestuous, desire for a Cleopatra figured as phallic mother. As Janet Adelman has pointed out, however, snakes in Renaissance mythographic tradition were frequently associated with women, particularly deceitful, seductive women such as Medusa or Spenser's Error. Mythologically, says Philip Slater, they are "always an oral symbol," perhaps more than a phallic one, and thus tend to signify questions of incorporation versus separation and to be associated with ambiguous boundaries. Because they shed their skins,

35. Constance Brown Kuriyama, "The Mother of the World: A Psychoanalytic Interpretation of Shakespeare's *Antony and Cleopatra*," *English Literary Renaissance* 7 (1977), 329–30, and, for the quotation, p. 333.

snakes are also linked with miraculous powers of regeneration and, because of their venomousness, with death.[36]

What such psychoanalytic interpretations of maternal figures have tended to omit, I suggest, are the historical valences that material practices inscribe in a sign like that of Cleopatra suckling the asp. The tableau is, in Kuriyama's nice phrase, "so condensed and richly ambiguous that a complete analysis seems impossible." She describes Cleopatra's monument as womblike and Antony's sleeplike death in it as a passive surrender to a wished return to infancy.[37] But its power, I prefer to say, comes less through fantasy associations with the womb than through familiar, even folkloric allusions to the hermetic female world and material practices of childbirth, which the snake, as baby substitute, works to support. If Cleopatra's monument becomes a symbolic representation of the womb, it does so indirectly by resembling the female enclosure of the birthing chamber, the parturient womb's outer envelope, a sealed-off space of temporary female empowerment surrounded—here literally—by patriarchal power. This theatrical birthing chamber, like actual ones, comes into being by the redefinition of a space given over to other representational uses. Here, as in birth, the redefinition is presided over by a culturally empowered woman acting apart from men, but in this anomalous imitation Cleopatra takes on both roles in the birthing drama. She is both the passive subject of the physical drama and the midwife, both the surrogate mother offering her breast and the woman who will die and leave her "real" children behind, both the central actor in a drama of physical mutability and the renouncer of womanly mutability:

> My resolution's plac'd, and I have nothing
> Of woman in me; now from head to foot
> I am marble-constant; now the fleeting moon
> No planet is of mine.
>
> (5.2.238–41)

Like the social space of childbearing, the monument is a hermetic enclosure belonging to and expressing female rule with a suffering

36. Janet Adelman, *The Common Liar: An Essay on "Antony and Cleopatra"* (New Haven: Yale University Press, 1973), pp. 64–65; Philip Slater, *The Glory of Hera: Greek Mythology and the Greek Family*, 2d ed. (Princeton: Princeton University Press, 1992), p. 97—a reference I owe to Adelman, p. 204 n. 29 and p. 226 n. 46. I should point out that Barbara J. Bono, too, finds the asp phallic. See *Literary Transvaluation: From Vergilian Epic to Shakespearean Tragicomedy* (Berkeley: University of California Press, 1984), p. 190.

37. Kuriyama, "The Mother of the World," p. 345.

but triumphant woman and her female attendants in its center. Some of the voyeurism that accompanies male entrance into ritualized female space and female practice, which I discussed in the last chapter, is perceptible here, as a final variation on the lovers' command of the gaze so insistent elsewhere in the play. Asking Iras for her robe, her crown, her best attire, Cleopatra is preparing herself for queenly, even necrophilic display to an importunate, collective male gaze, but not until *after* and *by means of* the suicidal nursing. The nursing itself is figured as an event occurring naturally within an exclusionary female space; it is a nostalgic, painful, last suckling of a weanling before the nurse passes beyond such bodily moments altogether. But this serpent, brought to her bosom by the queen whom "age cannot wither," is troped as a surrogate baby of subversive, carnivalesque power. Its suckling keeps the maternal body from paternal appropriation; it participates in a conspiracy that uses the nursing bond to defeat and embarrass father, to deny his disciplinary goals for the maternal body and its loyal suckling: "O, couldst thou speak, / That I might hear thee call great Caesar ass / Unpolicied" (306–8). Cleopatra's mimicry of the wet nurse's role after the great political events of the play is part of her insistent cultivation of ordinary experiences, "commanded / By such poor passion as the maid that milks / And does the meanest chares" (4.15.74–76). In taking the asp to her breast, she does act the part of hired labor, a surrogate body. But since her action is troped explicitly as mimicry, it also acknowledges and defers metadramatically to the bodily absence at the physical center of this moment—the boy actor with "nothing of woman" in him, not even a breast to offer a surrogate baby.

Like actual seventeenth-century childbirths, this last dramatic sign of Cleopatra's putting asps to her bosom is a ceremonial event related in political meaning and affect to carnival, most obviously to carnivalesque interpretation of the temporary empowerment of women in childbirth rituals. The scene is also carnivalesque in celebrating the material bodily principle and in deploying such verbal and theatrical motifs of carnival as the equivocating low character introduced like *Hamlet*'s gravediggers or *Macbeth*'s Porter to laugh at death.[38] The coming together of queen and clown, who is welcomed into space from which Caesar has been temporarily deflected, enacts a traditional motif of social leveling quite distinct from the lovers' witty play with

---

38. For a full discussion of these motifs, see Michael D. Bristol, *Carnival and Theater: Plebeian Culture and the Structure of Authority in Renaissance England* (London: Routledge, 1985), pp. 179–96.

hierarchical and gender distinctions in earlier parts of the play. From the clown's material point of view the queen is still a woman, indeed a bawdy and sexual woman; his quibbles make the queen a procurer of erotic delight like the "very honest woman—but something given to lie" who gave him "a very good report o' th' worm" (251, 255). For the country fellow, Cleopatra differs from other women in her social being, as a matter of rank, but not in her bodily being, where female desire works to collapse all difference: "You must not think I am so simple but I know the devil himself will not eat a woman. I know that a woman is a dish for the gods, if the devil dress her not. But truly, these whoreson devils do the gods great harm in their women; for in every ten that they make, the devils mar five" (5.2.271–77).

It will be clear that Cleopatra's suicide metaphorically reverses the ordinary meanings of the nurse with baby at her breast. She enacts an antinursing, but more crucial for my argument, she precisely inverts the customary structure of power relations in birth and wet-nursing. Here it is the nurse who has sought out the baby; it is the baby who separates the nurse from her reproductive bodiliness. It is death that this nurse desires of the baby, which the baby will bring to her. Here the source of bodily danger comes not from a nurse applying wormwood to her dug or from a murdering mother exchanging her milk for gall. It comes from a "baby" whose bite is a poison desired by its taker, a bite of desired aversiveness.

There is more to say of Cleopatra's comically inverted mimicry of the wet nurse's role: that instead of the baby's social movement out and down to its country environment, the country baby comes in a basket "up" to the queen and her women, only to disappear from view again. The nurse asks the bringer of the baby for guarantees of the baby's character: "Hast thou the pretty worm of Nilus there, / That kills and pains not?" (5.2.243–44). And the bringer of the baby here warns the nurse of her risk: "Look you, the worm is not to be trusted but in the keeping of wise people; for indeed, there is no goodness in the worm" (265–66). In her address to the "pretty worm," Cleopatra repeats the very terms Juliet's nurse applies to her weanling, calling it "mortal wretch" and "poor venomous fool" (5.2. 303, 305) in the language of endearment used indistinguishably for animals and babies.[39] As she coaxes it to take the breast and "with thy sharp teeth

39. The *OED* is particularly interesting in its treatment of *wretch*, a word that in its etymological journey in German retains the original connotations of an exile, one driven away from his or her native country, but in English becomes a more general word to describe one sunk in misery and distress. The connotations of the German for

this knot intrinsicate / Of life at once untie" (304–5), Cleopatra's desire for death is inextricable from a nurse's perhaps ambivalent desire for her nursling's erotic bite, itself figuring the lover's erotic violence: "The stroke of death is as a lover's pinch, / Which hurts, and is desir'd" (295–96). Like the puppies applied to the engorged breasts of a lactating woman, or the tame Macedonian dragon, the asp brings a desired relief from bodily tension to Cleopatra, a relief that the ubiquitous pun on "die" construes as erotic and here perhaps specifically as autoerotic since the asp is a cold, unknowing agent of bodily release which has to be coaxed into doing what comes naturally: "Be angry, and dispatch" (306).

But it is Cleopatra's use of the asp not only to commit suicide but to prevent a humiliating thralldom to Caesar which most legitimizes a carnivalesque interpretation of the scene and the asp-baby's mediation of its nurse's quietus. In Plutarch's description of Cleopatra's physical suffering after Antony's death, Shakespeare might well have recognized bodily inscriptions like those of the childbearing woman. In her grief, says Plutarch,

> she had knocked her brest so pitiefully, that she had martired it, and in divers places had raised ulsers and inflamacions, so that she fell into a fever withal: whereof she was very glad, hoping thereby to have good colour to absteine from meate, . . .
>
> [When Caesar visited her in this sickness] she sodainly rose up, naked in her smocke, and fell downe at his feete marvelously disfigured: both for that she had plucked her heare from her head, as also for that she had martired all her face with her nailes, and besides, her voyce was small and trembling, her eyes sonke into her heade with continuall blubbering: and moreover, they might see the most parte of her stomake torne in sunder.[40]

Plutarch suggests that Cleopatra's self-mutilation comes from two sources of grief, one of them maternal—the death of Antony and Caesar's threats against her children. The disfigurement, her "martir-

---

a word applied to a real or troped baby in figurative exile from its place of maternal origin are suggestive, but even as a term of endearment or pity in English the word is semantically rich as description of a nurse-child or weanling.

40. I quote from "The Life of Marcus Antonius," in *Plutarch's Lives of the Noble Grecians and Romanes*, trans. Sir Thomas North (1579), reprinted in *Narrative and Dramatic Sources of Shakespeare*, ed. Geoffrey Bullough (London: Routledge and Kegan Paul; New York: Columbia University Press, 1964), 5:313.

ing," isolates the bodily sites of reproductivity—breasts and especially the torn stomach—as the signifiers of psychic trauma. Compared to Plutarch, Shakespeare mentions Cleopatra's children only obliquely, and he omits details of Caesar's manipulation of Cleopatra through them. But he does figure the monument (Plutarch does not) as a female space where birth, death, and nurture converge and are resignified.

The moment profoundly genders the gaze, calls the gazer to a heightened sense of his/her own engenderment even as it recalls a symbiotic union with the mother which precedes the fall into gendered subjectivity. If the male gazer upon this scene feels both nostalgic and intrusive, both called to regressive reminiscence and warned away from it, a female gazer might well feel less intrusive and potentially more empowered through vicarious participation in the queen's defeat of Caesar. Perhaps both gazers are capable of a sense of discomfiture and trespass, however, at overhearing the nurse's intimate address to her nurse-child and her acknowledgment of its function as erotic surrogate when she puts a second asp, a twin nurseling, to her breast: "As sweet as balm, as soft as air, as gentle— / O Antony!—Nay, I will take thee too" (311–12). The asps are also a surrogate for Antony, whose lover's pinch they replace.

Cleopatra's carnivalesque embrace of troping, her bodily enactment of metaphor, collapses customary antitheses and structures of difference. To use the snake as baby is to eroticize fear as an aspect of desire. Poison becomes food, snake becomes baby, bite becomes kiss, absorption becomes lactation, death becomes erotic life, boundary becomes transit. Carnival subversiveness even survives Cleopatra herself because of the disappearance of the asp, escaping paternal detection and punishment. Only a trace of its physical conjunction with Cleopatra is visible, according to the onstage audience, and none at all, of course, to us, the only surviving witnesses of the carnivalesque moment. In this aspect of the asp is perhaps another clear link to oedipal fantasy of undetected union with the maternal body.

More to my point, however, is that once Cleopatra is dead and the monument has been penetrated by Caesar and his entourage, the monument itself is instantly, even violently transformed into a new kind of space, gendered male and public. The domestic quiet of female enclosure, here presided over by death, is invaded first by the guards and Dolabella, then by "Caesar and all his Train, marching," dominated by a new, rationalized gaze and a new empirical discourse.

Erotic death, fear, and desire succumb to forensic analysis. "Here, on her breast," says Dolabella, "there is a vent of blood, and something blown; / The like is on her arm" (5.2.348–50). "Most probable / That so she died," responds Caesar diagnostically, and he reductively literalizes Cleopatra's metaphorics of death into a kind of empirical project: "For her physician tells me / She hath pursu'd conclusions infinite / Of easy ways to die" (353–56).

Caesar's final entrance in the play symbolically marks the historical emergence of a new kind of collective discipline of mind and body, a demarcation of bodily distance, and an insistently unmetaphoric discourse. If this too seems voyeuristic, a call to imagine what could not be displayed for corroboration on the epicene body of the boy actor, the voyeurism has more to do with the forensics of the Renaissance anatomy theaters and their modes of bodily trespass than with the intimate and regressive participatory affect of the nursing scene for which no specialized knowledge, no professionalism of gaze is required. Cleopatra's suicide signifies the agency of death itself as a form of carnivalesque power against which Caesar and all forms of earthly power are conspicuously helpless, against which the analysis of forensic evidence seems merely a defensive, face-saving discursive back-formation. More than that, Cleopatra's suicide tropes on what—as we saw in the case of Juliet's nurse—is a cultural legacy of female empowerment in and through the reproductive body. Lactation begins as an involuntary bodily process, another conspicuous form of female effluence related to both woman's proneness to infirmity and her disruptive sexuality. But the key to a wet nurse's productivity, hence social power, is her control over her own milk giving and, through it, control over matters of death and survival. Cleopatra's metaphorics borrow some of that power to her own ends here. And in their sublime transmutations of fear and desire they seem to acknowledge the libidinal self-gratification contained within the hermetic enclosure of the nursing dyad.

ॐ

There are other social meanings to ascribe to the theatrical sign of a woman bringing an animal to her breast, particularly when that action is followed by the quasi-judicial inspection of her corpse by a political ruler. One is to be found in the Jacobean preoccupation with witches, particularly with the categorical differences between the bodies of witches and those of other women. A patriarchal order,

Christina Larner has argued, divides women on the grounds of conformity. I would add that in the witch-hunting patriarchal order in seventeenth-century England that conformity was in part bodily because patriarchy found in the apparent objectivity of bodily evidence a means of occluding the ideological grounds for social division. Thus, if Cleopatra's imitation of the wet nurse somatically expresses her commonality with ordinary women, whose lives were defined by domestic routines and physical obligations such as suckling babies, it also links her through metonymy with the bodily habitus of the witch—a woman out of the ordinary, in fact, one expelled from the ranks of ordinary women by a scapegoating process of social (mis)recognition.[41] Scholars for a long time have pointed out that Cleopatra's associations with mythological or literary witches such as Medusa or Tasso's Armida are never far from the surface of the play. Antony excuses his thralldom to Cleopatra by twice calling her a witch (4.2.37, 4.12.47), as does Pompey in calling for Cleopatra's destruction of Antony through witchcraft, by means of the old hero's regression to an infantile sensuality:

> Let witchcraft join with beauty, lust with both,
> Tie up the libertine in a field of feasts . . .
> That sleep and feeding may prorogue his honor.
> (2.1.22–26)

Such associations with witchcraft serve to magnify and mystify Cleopatra's sexual magnetism, making it both dangerous and excessive.[42] But in the early years of James I's reign, when witchcraft prosecutions were at their height, no use of the word "witch" may be seen as socially neutral or merely literary. Thus between Cleopatra's troping of her death as an intimate, ordinary form of female agency and Caesar's forensic gaze upon her breast exists a third possibility—that for an audience in early seventeenth-century England suckling an asp would resemble the hyperordinary erotic bond of a witch and her animal familiar.

Like the women accused in witchcraft prosecutions, Cleopatra from the Roman point of view is an Other perceived as possessing incom-

---

41. Christina Larner, *Witchcraft and Religion: The Politics of Popular Belief*, ed. Alan Macfarlane (Oxford: Basil Blackwell, 1984), pp. 87, 30.

42. Adelman discusses Cleopatra's links with various literary witches and temptresses in *Common Liar*, pp. 64–66.

prehensible and unwarranted kinds of agency, here that form of excessive sexual agency constructed as a female seductiveness fatal to manliness. Even her suicide becomes a sign of excessive agency in its troping upon the life-and-death power that maternity and lactation give to the maternal body—in her example a power turned, perhaps paradoxically, in upon itself. As a force perceived by the state to be its enemy, Cleopatra also serves another social function that we now ascribe to witches—strengthening a community's self-cohesion by the perception of her difference.[43] Perhaps even more to my point, Cleopatra could be said to share some demographic characteristics with seventeeth-century witches, all of whom were "by definition," says Larner, "abnormal" persons.[44] Like most of them, a mature widow, past childbearing, and admittedly "wrinkled deep in time," Cleopatra faces a future in which she would become increasingly dependent for her survival on those superior to her in strength and means. She kills herself rather than face the shame of capture, public display, and powerlessness and in death continues to resist the state's attempts to read and control the meaning of her body. In her suicide she escapes the fate of most of the women accused of witchcraft, who were searched, tortured, and executed and for whom a painless suicide at some point in their ordeal would have seemed fortunate. Where Cleopatra's theatrical body most differs from those of the poor women caught up in the Jacobean witch-hunt is in its opacity, its near illegibility to the forensic gaze: Caesar says he can find no "external swelling" to suggest the *swallowing* of poison; where Cleopatra's body has taken in poison is visible only by the "vent of blood, and something blown," which appears on her breast and arm (5.2.346, 349). For Caesar her death is a signifier of limit, and a discursive turn to probability is his only recourse: "Most probable / That so she died" (353–54).

But the body of an English witch was made to speak out, to betray its female subject far more visibly than Cleopatra's. Torture and interrogation were functions of a judicial power that took these bodies,

43. See Mary Douglas's introduction to *Witchcraft: Confessions and Accusations* (London: Tavistock, 1970), p. xxv: "The witch-image is as effective as the idea of the community is strong." See also Peter Stallybrass, "*Macbeth* and Witchcraft," in *Focus on "Macbeth,"* ed. John Russell Brown (London: Routledge and Kegan Paul, 1982), p. 190.

44. Larner, *Witchcraft and Religion*, p. 45. The social profile comes from the work of Alan Macfarlane on the Essex witches, *Witchcraft in Tudor and Stuart England: A Regional and Comparative Study* (London: Routledge and Kegan Paul,1970), pp. 158–66; and the explicitly feminist revision of that work in Christina Larner's *Enemies of God: The Witch-Hunt in Scotland* (London: Chatto and Windus, 1981), pp. 1–28.

unlike Cleopatra's, beyond the reach of dramatic, if not discursive, representation. One irony of this painful chapter in women's history is that if, as Elaine Scarry has argued, the structure of torture works to display the excessive agency of the torturer, to confirm the torturer in his self-experience *as* agent, then torture of the English witch seems determined to confer agency where one would least expect to find it in patriarchy—in old, impoverished village women.[45] More crucial for my purposes here, a major difference between English and virtually all other national forms of witchcraft prosecutions was the almost obsessive attention that English authorities paid to the presence on the witch's body of a "bigge," or mark, the site where the familiar was said to suck the witch's blood in payment for his services.[46] A key step in the prosecution of an English witch came when local matrons searched her body for any unusual mark, pap, or teatlike growth. Such marks cannot have been hard to find on the bodies of old women, as skeptics in the matter kept pointing out. In the witchfinder Matthew Hopkins's dialogic pamphlet, "The Discoverie of Witches," several skeptical queries point out the kind of blemishes likely to be found, especially on the bodies of the poor or aged: "Many poore People are condemned for having a Pap, or Teat about them, whereas many People (especially antient People) are, and have been a long time troubled with naturall wretts [warts] on severall parts of their bodies, and other naturall excressencies, as Hemerodes, Piles, Childbearing, &c. and these shall be judged only by one man alone, and a woman, and so accused or acquitted."[47]

But Hopkins insists that forensic interpretation of the accused witch's body never relied on "private judgments alone," depending instead on a consensus, what we would call a social classification:

> For never was any man tryed by search of his body, but commonly a
> dozen of the ablest men in the parish or else where, were present, and
> most commonly as many ancient skilfull matrons and midwives present

45. Scarry writes: "Torture systematically prevents the prisoner from being the agent of anything and simultaneously pretends that he is the agent of some things. Despite the fact that in reality he has been deprived of all control over, and therefore all responsibility for, his world, his words, and his body, he is to understand his confession as it will be understood by others, as an act of self-betrayal." See *The Body in Pain: The Making and Unmaking of the World* (Oxford: Oxford University Press, 1985), p. 47.

46. Larner, *Witchcraft and Religion*, p. 76; and Barbara Rosen, ed., *Witchcraft*, Stratford-upon-Avon Library, no. 6 (London: Edward Arnold, 1969), p. 30.

47. Matthew Hopkins, *The Discovery of Witches* (London, 1647; Wing H 2751), p. 3; also quoted in *The Witchcraft Papers: Contemporary Records of the Witchcraft Hysteria in Essex, 1560–1700*, ed. Peter Haining (London: Robert Hale, 1974), p. 179.

when the women are tryed, which marks not only he, and his company
attest to be very suspicious, but all beholders, the skilfulest of them, doe
not approve of them, but likewise assent that such tokens cannot in their
judgements proceed from any the above mentioned Causes.[48]

A body under interrogation whose warts and excrescences are
"tokens" is one already deeply inscribed with social expressiveness,
already overcoded. Even before judgment is passed, such a body has
already been made to count in a culture's ongoing, always contested
classification of what is and is not natural. The teat becomes a
metonymy of awesome determinacy, as the skeptic's language suggests: "People are condemned for having a Pap, or Teat about them."
  When the skeptical countervoice remains unconvinced of visible
difference between the devil's marks and "naturall excressencies," the
apparent gender neutrality of Hopkins's first exchange gives way to
the underlying misogynistic paranoia that fueled the European witch-
hunts.[49] He responds in terms of a "natural" norm, an ethical map-
ping of the body from which the body of the witch is said to depart.
Devil's marks are "farre distant from any usuall place, from whence
such naturall markes proceed"; they lack ordinary sensitivity to pain;
and unlike natural marks, on which he confers stability, they are subject to change. In fact, he says, because witches will find surrogate
nurses for their imps, the investigator should allow the teats to become engorged and thus reveal their (un)natural function: "Keepe
her 24. houres with a diligent eye, that none of her Spirits come in any
visible shape to suck her; the women have seen the next day after her
Teats extended out to their former filling length, full of corruption
ready to burst, and leaving her alone then one quarter of an houre,
and let the women go up againe, and shee will have them drawn by
her Imps close againe: *Probatum est.*"[50]
  Particularly revealing of the witch-hunter's fear of maternal power
is this vision of a wet-nurse cooperative, with witch wet nurses trading
their imps back and forth in order to escape detection. For Hopkins,
the dyadic bond between the witches and their animal nurselings
stands in a complex relation of similarity and difference to the dyadic
bond of nurse or mother and her baby. In being capable of engorge-

48. Hopkins, *Discovery of Witches*, p. 3.
49. Larner has convincingly made the case that witch-hunting was more or less
synonymous with woman-hunting in *Enemies of God*, pp. 3–4, 89–102.
50. Hopkins, *Discovery of Witches*, p. 4.

ment, the teats of Hopkins's hypothetical witches clearly resemble the breasts of lactating women. The body of the witch, like the body of the lactating mother accustomed to the sucking action, would seem to depend for relief on the presence of the suckling familiar. But because the content of the witch's body must be defined as antithetical to that of ordinary women, her engorged teat is full not of breast milk but "of corruption ready to burst." That is, her teat is like the ulcerated or infected breast of a lactating woman, full of matter which was thought to harm the nurseling.

We could argue that, as a mark of difference, the idea of the witches suckling their own and each other's familiars works to reinforce the normalcy of the wet-nursing culture and its surrogate mothers. But some slippage in the other direction may also be taking place, especially if we include in our thinking the female secrecy and hermetic enclosure of seventeenth-century birth practices. Not only do witches resemble lactating mothers, but thanks to the witch-hunters' fetishistic attention to the witch's teat, lactating mothers come to resemble witches. It is a resemblance that rests upon the identification of any female body as grotesque but the maternal body as particularly so. The maternal teat on the witch's body was systematically rezoned downward, from above to below the waist, from the breast, where suckling would be visible, to the privy parts, deep within the enveloping darkness and privacy of the witch's skirts. The nearness of this teat to the birth site is clearly not gratuitous, especially since "childbearing" (reproductive cause substituting for bodily effect) was one source of "naturall excrescencies." Searchers were careful to insist that such teats, though they resembled hemorrhoids, were not: one Essex informant reported finding "three long teats or bigges in her secret parts, which seemed to have been lately sucked; and that they were not like pyles, for this informant knows well what they are, having been troubled with them herself."[51]

The defensiveness of the searchers is particularly evident in their repeated denials of the resemblance between their own piles and the witch's "bigge." And such defensiveness is understandable: one source of psychological terror in this kind of examination, for the witch and perhaps for the "grave matrons" and midwives who were

51. "The Information of Francis Milles, taken upon oath before the said Justices, April 29, 1645," from *A True and Exact Relation of the Several Informations, Examinations, and Confessions of the Late Witches* (London, 1645), reprinted in Haining, *Witchcraft Papers*, pp. 162–63.

asked to search her, is precisely that the witch herself could not have seen or known her body's secret parts as her searchers did. Before the search, her warts and blemishes were not yet "tokens" either to herself or to anyone else, But in the course of the search her body underwent a shameful transformation, since one step involved shaving the accused woman's body hair.[52] Afterward, the witch might well have discovered not only a terrifying new body image but also sudden alienation from a body whose social meanings she could no longer control. Thus, poor Mary Greenleife, asked "how she came by those teats," replied "she never knew she had any such untill this time, they were found in those parts upon the said search."[53] It cannot be surprising that Mother Sawyer, the witch of Edmonton, tried desperately to resist the search by the "grave matrons" whom the court's officers had brought in off the street: "Fearing and perceiving she should by that search of theirs be then discoverd, behaved herself most sluttishly and loathsomely towards them . . . yet nevertheless niceness they laid aside."[54] As Eve Sedgwick has pointed out, the back of the body and especially the hind parts are the least subject to ocular control and, as a place of non- and misrecognition, the least easily defended. Hence they are the site of greatest psychic vulnerability, shame, and punishment, holding the "potential for a terrifying involuntarity of meaning."[55] To this involuntarity the executed bodies of the Jacobean witches attest.

Even before the imposition of any judicial pronouncement of guilt or innocence, the presence on her body of these demonic warts and nipples worked to class the witch with other kinds of deviant women, particularly sexually deviant ones: these were marks "which honest women have not."[56] Indeed Hopkins's introduction of the witch into the category of the sexually deviant and transgressive female suggests the kind of discursive transformation continually and necessarily at work in the witchcraft materials—the compulsory conversion of involuntary bodily events into the voluntary transactions of desire. In the ordinary meaning of the terms, sexual honesty or dishonesty in wom-

52. Rosen, *Witchcraft*, p. 17.
53. Quoted in Haining, *Witchcraft Papers*, p. 156.
54. I quote here from Henry Goodcole, *The Wonderful Discoverie of Elizabeth Sawyer a Witch* (London, 1621; STC 12014), reprinted with modernized spelling in *The Witch of Edmonton: A Critical Edition*, ed. Etta Soiref Onat (New York: Garland, 1980), p. 387.
55. Eve Sedgwick, "A Poem Is Being Written," *Representations* 17 (Winter 1987), 126. Her specific reference here, interestingly enough, is to the body of the child.
56. I am quoting from Hopkins, *Discovery of Witches*, p. 2, here but the phrase recurs in witchcraft materials.

an was thought to be a faculty of her will—to obey or transgress patriarchal strictures on female chastity before, during, and after marriage. Sexual honesty was a function of will mastering desire, but imputations of sexual dishonesty also assumed responsibility and free will in the female transgressor. The charges of witchcraft, too, necessarily depended on, presumed free will and responsibility on the part of the witch, for whom the taking up of witchcraft, the doing of *maleficium* was—like sexual transgression—thought to be a matter of choice. In the handy-dandy of grammatical transposition, a much-quoted phrase from Scripture—"Rebellion is as the sin of witchcraft" (I Samuel 15:23)—precisely makes the point.[57] Indeed Christina Larner has linked the emergence of witch-hunting to the newly ambiguous, deeply contradictory status of women in post-Reformation culture, which gave women a new personal responsibility for their actions while continuing to inform them authoritatively of their "ritual and moral inferiority."[58] At moments of such ideological uncertainty, questions of voluntarity and involuntarity would make the crucial and bodily metonymies of that opposition deeply meaningful or, as in the case of the witch's teat, turn the involuntary bodily blemish into the symptom of freely chosen malevolence. Perhaps even more rebellious, offering the blood of one's body to be sucked by the devil's creatures inverts the symbolism of the Eucharist, especially in the context provided by the lactating Christ of medieval symbolism.[59] Like Christ, the witch would offer her blood voluntarily and as the expression of her allegiance to the Devil. Her motives—malice and revenge—would invert the merciful motives of Christ, and presumably the system of reward and punishment which led to the suckling of imps would parody the supernatural Christian economy. Furthermore, the suspicion of a forbidden eroticism which seems to haunt the inquisitors would also invert the sublimations of properly ordered and regulated forms of Christian love.

❧

Thus what was thought to take place physically between a witch and her familiar imagines a crucial change in ordinary bodily procedures, a morally weighted transformation from the involuntary to the volun-

57. For the contemporary reliance on this verse, see Stuart Clark, "Inversion, Misrule, and the Meaning of Witchcraft," *Past and Present* 87 (1980), 118–19.
58. On this issue, see Larner, *Enemies of God*, p. 101.
59. Caroline Bynum, "The Body of Christ in the Later Middle Ages: A Reply to Leo Steinberg," *Renaissance Quarterly* 39 (1986), 422–27.

tary. Lactation, obviously, is an involuntary consequence of parturition, but given a sufficient sucking stimulus it can be maintained long afterward. In other words, lactation begins involuntarily but is highly responsive to management. Maintaining lactation through demand suckling was (as we have seen) a relatively effective and presumably well-known form of contraception, and it had the benefit of conferring substantial personal and social power on some women by giving them a measure of control over their own reproductivity. To the degree that effective contraception through suckling necessarily implies planning, self-management, and purpose, it may have symbolized female self-sufficiency in the socially crucial arena of fertility and reproduction. It is ironic, as I noted in the last chapter, that wet-nursing endowed lower-class women with this form of bodily self-management only by systematically taking it away from the mothers socially above them. Perhaps just as threatening for a jealous and sexually insecure patriarchy, prolonged suckling and the extension of the nursing dyad to include a succession of nurse-children would also have given women a reliable source of physical pleasure, obtainable apart from or even despite a male presence. It is just this possibility that underlies the force of Cleopatra's conspiratorial whisper to her asp-baby to call Caesar an "ass / Unpolicied."

Thus a witch's bodily bond with her familiar would both resemble and invert the structure of relations within the nursing dyad, much as Cleopatra's taking up of the asp-baby does. It becomes a form of the carnivalesque which works to "decarnivalize" ordinary nursing relations. Barbara Rosen has sought to rationalize this aspect of the English witch-hunt by arguing that neighbors "*did* see old women with pets," and expressed the forbidden affection between the witch and her familiar by means of the "cosy, slightly perverted relationship of a lonely and poverty-stricken woman to her pet animal."[60] But this recourse to common sense does not explain the interrogators' fascination with the image of an old woman, usually past her reproductive and lactating years, giving suck; nor does it take into account the fact that cross-species suckling—such as the puppies drawing out engorged breasts—was known either in theory or in practice in early modern bodily culture. To me, the cultural preconditions for this aspect of the witch-hunt interrogation would seem to include fear of erotic self-sufficiency and suspicion of a female sensuality outlasting reproduction and marriage—both metonymized by the nursing dyad.

60. Rosen, *Witchcraft*, p. 32.

The witch-hunters' imagination focuses with intensity upon the imaginary erotic spectacle of the witch and her familiar. When the dialogic voice in Hopkins's pamphlet asks why a spirit like the Devil, wanting "no nutriment or sustentation, should desire to suck any blood," the barely suppressed eroticism of Hopkins's response suggests a kind of identification with the corporeal intensity and intimacy of the Devil's attachment to the witch's body: "In this case of drawing out of these Teats, he doth really enter into the body, reall, corporeall, substantiall creature, and forceth that Creature (he working in it) to his desired ends, and useth the organs of that body to speake withall to make his compact up with the Witches."[61] Minister Henry Goodcole's interrogation of Mother Sawyer, the witch of Edmonton, is even more fixated on the old woman's bodily practices, particularly on questions of sexual initiative, pleasure, and voluntarity: "In what place of your body," he asks, "did the Devil suck of your blood, and whether did he choose the place, or did you yourself appoint him the place? . . . and tell the reason if that you can, why he should suck your blood." The specificity of the question, according to Goodcole, was intended "to confirm the women's search of her, concerning that she had such a mark about her," which he then goes on to describe in length, breadth, location ("a little above my fundament"), conformation, and color. He also asked the witch if she pulled up her coats for the Devil, how long the sucking would last, whether or not it was painful, whether she handled the Devil when he came to her—questions that seem to an alienated modern reader distinctly voyeuristic, enhancing Goodcole's and his readers' vicarious enjoyment and graphic mental staging of her forbidden act. Goodcole's preface confirms this impression, for to a suspicious reader, it seems both to eroticize his own relation as writer to his audience of reader-suitors and to conceal from himself and them their erotic investments in his material. Thus he reports without any sign of textual unease that the suspicions of the local magistrate were confirmed "by some of her neighbours, that this *Elizabeth Sawyer* had a private and strange mark on her body."[62]

From Goodcole's secure place within the ideological framework of witchcraft belief, the vividness of his evidence and the specificity of

---

61. Hopkins, *Discovery of Witches*, pp. 4–5.

62. Goodcole, *Wonderful Discoverie*, pp. 392, 386. Kathleen McLuskie has argued that Goodcole, sensitive to the long-standing disbelief in witchcraft or to the scruples of many jurists involved in prosecution and sentencing, wants to "emphasize the importance of human agency in calling up the devil." See *Renaissance Dramatists* (Atlantic Highlands, N.J.: Humanities Press, 1989), p. 64.

his questions are probably a form of legal realism intended to deflect negative judgment or skepticism. Though clearly the question of the mark's actuality—which might be substantiated by this kind of detailed textualization of Elizabeth Sawyer's body—is less relevant than the mark's function, about which the women searchers can only speculate: it "seemed as though one had sucked it." Thus Goodcole writes that the publication of the pamphlet has been "importunity extorted from me, who would have been content to have concealed it. . . . For my part I meddle here with nothing but matter of fact. . . . And the rather do I now publish this to purchase my peace, which without it being done, I could scarce at any time be at quiet for many who would take no nay." One should note (apart from the anarchic potential in a bawdy accidental pun on "meddle") his repetition of the verb *extort*, when he describes Elizabeth Sawyer's confession as having been "with great labour . . . extorted from her." Despite Goodcole's insistence that the confession is hers "*verbatim* out of her own mouth delivered to me," it is clear that the voice of Elizabeth Sawyer's confession belongs to her interrogator, part of the externalization of agency which is effected in the intimacy of torturer and tortured.[63] It does not matter that Goodcole was not Sawyer's torturer. (In England torture mostly involved deprivation of food and, especially, sleep.) The point is rather, as Scarry says, that in torture "one's own body and voice now no longer belong to oneself."[64] When Elizabeth Sawyer, having been convicted, is asked why she denied at her trial the practices she confesses to in Goodcole's pamphlet, she says simply, "I did it thereby hoping to avoid shame." But it is the imposition of shame on which Goodcole seems most intent, dismissing the "ridiculous fictions of her bewitching corn on the ground, of a ferret and an owl daily sporting before her" so that he can draw from her like a prosecutorial familiar the details of her intimacy with the Devil.[65] Thus the question of whose autoeroticism is being defended against here arises particularly in the context of a publication whose delivery to the importunate public is said to purchase its writer's peace.

In Thomas Dekker, John Ford and William Rowley's *Witch of Ed-*

---

63. Goodcole, *Wonderful Discoverie*, pp. 387–88, 381, 388. See Keith Thomas's discussion of Goodcole's and Hopkins's interrogations in *Religion and the Decline of Magic: Studies in Popular Beliefs in Sixteenth- and Seventeenth-Century England* (1971; rpt. Harmondsworth, England: Penguin, 1978), pp. 617–18.

64. Scarry, *The Body in Pain*, p. 53.

65. Goodcole, *Wonderful Discoverie*, pp. 397, 382.

monton, the themes of the witch's shameful self-agency, which Good-cole defines narrowly and treats with obsessive detail, are imbricated in what Anthony Dawson has aptly called "a sharply delineated material context."[66] But Dawson underestimates, I think, the powerful social valences of the physical relationship hinted at between the witch and Dog, her familiar. Despite the playwrights' surprising measure of sympathy for and understanding of the witch's unfortunate role in her visibly imperfect, hypocritical community, Mother Sawyer also becomes the vehicle for a comic exposure of female bodiliness not unlike what we have already seen in *A Chaste Maid in Cheapside* or even *A Midsummer Night's Dream*. Mother Sawyer's powerful opening speech, for example, plays upon the coarse trope of the degraded female body as privy:

> Why should the envious world
> Throw all their scandalous malice upon me?
> 'Cause I am poor, deform'd and ignorant,
> And like a Bow buckl'd and bent together,
> By some more strong in mischiefs then my self?
> Must I for that be made a common sink,
> For all the filth and rubbish of Men's tongues
> To fall and run into?
>
> (2.1.1–8)[67]

At the moment when the witch bitterly recognizes the recursive processes of scapegoating in which communal rejection makes her participate, the playwrights give her a complex trope that effects a violent, carnivalesque reversal of bodily strata: men's words, displaced downward, become excreta and the body of the old woman is encoded as a site of evacuation. We have seen this trope before in relation to the prostitute whose vagina is metaphorically a common receptacle for seminal evacuations. Here Mother Sawyer is the de facto product of her community's hypocritical social engineering—since filth must run off somewhere—but the metaphor of the "common sink" links her with another recognized form of deviant woman as homologous objects of deeply ambivalent desire, fear, and social utility.

66. In Anthony Dawson, "Witchcraft/Bigamy: Cultural Conflict in *The Witch of Edmonton*," *Renaissance Drama* n.s. 20 (1989), p. 77. Dawson's argument anticipates mine at many points.

67. Quotations from *The Witch of Edmonton* refer to *The Dramatic Works of Thomas Dekker*, vol. 3, ed. Fredson Bowers (Cambridge: Cambridge University Press, 1958).

It is difficult to decide how aware the playwrights might be of this circulation of meanings, but their decision to join the Mother Sawyer plot with the bigamy plot of Frank Thorney, as Dawson argues, does suggest their detailed awareness of social and ethical comparisons to be drawn up and down the Jacobean social hierarchy—in particular the illegal contracts on which both bigamy and witchcraft are based.[68] Certainly the play is very clear that its characters do not know, cannot know the real power relations in which they are enmeshed, in part because of sudden changes of desire and circumstance, in part because social and personal agency here is always complexly a function of specific material and symbolic variables that the characters cannot control. But despite, or perhaps because of, the play's social complexity, the power structure and the libidinal economy of this rural society do in fact overlap: Sir Arthur at the top of the social pyramid initiates the chain of events leading to Frank Thorney's bigamy; Mother Sawyer at the bottom occupies a place at the end of the libidinal economy as the "common sink." She is the site not of desire but of fear, revulsion, ridicule, and she partly understands the nature of her ideological interpellation and function as witch: "This [malediction] they enforce upon me: and in part / Make me to credit it" (2.1.14–15). All the other characters of the play are placed, with varying degrees of irony, somewhere between these poles of desire, agency, and reward. And at the end of the play, Sir Arthur has not been caught or punished for his sexual transgression, but Mother Sawyer is led off to trial.

Despite the playwrights' brilliant deconstructive exposure of the social mechanisms that victimize Mother Sawyer, however, their representation of the old woman's relationship to Dog continues to draw upon the kind of voyeuristic, misogynistic fantasy about the bodily secrets and occult powers of maternity we have already seen in Goodcole and before that in the Amazonian obsessions. Furthermore, they draw upon the comic potential of an absurd relation to the dug which we have already seen in Juliet's weaning and Osric's ridiculous "compliance." Not only is the relationship with a familiar peculiar to women accused of witchcraft, but it seems to be an occult part of a self-perpetuating culture identified as female. Mother Sawyer at first seems alienated from even this aspect of her society, since she does not know what other old women know:

68. Dawson, "Witchcraft/Bigamy," pp. 79–80.

I have heard old Beldames
Talk of Familiars in the shape of Mice,
Rats, Ferrets, Weasels, and I wot not what,
That have appear'd, and suck'd, some say, their blood.
But by what means they came acquainted with them,
I'm now ignorant:

(2.1.97–102)

In the case of so isolated a woman, cursing rather than gossip seems to be the immediate means of coming by a familiar. "Ho! have I found thee cursing?" says Dog, "now thou art mine own" (116). But cursing in this context seems to signify as an attribute of womanhood, particularly in a period when, even apart from the witchcraft prosecutions, socially disruptive female speech was increasingly criminalized.[69]

In addition, then, to the fear of maternal nurture the fear of witches also reflects an even more paranoid anxiety about maternal conspiracy, which the witchcraft depositions seem to confirm. Perhaps it can be linked to the female hermeticism of birthing practices, and it certainly is related to the high incidence of midwives among both the women appointed as searchers and those accused.[70] The witchcraft depositions represent women who have received familiars from their mothers, passed them on to their daughters, or (as we saw in Hopkins's pamphlet) temporarily given them to another witch to suckle. One Anne Cooper confessed that she "offered to give unto her daughter Sarah Cooper an impe in the likenes of a gray kite, to suck on the said Sarah; . . . and told the said Sarah, there was a cat for her." Another Essex woman confessed to four familiars, "which shee had from her mother, about two and twenty yeeres since." In one case, the teats themselves seemed hereditary, for the daughters of one suspected witch were searched and an informant reported "that two of them had bigges in their privy parts as the said Margaret their mother had."[71] Such fears of maternal conspiracy may appear particularly ironic to the modern reader in view of the testimony elicited from women and girls against their own mothers and sisters. The

69. See Lynda E. Boose, "Scolding Brides and Bridling Scolds: Taming the Woman's Unruly Member," *Shakespeare Quarterly* 42 (1991), 184–85.

70. There is a somewhat outdated account of this preponderance in Thomas Rogers Forbes, *The Midwife and the Witch* (New Haven: Yale University Press, 1966), pp. 112–32. Larner discusses the connection somewhat skeptically in *Enemies of God*, p. 101.

71. Quoted in Haining, *Witchcraft Papers*, pp. 158, 172, 163.

withchcraft depositions testify not so much to female conspiracy as to the virulence and durability of village quarrels, particularly among women. A number of the village quarrels that led to witchcraft accusations revolve around the sudden deaths of young children or, in at least one recorded instance, around a quarrel over the wet-nursing of a child.[72]

Mother Sawyer signs her unholy compact by giving Dog her arm to suck; the more intimate relationship revealed in the sources is beyond the bounds of dramatic representation. With Dog's services, her power now seems to extend to the humiliation of her enemy, Old Banks, who confesses to a terrifying involuntarity of meaning in his own bodily behaviors and his own unnatural dependence on an animal: "I cannot chuse, though it be ten times in an hour, but run to the Cow, and taking up her tail, kiss (saving your Worship's Reverence) my Cow behinde; That the whole Town of *Edmonton* has been ready to be-piss themselves with laughing me to scorn" (4.1.53–58). This too is beyond the reach of dramatic representation. The anal kiss, enjoined by Satan, was a conventional ritual act, which, says Stuart Clark, inverted "religious worship and secular fealty."[73] Here the bovine instrument of Mother Sawyer's revenge seems to stand specifically for Mother Sawyer herself, who shares with the cow the critical attribute of femaleness. The even bawdier analogy—visible beyond this metonymic chain—of Banks's anal kiss to cunnilingus is made clear by Banks himself: "I, no lips to kiss but my Cows—" (4.1.67). Mother Sawyer's teat, we recall from the source in Goodcole, was "a little above my fundament." Furthermore, the nature of Banks's obsession collapses the otherwise clear distinctions between the wealthy old farmer and Mother Sawyer's familiar. Immediately after the witch has called her enemy a "black Cur, / That barks, and bites, and sucks the very blood / Of me, and of my credit" (2.1.111–13), the black Dog appears to enact the old widow's revenge.

The later reunion in act 4 of Dog and witch demonstrates the development of their mutual intimacy and dependency when Dog's demands to have the teat "now" (4.1.152) have to be denied. The play does invest this relationship with a remarkable, if finite, degree of sympathy, even while representing it as a parody of "both sexual and

72. See the information of Grace Thurlow against Ursula Kemp in *Witchcraft*, ed. Rosen, pp. 107–8.
73. Clark, "Inversion, Misrule, and the Meaning of Witchcraft," p. 126.

maternal tenderness."[74] The playwrights' ability to construct Mother Sawyer as a complex, persecuted, and lonely old woman could well have worked to enhance sympathy for the women caught up by the witch craze. But to the extent that a parody of maternal tenderness works to satirize not just old women but all women, the witch is functioning not simply as the representative of a particular, even extreme kind of social outcast but also as the emblem of universal and, not coincidentally, somewhat ridiculous female affectionateness and sensuality. We might imagine the Dog pawing her skirts, wanting access to the enveloping and apparently suggestive darkness beneath. She redirects his desire to the upper body instead: "Stand on thy hind-legs up. Kiss me, my *Tommy*" (155). And she equates her desire for his affection with the affection of ladies for "Hound, / Monkey, or Parakeet" (161–62).[75]

Lacking metadramatic awareness of her fictionality, Mother Sawyer does not tell Dog she cannot offer him her teat because such behavior is beyond the reach of dramatization. She excuses herself instead on the physiological grounds that her body works just like any lactating woman's. Her supply of blood, like theirs of milk, is affected by changes in her psychological state, here the humoral drying caused by heat:

> I am dri'd up
> With cursing and with madness; and have yet
> No blood to moysten these sweet lips of thine.
>   (4.1.152–54)

My point is that any witch's reported relationship with her familiar was an extreme manifestation of suckling behaviors, even cross-species suckling, common to, or at least possible for, all childbearing women.

74. Dawson, "Witchcraft/Bigamy," p. 87.

75. The possible range of Dog's behaviors here may be more revealing of the modern critic's preoccupations than of anything else. Onat praises the dramatists for their restraint in detailing the relationship: "Had they been intent only upon capitalizing upon the sensationalism of the event, they might very well have emphasized such features" (gloss to 4.1.151, *Witch of Edmonton: A Critical Edition*, p. 345). My own argument leads me to imagine somewhat broader or at least more "sensationalistic" stage action here. My sense of the suggestiveness of the enveloping dark of a woman's skirts comes not only from my reading of the birth materials in Chapter 4, but also from Jonson's treatment of Dapper and the Queen of Fairy in *The Alchemist*. It is also worth pointing out that ladies and their pets were satiric targets well before Pope's Belinda.

We have seen the revulsion inspired by old women's dugs. If witch-hunts *were* woman-hunts, then the English fascination with the bodily features of witches, with the witch's teats, brings the bodies of all sexually mature women into a dangerous hermeneutic circle, into a zone of paranoid expectation. That this may be the case in *The Witch of Edmonton* is also suggested by the fact that Dog appears not only to the witch but also to Cuddy Banks. There, as in his relation to Mother Sawyer, Dog seems clearly to function as a projection of the character's desires, even desires for mischief. But Cuddy's affection for Dog is a function of the fact that even though he perceives him to be a devil, he always treats him and even protects him like a dog. He has "given him a bone to gnaw twenty times. The Dog is no Court foysting Hound, that fills his belly full by base wagging his tayl; neither is it a Citizens Water-Spaniel, enticing his Master to go a-ducking twice or thrice a week, whilst his Wife makes Ducks and Drakes at home: this is no *Paris*-Garden Bandog neither, that keeps a Bough, wough, woughing, to have Butchers bring their Curs thither" (4.1.230–36). In other words, Cuddy's "normal" relationship with Dog, set in a gallery of other man-dog relationships, works to mark a difference—at least in part of gender—from the witch's relationship with her familiar. Thus in the image of the teat the witch offers to her familiar is a memorial rejection, even a defiance, of a maternal dug that will *not* be complied with or sucked any longer.

ᏒᏆ

There are no witches per se in *The Winter's Tale*, no images of women putting animals to their breast, no narratives of a baby's late weaning. But I want to conclude my discussion of the new disciplinary regime for the maternal body by turning to its emplotment in this late Shakespearean romance. In it the meanings I have constructed for the figures and events of the birthing narrative converge in an extended familial and political crisis. Early modern patriarchy's suspicions about pregnancy, birth, maternal surrogacy and nurture are embedded here in a strikingly discontinous narrative, broken in two by the "wide gap" of sixteen years between acts 3 and 4.

I want to center my discussion on Perdita's key position in this two-part narrative. In its experience of the play's discontinuities, the audience finds in her its most reliable and meaningful counterpart within the fictional frame, though Perdita herself, of course, has no subjective awareness of the discontinuities of her experience. Alone among the characters, she belongs to and reconciles both of the play's sharply differentiated environments, one inhabited by her "blood" parents and the other by her "milk" parents. (Until Hermione's return, of course, both sets of parents are represented only by the paternal half, since the Old Shepherd's wife dies sometime before the events of act 4.) In her movement through the cyclical pattern of extrusion and return Perdita undergoes the common experience of the romance protagonist and also, as my imagery of blood and milk implies, the traumatic experience of the seventeenth-century nurse-child, sent away from home soon after birth and returned months or years later. The play enacts a narrative that roots the infant's trauma—its rage and oral deprivation—in its father's own infantile rage and jealous desire for a place near the maternal body. It is the recognition of this element of her experience, I suggest, which would resonate most profoundly for those members of a Jacobean audience who were themselves nurse-children. In the narrative discontinuities of the play, in its spatiotemporal derangements, the archaic content of their own repressed memories and wishes would be represented.[76]

Peter Erickson has formulated the play's motivating disturbance most succinctly and helpfully for my purposes:

> The most obvious disturbance in male control is the abrupt manifestation of Leontes' alienation from Hermione. Hermione's visible pregnancy activates a maternal image that seems in and of itself to provoke male insecurity. . . . To adapt Melanie Klein's language, what is called into question here is the "good breast" ("fertile bosom"): the "bounty" provided by maternal "entertainment" is suddenly suspect and inherently untrustworthy.[77]

But Erickson sees in Leontes' alienation from Hermione the *symptom* of a disruption in male relationships based upon a complex structure

76. I borrow the term "spatiotemporal derangement" from Michael D. Bristol, who connects it with the psychoanalytic trajectory. See "In Search of the Bear: Spatiotemporal Form and the Heterogeneity of Economies in *The Winter's Tale*," *Shakespeare Quarterly* 42 (1991), 145.

77. Peter B. Erickson, "Patriarchal Structures in *The Winter's Tale*," *PMLA* 97 (1982), 819. Erickson's argument dovetails with mine at many points, particularly in the emphasis we both place on maternal nurturance, and it has been helpful in clarifying my thinking about the play. But he is much less interested than I am in contextualizing the play within the material practices of a wet-nursing culture. Carol Thomas Neely, too, has centered her feminist discussion of the play on maternity, but again without siting it in the specific practices of childbearing. See "Women and Issue in *The Winter's Tale*," *Philological Quarterly*, 57 (1978), 181–94.

of exchange—the relentlessly competitive gift economy characteristic of aristocratic society. That is, Erickson sees flaws fundamental to, inherent in the governing relations *within* patriarchy as the root cause of the play's opening crises. In this, the pregnant Hermione, whose feminine bounty is subject to extreme idealization by both kings, functions as more or less innocent victim since, according to Erickson, the initial tension "is a product of male interaction rather than of female intrusion."[78] But without putting such interpretations completely aside, it is also possible to construe Leontes' sudden jealousy by reference to the material practices of child rearing, specifically to surrogacy as the institutional model for parenting. Leontes' jealousy, in such a reading, is explicable as the product of his own personal history, however incompletely that history is detailed in the opening dialogues. The history itself is to be understood as produced within the sedimented ensemble of cultural practices, including the practice of wet-nursing. Leontes' history, then, is a typical, not a unique case— indeed, so typical that it is virtually replicated in his foster-brother Polixenes.

Earlier I discussed the traumatic effects on the subject of the inconsistent or ruptured nurture occasioned by the practice of wet-nursing, and the shamefulness of prolonged dependency on the breast, particularly for males ("His mother's milk is scarce out of his nose"). In Juliet we saw the potential for ambivalent class identification because of the gap in nurturance which opens up between the two socially differentiated mothers. In *The Witch of Edmonton*, the "real" body of the accused witch—bountiful where and to whom it should not be, actively maternal beyond the years of reproduction—bears a burden of cultural paranoia not unrelated to wet-nursing and the female hermeticism of birthing.

What I find at play in *The Winter's Tale*, concentrated in but not exclusive to Leontes, are the signifiers of a virtually overwhelming oral deprivation and jealousy that subtends the relations among the three principals virtually from the opening exchanges. Explanations of the rivalry between the two kings have tended silently to assume that competition is the structural means for expressing their

78. Erickson, "Patriarchal Structures," 819. The classic treatment of the gift economy is Marcel Mauss, *The Gift: Forms and Functions of Archaic Society*, trans. Ian Cunnison (New York: Norton, 1967). Mauss's work has been very influential among Shakespeareans, including Erickson and Bristol, to whose essays on the play I am much indebted.

relationship—even for *having* a relationship at all—as adults and rulers. The affective and ethical tensions of the guest-host bond operate only between equals, but presuppose their status as adults as well. We learn that the relationship between Polixenes and Leontes began during a period in childhood which is retrospectively subject to extreme idealization by both kings and their retainers:

> What we chang'd
> Was innocence for innocence; we knew not
> The doctrine of ill–doing, nor dream'd
> That any did.
>
> (1.2.68–71)

But such idealizations of childhood are no more trustworthy than the idealizations of female bounty to which Erickson alerts us, and both are profoundly linked in a hermeneutic of suspicion or in the textual indeterminacies that riddle the play's opening events.[79]

The famous image of Leontes and Polixenes as "twinn'd lambs that did frisk i'th'sun, / And bleat the one at th' other" (67–68) seems to signify the lack of visible difference between the two as boys. Twinness, Polixenes implies, is an ideal equality and echoing reciprocity where neither partner begins or ends the exchange. Their unity—so Polixenes seems to imply—was based on being boys together, gendered alike, separated from the company of the opposite sex: "In those unfledg'd days was my wife a girl; / Your precious self had then not cross'd the eyes / Of my young playfellow" (1.2.78–80). Thanks in part to the conventional association of lambs with Christian innocence, this is an image of mutuality without competition between "playfellows" who are not, after all, biological brothers and thus do not stand in each other's way in the ferocious primogenitary sweepstakes.[80] Both inherit crowns and kingdoms comfortably remote from

---

79. Howard Felperin sees the play, particularly the questions raised at the opening by Hermione's seductive behaviors, as an "extreme case" of textual indeterminacy and uses it as a test case of deconstruction in "'Tongue-tied Our Queen?' The Deconstruction of Presence in *The Winter's Tale*," in *Shakespeare and the Question of Theory*, ed. Patricia Parker and Geoffrey Hartman (London: Methuen, 1985), pp. 3–18.

80. On the structural importance of this source of fraternal rivalry, see Louis Adrian Montrose, "The Place of a Brother in *As You Like It*," *Shakespeare Quarterly* 32 (1981), 31–37. Recently Kay Stockholder has seen in the "twinn'd lamb" image a covert reference to childhood homoeroticism, an interpretation with which I clearly take issue since I construe the absent mother here as the object of desire. See *Dream Works: Lovers and Families in Shakespeare's Plays* (Toronto: University of Toronto Press, 1987), p. 185.

each other, marry fertile women, produce male heirs. Wherever we are to assume that the two princes were raised together—and here the play is silent—they presumably were groomed for parallel royal destinies. The objective sources of male conflict in early modern culture are conspicuously removed, leaving behind the symbolic, though severe competition of hospitality. Thus we infer that their competition—like the erotic temptations of which Polixenes goes on to speak in this conversation with Hermione—began at maturity in a fall from childhood union.

But the image of "twinn'd lambs," taken somewhat more literally, offers itself to another reading that allows us to move the competition between the foster brothers back to an earlier time in their lives and to see how that competition would be restimulated by Hermione's pregnancy. Twins issue from a single maternal body—more often for ewes, of course, than for human mothers, then as now; we can imagine them engaged from birth in a competition for maternal resources. As I reported earlier, the mother of twins was routinely told she could not expect to have enough milk to suckle both; a wet-nurse, too, might have suckled a succession of children but, officially, never more than one at a time. Moreover, because twins issue from the maternal body separately, one after the other, they only *seem* to challenge the exigency of birth order, though identical twins, especially *male* twins, would confound such crucial difference by their doubleness. (Shakespeare's own evident, well-founded interest in twins never minimizes the difficulty, the eeriness of such human duplication, or the possibility of parental preferences: the mother in *The Comedy of Errors* chooses to take the younger twin.)[81] This kind of ambiguous blurring of sequence and distinctions surfaces elsewhere in this play, as when Perdita's brother tells a Sicilian courtier he was "a gentleman born before my father" (5.2.139–40).[82] Polixenes' sentimental implication that lack of difference was a feature of childhood unity between "twinn'd lambs" fails to account for the rivalry of twins, particularly for the possibility that one would usurp the place of the other or that only one place *in relation to the maternal body* would be available.

Thus it is the visible invisibility of Hermione's second pregnancy, coinciding with the visit from Polixenes, which triggers Leontes' psychic break. He retreats into an identification with Mamillius in which,

81. For other examples of what she calls Jacob and Esau figures, see Patricia Parker, *Literary Fat Ladies: Rhetoric, Gender, and Property* (London: Methuen, 1987), p. 247 n. 4.
82. Ibid., pp. 67–69, for a discussion of the figure of reversal, *hysteron proteron*.

Erickson says, Mamillius becomes his new "twinn'd lamb,"[83] Hermione and Polixenes a pair of treacherous parents reenacting his displacement. This regressive identification is driven not only by Leontes' desire to escape from an intolerable present suspicion of Hermione's fidelity into the childhood embodied in Mamillius. It could also be driven, I suggest, by Leontes' memory of his own early displacement from the maternal body, activated by the little boy's imminent displacement from his exclusive relation to his mother and by the semiotic links to the breast in the little boy's name.[84]

It is significant that Mamillius is as yet "unbreech'd," still in the world of women and wearing the skirts of infancy. Perhaps he is about to be transferred to the more overtly competitive male domain, but this change would underscore the precariousness of his current place and the momentousness of the changes symbolized by Hermione's swollen womb. His situation recalls the struggle between Titania and Oberon over the changeling boy in *A Midsummer Night's Dream*, because the displacements implied by the transition—there, of course, sharply contested—are similar: Titania, not lactating, is nonetheless surrogate mother of her dead gossip's baby. (She ends up, as we know, with a baby, doubly surrogate, in Bottom.)

We can construe the relationship of Polixenes and Leontes, then, in terms of the suggestive French phrase, *freres de laict*, or "milk brothers,"[85] since competition for the nurse's body was understood as a feature of parental surrogacy. Joubert, arguing for maternal breast-feeding, offers as inducement a vivid picture of the nurseling's attachment to its surrogate mother:

> Is there not pleasure and enjoyment . . . when they will not allow their nurse to hold another child in their presence or to nurse it? When they begin to defend her if someone bothers her or pretends to beat her, how they are the first to weep and to become violent in order to vindicate the outrage? This great love, bordering on jealousy, is so pleasant and enjoyable that it thrills the heart of the nurse if she is of a good, human, and

83. Erickson, "Patriarchal Structures," 821.

84. In his dictionary Cotgrave defines *Mamillaire* as "of, belonging to the breasts, paps, or dugs." Given Leontes' smug satisfaction that the boy was wet-nursed, the name may sound ironically. See *A Dictionarie of the French and English Tongues* (London, 1611; STC 5830; rpt. Menston, England: Scolar Press, 1968).

85. Cotgrave elides this suggestiveness by translating the term merely as "foster brothers." Perhaps that relationship implied the kind of competition we find thematized in *freres de laict*.

gracious nature. In fact, she will not love her own children more than the outsider she is nursing.[86]

The early relationship of Leontes and Polixenes can be understood as rooted in an identity of relation to and competition for a maternal body.[87] Though this body is occluded in the figure of the "twinn'd lambs," it returns, overcoded, in the pregnancy writ large in Hermione, another maternal object of desire who is not their mother. But the maternal body's occlusion by Polixenes here seems to me to suggest the extent to which the presence of presocial rivalry for the maternal body, hence of *need* for the maternal body, has to be repressed in favor of a later narrative of female seduction: "O my most sacred lady, / Temptations have *since then* been born to 's" (1.2.76–77). But even Polixenes' figurative use of "born" seems to give the game away: it is to the specter of birth, the birth of the Other, that this rivalry may be linked. Leontes' rage seems, both to himself and to us, the jealousy of a grown man, the result of one temptation born "since then." The rage presupposes and is naturalized by the exclusiveness of genital sexuality, a man's property in his wife. But it can also be understood to have a regressive component, stimulated by the arrival of his foster brother but capable of being directed at anyone, including Mamillius and the new baby, who would deflect Hermione's attention and compete legitimately for her bounty as wife and "good breast."

In employing psychoanalytic paradigms to describe Leontes' jealousy, I do not mean to imply an acceptance of him as a fully represented consciousness; the suddenness of his manifestation of full-blown affective states has always seemed to defy the canons of "realistic" psychological portraiture, even in early modern drama. To the contrary, I think the text provides enough details of the cultural environment to make Leontes, Polixenes, and even Mamillius *representative* products of specific modes of enculturation and engenderment, key among them wet-nursing and a discontinuous relationship with two maternal bodies. Leontes' jealousy, in such terms, is structural, not

86. Joubert, *Popular Errors*, p. 197.

87. Thus Bristol says, "Despite their protestations of love and friendship, then, and despite the imagery of the 'twinn'd lambs,' Leontes and Polixenes are in fact engaged in a bitter and potentially deadly struggle for honor and prestige" ("In Search of the Bear," p. 156). My point has been to show that, far from denying the competition, the imagery of "twinn'd lambs" can be seen to underwrite and even ground it.

idiosyncratic, his subjectivity social rather than individual. Thus the opening scenes are full of the affective paradoxes and contradictions of early modern child-rearing practices. Like their representatives Leontes and Polixenes, the English upper classes invested enormous economic, social, and psychic stakes in succession and inheritance, privileging continuousness of name and race. Aristocratic mothers were urged to breast-feed their children, and yet, they continued to give their children away at crucial developmental stages throughout childhood or—as is the case with Polixenes here—had reasons to leave them for long periods of time. This argument seems but is not anachronistic. Hermione herself makes Polixenes' silence about his son a striking omission:

> To tell he longs to see his son were strong;
> But let him say so then, and let him go;
> But let him swear so, and he shall not stay,
> We'll thwack him hence with distaffs.
>
> (1.2.34–37)

Indeed, the threat of a shaming punishment and return home at the hands of distaff-bearing women here suggests a double-binding power in maternal shame and disapprobation to which Polixenes would hardly want to accede: he is obliquely reproved for not missing his son, but had he admitted to such longing, he would have been beaten home by the women, shamed in a classic image of female rule. In response to Leontes' question—"Are you so fond of your young prince, as we / Do seem to be of ours?" (164–65)—Polixenes describes Florizel, the son we later meet, as "now my sworn friend, and then mine enemy" (167). The assertion of intense interest in his son—"He's all my exercise, my mirth, my matter" (166)—is ironized by its opening qualifier, "*If* at home, sir" (165). This is a king who has failed to cite his son as a pretext for returning home and has just extended his royal visit for a month; and his *wife*, the *mother* of his son, turns up missing from all these exchanges.

In part, my point is that the play thematizes the measure of affection between parent and child even as its male characters appear, defensively, to idealize the affection *between* children. But as Leontes imagines Hermione's adulterous liaison with Polixenes, what issue most strikingly as delegates from the (cultural) unconscious are the signifiers of oral rage, deprivation, and betrayal, directed at the pregnant woman and the surrogate brother. It is as if the most threatening aspect for Leontes in Polixenes' presence at his court is that it reenacts Leontes' displacement from a female bounty he imagines more in oral than in sexual terms. Thanks to Polixenes' timely arrival, woman's treachery in the feeding situation has been triangulated.

Even worse, Hermione herself seems to participate in this oral recoding of infidelity. She describes the hearing of praise as a sublime satisfaction in which oral and sexual pleasures commingle. It "cram's with praise," she tells Leontes, "and make's / As fat as tame things" (1.2. 91–92). The woman fattened by pregnancy mirrors herself as fattened by praise. For Leontes, sexual humiliation is imagined as an oral defeat, a theft of the food literally embodied in the full body of pregnancy. To be cuckolded is thus to have one's "pond fish'd by his next neighbor" (1.2.195). Not only is such a theft by its nature invisible, but the image represents the "full" Hermione as a stocked pond, her fetus as a fish, oddly, put in rather than taken out by Polixenes. For such a possessive imagination, cognition becomes a form of eating or ingestion, ignorance a form of starvation: "'Tis far gone, / When I shall gust it last," he tells Camillo (218–19). Knowledge of infidelity is like a court feast, where places at the table and shares of food are distributed hierarchically: "Lower messes / Perchance are to this business purblind?" (227–28). Amid such full-blown oral paranoia, anyone else's satisfaction is a form of treachery, a specific deprivation: "Satisfy? / Th' entreaties of your mistress? Satisfy? / Let that suffice" (1.2.233–35). It is not surprising that Leontes turns to Camillo not only for corroboration but, in his capacity as Polixenes' cupbearer, for a revenge by means of poison fitted to the crime of theft of nurture. Or that the subsequent knowledge of Camillo's desertion and Polixenes' escape is a cognitive poison—"I have drunk and seen the spider" (2.1.45)—which leaves Leontes malnourished, "a pinch'd thing" (51), until he defends against it by declaring himself "satisfied," needing "no more" (2.1.189) in his certain knowledge of the treachery.

The oral component of male jealousy here seems specifically regressive. More crucial for my larger argument about the disciplinary regimes of pregnancy, that orality cannot be separated from the cultural ascription of grotesqueness attaching to the female body in maturity, once it is "opened" by sexual experience and swollen by pregnancy. Thus the extremity of Leontes' psychic disturbance may be measured by how overtly his preoccupation with the signifiers of female grotesqueness is made manifest. Hermione is a sluiced pond, she is slippery, her womb is a thoroughfare not only for an enemy but for all his train, here bawdily his phallic equipment:

> No barricado for a belly. Know't,
> It will let in and out the enemy,
> With bag and baggage.
>
> (1.2.204–6)

Even apart from Leontes' own paranoid utterances, the play's rhetoric constructs figurative links between pregnancy and displacement which seem to draw upon the rituals of birth and the wet-nursing culture. Polixenes, describing Leontes "as he had lost some province and a region / Lov'd as he loves himself," says he is left "to consider *what is breeding* / That changes thus his manners" (1.2.369–70, 374–75, emphasis added). Leontes violently separates Mamillius from the company of his mother, as if to reenact, almost vengefully, their earlier separation in infancy: "Give me the boy. I am glad you did not nurse him" (2.1.56). He allows himself the retrospective celebration of disconnection between mother and son at the breast, as if that decision, now proved to have been well made, had been his own and as if Mamillius had never been a recipient of Hermione's bounty in that privileged form: "Though he does bear some signs of me, yet you / Have too much blood in him." (2.1.57–58). He conspicuously leaves Hermione, doubled back upon herself, condemned by the plenitude of pregnancy, companioned perhaps erotically by the infant within: "Let her sport herself / With that she's big with" (2.1.60–61). But Hermione's ladies have already threatened Mamillius with his own displacement from his mother and even from themselves:

> The Queen your mother rounds apace: we shall
> Present our services to a fine new prince
> One of these days, and then you'ld wanton with us
> If we would have you.
>
> (2.1.16–19)

More important still, Shakespeare alters the timing of the queen's pregnancy and delivery from that given in Robert Greene's *Pandosto* in ways that connect Leontes' jealousy and sense of displacement from the maternal body with the early modern practices of birth. In *Pandosto*, the enforced departure of Polixenes' counterpart Egistus and the queen Bellaria's imprisonment occur before the queen discovers herself to be pregnant. The nine or so months of her pregnancy and delivery take place in prison, presumably away from the sight of Pandosto, and thus those events are separated from the earlier onset of his jealousy. Here, as we learn retrospectively, the duration of Polixenes' visit and Hermione's pregnancy coincide. Shakespeare has timed the opening events of his play to mark the end of Hermione's pregnancy. And in fact, as the Lady's teasing remarks to Mamillius, just quoted, imply, had Leontes not separated Mamillius so violently from his mother, Hermione's lying-in would have done so by force of custom. However temporarily, Mamillius would have been displaced from his mother's quarters in the reconstitution of domestic space which occurred with the onset of labor.

Here, by ordering Hermione to prison and causing his baby to be born there, Leontes, we could argue, retains patriarchal control over events and space customarily in the charge of women. Hermione asks for the company of her women because of her approaching delivery:

> Beseech your Highness
> My women may be with me, for you see
> My plight requires it.
>
> (2.1.116–18)

Here, as in *Measure for Measure*, where Juliet also gives birth in prison, birth becomes an activity the state seeks to control and monitor as an extension of its desire to control sexuality. Thus, the power of a jealous patriarchy encloses the female hermeticism of birth within and makes it a function of the disciplinary hermeticism of the prison. Female empowerment has been contained and the practices of birth, in effect, decarnivalized. Furthermore, since Leontes' formal accusation of Hermione for treason and infidelity precipitates labor "something before her time" (2.2.23), Leontes becomes identified not only with the reinscription of the childbirth space but as the usurping principle of authority over its temporal management.

But it is also possible to put the case the other way round: Leontes may imprison Hermione and disenfranchise her, but once her labor has begun he cannot prevent the prison from being reconstituted as a birthing chamber or the delivery of Hermione's baby from taking place, as Paulina points out:

> This child was prisoner to the womb, and is
> By law and process of great Nature thence

Freed and enfranchis'd, not a party to
The anger of the King, nor guilty of
(If any be) the trespass of the Queen.
                                                     (2.2.57–61)[88]

The play inscribes a symbolic contest over childbirth, but the result of that contest is left indeterminate. Paulina, by showing Leontes the baby, seems also to show him the limits of patriarchal control over the female body—a limit effectively delineated by the practices of birth. But it is the tyrant Leontes who, in effect, decides upon the baby's nurture. Paulina's gesture of "freeing" the baby from its mother's imprisonment—acting as its midwife into the patriarchal world of culture—makes clear the inseparability of events within the birthing chamber from events outside it or, alternatively, the impossibility of sealing off either the birthing chamber *or* the prison from competing sources of authority. Paulina's own authority is that which cultures often informally vest in older women past the years of childbearing, the "grave matrons" who searched for the witch's teat, for example, or who were charged to ask a bastard-bearer in labor who was the father of her child.[89] Leontes' paranoia sees in *her* all the myriad forms of female disorderliness which were becoming criminalized during this period and hence the proper business of the state. He calls her "a mankind witch," "a most intelligencing bawd," a "callat / Of boundless tongue, who late hath beat her husband" (2.3.68, 69, 91–92).

It is precisely the nature of Leontes' tyranny, however, to insist upon his power over the customary forms of female agency and management in birth, to effect his personal will even against local privilege— here metonymized by the privilege of childbed from which he hales Hermione for her trial. Lying-in, remember, customarily proceeded by stages—the upsitting, going out of the chamber into the rest of the house, and the going abroad to church. A queen's lying-in would have been far more elaborate but presumably would replicate the stages

88. A 1619 sermon of Donne's suggests that such a disciplinary inscription of birth was a convention of theological discourse: "Wee are all conceived in close Prison: in our Mothers wombes, we are close Prisoners all: when we are borne, we are borne but to the liberty of the house." See *The Sermons of John Donne*, ed. George R. Potter and Evelyn M. Simpson (Berkeley: University of California Press, 1955), 7:197. I discuss this image in *The Idea of the City in the Age of Shakespeare* (Athens: University of Georgia Press, 1985), p. 215.

89. See Karen Ericksen Paige and Jeffery M. Paige in *The Politics of Reproductive Ritual* (Berkeley: University of California Press, 1981), p. 211, on the authority often invested in the postmenopausal woman.

from childbed to church. Hermione's trial displaces the churching ceremony, which even for queens, was the proper form of public reincorporation into the social body because it represented an affirmation of the bodily recovery and purgation that traversed all gradients of rank.[90] What Hermione experiences is precisely the public shame that the churching ceremony, however implicitly, sought to contravene for any newly delivered woman. She is forced into public, "i'th'open air," and out of the enclosed birthing chamber before time, "the child-bed privilege denied, which 'longs / To women of all fashion" (3.2.103–4). She calls Leontes' hatred "immodest" (102), thus, because it has exposed her to public view too soon after birth and questioned her reincorporation into the social body not on physical but on moral grounds.[91]

In *Domesticall Duties*, William Gouge singles out for severe reproach the husband who accuses his wife of infidelity at or near her lying-in, whether or not the charge is just: "To lay this to a wives charge unjustly, is at any time a most shamefull and odious reproach: but in the time of childebirth whether just or unjust, a thing too too spightfull and revengeful. Some wives are so farr overcome thereby, (especially in the time of their weaknesse) as they are not able to beare it, but even faint and die under the reproach: others more stout vow never to knowe their husbands againe."[92] The new mother needed physically to be kept from emotional distress, for a dangerous flow of the lochia during the lying-in period, Guillemeau suggests, "may arise from passions of the minde, . . . or from some other ill government in her childe-bed." He somewhat redundantly advises: "Let her shun anger, melancholy, griefe, and other such passions of the minde: Let her keep her selfe quiet, not much stirring or troubling her body."[93]

Important to note here is that Guillemeau assumes the birthing chamber to be an agential space for women, the new mother an agent or coagent within it: "Let her *keepe her selfe quiet*." Gouge's manual goes

90. I owe this information to conversations about Queen Anna's churchings with Leeds Barroll.

91. *Immodest* is usually glossed "immoderate, excessive," but Shakespeare elsewhere uses it to mean inappropriate or indecorous. The senses may play together here in the relatively recent transfer of the word from Latin.

92. William Gouge, *Of Domesticall Duties* (London, 1622; STC 12119; rpt. Amsterdam: Theatris Orbis Terrarum; and Norwood, N.J.: Walter J. Johnson, 1976), pp. 401–2.

93. Jacques Guillemeau, *Child-birth, or The Happy Deliverie of Women* (London, 1612; STC 12496; rpt. Amsterdam: Da Capo Press, 1972), pp. 223, 224.

even further, inscribing a childbed privilege homologous with the broad license of carnival. Even the woman who could *justly* be accused of bearing a bastard is to be relieved from moral judgment for the duration of her recovery. For Leontes to abrogate Hermione's rights in childbed is, among other things, a clearly unwarranted intrusion of patriarchal power—at least for the duration of her lying-in—into an arena formerly assigned to women's control. That is, Leontes' tyranny is constituted not only by his *mistake* in suspecting Hermione but also by his violation of what is due to her and all women in the management of their "great pain and peril."[94] In addition, by separating her at this moment from her children "like one infectious" (3.2.98), Leontes seems to collapse the never very stable distinction between two categories of pollution—the ineradicable stain of moral pollution and the temporary, if exigent, bodily pollution that still attached to parturience: "As *Fernelius* saith, The place from whence comes life, is also the breeder of the most deadly poison."[95]

All these traumas of separation and suspicion are most vividly signified by the abrupt and violent weaning of Perdita, "the innocent milk in it most innocent mouth" (3.2.100). But this suddenly orphaned baby's experience should not be understood as the pathetic fate of the exceptional subject. It is rather a version, romantically heightened, of what happened soon after birth to countless babies in the wet-nursing culture, though in most cases without so explicit an infanticidal motivation. This baby, like those, suffered inexplicable extrusion from the birthing chamber, enforced alienation from the maternal breast, and a journey to the unknown rural environment of a foster family lower in station than its own. Even though the birth parents knew where they had placed their baby and occasionally visited it, the physical and social separation of the two environments was virtually as complete as it is here. In the play social disjunction is expressed as a shift in genre from the opening tragic action to the romance plot of acts 4 and 5.[96] In terms of modes of identification for

94. I am quoting from the language of the churching ceremony from *Book of Common Prayer, 1559: The Elizabethan Prayer Book*, ed. John E. Booty (Charlottesville: University Press of Virginia, 1976), p. 315.

95. I quote here from Culpeper, *Directory for Midwives*, p. 114.

96. Like Bristol, I find the most satisfactory brief accounting of the genre in this part of the play in Mikhail Bakhtin, "Forms of Time and of the Chronotope of the Novel," in *The Dialogic Imagination: Four Essays by M. M. Bakhtin*, ed. Michael Holquist, trans. Caryl Emerson and Holquist (Austin: University of Texas Press, 1981), pp. 86–110.

the audience or reader, however, that shift also changes the focal subject positions implied by the narrative—from the intrafamilial concerns of the disunited parents to the individualistic desires of the children. Such a shift implies that the romance plot is not a story of lost children—a story privileging the parental perspective—but a story of lost *parents*. Events are seen from the perspective of the child, who knows where she is but not where she comes from. More specifically, I see the later events of *The Winter's Tale* as the masterplotted representation of the generic desires and intrapsychic traumas of wet-nursed children.

Perdita is luckier than her counterpart in *Pandosto*, since that baby, put out to sea alone, starves for two days before being rescued. When she is finally picked up by a naïve shepherd who mistakes her for a god, her instinctual search for the breast becomes the decisive token of her humanity (or, alternatively, of its having been born of woman): "The Sheepeheard, who before had never seene so faire a Babe, nor so riche Jewels, thought assuredly, that it was some little God, and began with great devocion to knock on his breast. The Babe, who wrythed with the head, to seeke for the pap, began againe to cry afresh, whereby the poore man knew that it was a Childe."[97] The key moment in this shepherd's first nurturing relation to the baby is when he recognizes it to be animal life—we could say *mammalian* life—because of its need for the breast. To take up the baby means to undertake to find it a breast or breast substitute, to reverse through surrogate nurture the violent action of its biological father to deprive it of the breast, "the innocent milk in it most innocent mouth."

In *The Winter's Tale* revenge against the violence of the biological father is exacted by the bear that devours Antigonus, chosen to be the executor of the harsh paternal will because of collusion with "Lady Margery, your midwife there, / To save this bastard's life" (2.3.160–61). Early modern culture associated bears with a complex of meanings, including tyrannous power, aggressive sexuality, and—most in-

97. I quote here from Robert Greene, *Pandosto: The Triumph of Time* (1588), reprinted in *Narrative and Dramatic Sources of Shakespeare*, ed. Geoffrey Bullough, vol. 8 (London: Routledge and Kegan Paul; New York: Columbia University Press, 1975), p. 173. It is worth pointing out, particularly given the role that the Nurse's husband plays in *Romeo and Juliet*, that Greene includes details of Perdita/Fawnia's rearing which Shakespeare omits, notably the old shepherd's affectionate playfulness with the little girl: "The shepheard every night at his comming home, would sing and daunce it on his knee, and prattle, that in a short time it began to speake, and call him Dad, and her Mam" (p. 175).

teresting for my argument—generativity and nurture. Living outside the human sphere of patriarchal culture, she-bears need not answer for the parentage of their cubs, and the hermeticism of their birthing practices is complete, purposeful, and uncontested. Michael Bristol notes: "The infant takes shape outside the womb as a purposeful action of a mother who is herself inside the womb or den."[98] Edward Topsell declares that male bears, despite their lustfulness, "give great honor to the females great with young, during the time of their secrecie." Though they hibernate together in the cave, male bears lie apart and abstain from carnal relations—presumably because of the pregnancy. The emergence of the she-bears from the caves takes place, according to Topsell, when "their young ones be thirtie daies old at the least."[99] Presumably the mother bear herself decides when the "lying-in" is completed.

That the she-bear's control over her own reproductive practices is an equivocal analogue, at best, for reproduction in the human sphere may be implied in the notorious tonal oddity of the scene in which this bear briefly appears. It is certainly possible to argue that Leontes' oral rage against the treacherous breast here finds its ironic fulfillment. The ostensible cause of that rage has been both exonerated and avenged; the infantile wish has achieved the punishment it desires when the two shepherds reveal their indecent fascination with the extent and state of the bear's leftovers: "If thou mayest discern by that which is left of him what he is, fetch me to th'sight of him" (3.3.133–35). But to the extent that the bear *is* identified with Hermione and becomes—with comic literalness—a symbol of natural appetite, woman is thereby reinscribed in the abjected place of nature, reidentified with the comic grotesque, and removed from effective cultural agency in matters of her own reproductivity. From this point of view, Leontes' tyranny is relevant to the mechanisms of the narrative, the affective engine that sets it in motion, and relevant even to the representation of jealousy. But his tyranny is not at all relevant to the ideologically charged representation of childbirth and nurture and the structure of gender relations within it, for his jealous containment of the birth-

98. Bristol, "In Search of the Bear," pp. 160–61. Bristol's interpretation of the meanings to be drawn from the folklore of the mother bear parallels mine, and I am indebted to him for the reference to Topsell in the next note. Bristol does not, however, connect this lore, as I do, with the actual material practices of the birthing chamber.

99. Edward Topsell, *The Historie of Foure-Footed Beastes* (London, 1607; STC 24123), p. 37.

ing scene in prison is a way of signifying larger cultural contests over the maternal body and its possible need for disciplinary structures.

The text of *The Winter's Tale* omits the details of Perdita's early nurture by the shepherd family, included in *Pandosto*. What the play offers instead is a narrative that powerfully defends against the kinds of paranoia endemic to wet-nursing cultures, particularly those concerning ambivalent class identifications. To the shepherd, the inexplicable opportunity to rear a "squire's child" (3.3.115), long past the days when his wife could have expected to take in a nurse-child close in age to their own son, is the means to local advancement. Their adoption of the baby is another significant fictional intensification of the financial windfall that a nurse-child could have brought to its family, though nothing resembling the wealth that Perdita brings. Perdita becomes, in a sense, the agent of her own security, as the provident, if unlucky, Antigonus hopes. "There these," he says, laying down the gold, "Which may, if Fortune please, both breed thee, pretty, / And still rest thine" (3.3.47–49). It is Perdita's own gold—the metonymy of her origins—that enriches and secures her early environment; but significantly, the gold does nothing to obscure the evident social differences between her and her foster family.

That Perdita remains a member of her own class within the foster environment is often taken as Shakespeare's late affirmation of "great creating Nature" (4.4.88). Conceptualizations of "Nature," however, are never simply a cultural given but always the representation of social interests. Thus we need to wonder why and on whose behalf Nature is being invoked here and why Perdita's "difference" serves to endorse the social practices of parental surrogacy. The contradictions of a wet-nursing culture that advocated but failed to practice maternal breast-feeding may provide an answer. In terms of the play's reenactment of the nurse-child's experience of extrusion and return, the essentialist difference persisting between Perdita and her foster family offers a powerful counternarrative for the specific fears and repressed anxieties of the wet-nursed child, a powerful defense against threatened fantasies of irreplaceability and worth. Perdita in speech and action becomes the sign that the child who went out is the child who returns, unchanged in the essentials of bearing and grace that identify her as a "natural" member of the ruling class. She is, in this sense, the opposite of Juliet, to the degree that we find in Juliet's reckless sexuality the effects of plebeian enculturation and ambivalent class identification. Unlike the Nurse, the Old Shepherd's wife never appears onstage to claim some part in her foster child's affection, and the question of who actually breast-fed Perdita—if not the shepherd's wife—is never mentioned. Instead, the wife enters the text only posthumously, as the idealized antidote to what I alluded to earlier as "woman's treachery in the feeding situation," the symbol of rural bounty, the tireless server of the communal feast as "pantler, butler, cook, / Both dame and servant; welcom'd all, serv'd all" (4.4.56–57). It is Perdita whom the play allows to have it both ways—two kinds of idealized dead mothers, one of whom can return to life once physical nurture has been achieved. The blood parents' loss of their child has created a gap, a structuring absence in the society that has sent it away, so great a gap that the social order cannot be repaired or even continued except by this child's return. The extruded child is an agent, in effect a signifier, even within the family that has sent it away. This is the exiled child's fantasy made authoritative by Apollo's oracle: "The King shall live without an heir, if that which is lost be not found" (3.2.135–36). The child's absence is coterminous with the mother's absence because here the child's loss has *caused* the mother's absence (as it would, from the point of view of the extruded nurse-child). The mother who returns is a mother whom the child's absence has spared the further indignities of reproduction, if not the further indignities of time, in a patriarchal society so clearly jealous of the child's claim on and hunger for the maternal body.

The absence of his wife and daughter has allowed Leontes to recover from the worst effects of his paranoia, to recover his desire for the body of his wife and to submit to the discipline of an endlessly deferred gratification, which, however, remains more oral than phallic in character. Leontes remembers Hermione as a vessel, with eyes full of tears and a mouth full of treasure:

> O, that ever I
> Had squar'd me to thy counsel! then, even now,
> I might have look'd upon my queen's full eyes,
> Have taken treasure from her lips—
>
> (5.1.51–54)

Paulina is both the placeholder of Leontes' desire and the agent of his discipline, embodying desire's memory without being its object. (Perdita, I would argue, is her own placeholder but threatens to become her mother's in the awakening of incestuous desire in Leontes.) Hermione needs to be resurrected, in the terms of this argument, to take Paulina's place next to her husband, to stand between her husband and her returned daughter as mother and wife, the legitimate object of desire in two similar but now separable forms.

This necessity suggests one reason why Hermione returns first as a literal placeholder, the cipher of herself, and only gradually takes on significance and dimensionality as a totemic object. But it is also true, I think, that the ritualistic character of her unveiling symbolizes its function as a reminder of the churching ceremony that Leontes' trial prevented; accompanied by her gossips, the woman to be churched entered under a white veil. Here the figure of a no longer reproductive Hermione reconciles the play's oppositions between oral deprivation and oral fulfillment without ever offering herself—as a woman does while she is pregnant, as Hermione did at the opening of the play—as food.[100] "If this be magic," says Leontes, "let it be an art / Lawful as eating" (5.3.110–11); but as I have maintained, eating in hunger is now safe only because the threat represented by Hermione's too-present maternity no longer obtains. This may be why Hermione does *not* recall the details of Perdita's birth, as does the Abbess at a similar moment at the end of *The Comedy of Errors*, describing the restoration of her two sons as the end of a grotesquely prolonged labor: "Thirty-three years have I but gone in travail / Of you, my sons, and till this present hour / My heavy burthen ne'er delivered" (5.1.401–3). Hermione focuses instead on the details of Perdita's foster care: "Where hast thou been preserv'd? where liv'd? how found / Thy father's court?" (5.3.124–25).

Crucially for this argument, the double-sided representationality of the tableau vivant—the statue as Hermione, Hermione as the statue—transcends the oppositional forms of maternity available to a wet-nursing culture.[101] As a living statue, she fills the space between the two forms of motherhood outlined in *Romeo and Juliet*, reconciling warm/cold, present /absent, responsive/demanding, active/passive. Even more to the point, perhaps, as statue she is all surface and no content, all opacity and no concavity (read womb), an object that can

100. C. L. Barber described the statue as "a sacred or taboo figure" in "'Thou That Beget'st Him That Did Thee Beget': Transformation in *Pericles* and *The Winter's Tale*," in *Shakespeare Survey* 22 (1969), 59. These suggestions of taboo I would connect with the cultural anxieties surrounding pregnancy in this play.

101. In making this case I implicitly take issue with arguments such as Carol Thomas Neely's in "Women and Issue," pp. 191–92, in which the statue scene is regarded as emblematic of patriarchal acceptance of full female sexuality.

represent physical change without being so threateningly immersed in it. She is no longer a "without door form," no longer a female grotesque too visibly representing the invisible forces of reproduction. She is a mother in the full social sense—longed for by husband and child—without being subject any longer to the shame and the juridical disciplines that attended motherhood in the tragic action. This Hermione moves, breathes, is warm to the touch, utters a few lines of verse; she is "stone no more" (5.3.99). But to suggest that these attributes of bodiliness return her to sexual being and demand acceptance by her husband of the meaning of female sexuality and reproductivity is to miss the key point that this Hermione is visibly altered and diminished by her experience of patriarchal discipline, as may be suggested by the silence in which she embraces Leontes. Indeed, as a living statue she is herself the subject of an evidently successful, self-imposed discipline of shame, and thus a perfect exemplar of the new bodily regimes of early modern selfhood.

Hermione's rescue from the embarrassments of the reproductive life she was prevented from having in full as well as those of the grave to which Leontes, his court, and his audience have consigned her may stand as final icon to this study of the early modern body's formation in the disciplines of shame. Her revelatory transformation from pregnant and parturient mother to statue—in Bakhtinian terms, from grotesque to classical body—is produced by narrative displacements in service to Leontes' hyperactive disciplinary regime. For my purposes however, what is crucial to a recognition of the practical significance of Hermione's bodily overdetermination here is the role of theater in inculcating the disciplines of bodily technique and affective self-regulation. The emotionally engaged spectator of *The Winter's Tale* is brought to an awareness of the narratively charged affective properties of theater—the metadramatic significance of the tableau vivant. But that metadramatic awareness probably does not, nor should it, extend to an awareness of the body of the young male actor, protected here by convention and required by the conditions of this heightened display of mimetic self-control to deny its humorality, its ongoing engenderment, its physical indeterminacy, its potential for mundane transgression, the trajectories of its own possibly uncertain desirings, even its emerging claim to the cultural prerogatives of the phallus. That he enacts such denial testifies, from one point of view, to the possibly coercive power of his employment as apprentice actor. But from another—that of the history of early modern bodily practices—his requisite physical and affective self-management signifies the potential responsiveness of the body "natural" to the most exigent of professional and cultural regimes, here represented in the specific entrepreneurial and mimetic protocols of the Jacobean stage. In the celebration of classical bodiliness which it is the queen Hermione's finally to claim, the boy Hermione is thus doubly, if temporarily, rescued from the embarrassments of *his* own bodiliness—the embarrassments created in the civilizing process of which he stands, for an Erasmian moment, as symbolic and material representation.

INDEX

Library of Congress Cataloging-in-Publication Data

Paster, Gail Kern.
   The body embarrassed : drama and the disciplines of shame in early
modern England / Gail Kern Paster.
      p.   cm.
   Includes bibliographical references and index.
   ISBN 0-8014-2776-2 (alk. paper). — ISBN 0-8014-8060-4 (pbk. : alk.
paper)
   1. English drama—Early modern and Elizabethan, 1500–1600—
History and criticism.   2. English drama—17th century—History and
criticism.   3. Body, Human, in literature.   4. Shame in literature.
I. Title.
PR658.B63P37   1993
822'.309356—dc20   92-36855